U0294772

The Chinese Medicine Study Guide Series

Fundamentals

Diagnostics

Acupuncture and Moxibustion

Medicinals

Formulae

Chinese Medicine Study Guide

Fundamentals

Project Editor: **Wang Li-zi**

Copy Editor: **Wu Heng**

Book & Cover Designer: **Yin Yan**

Typesetter: **Wei Hong-bo**

Chinese Medicine Study Guide

Fundamentals

Zhou Xue-sheng
Prof. of Chinese Medicine, Nanjing University of CM

Translated by

Hong Mei, Ph. D. CM   **Zhang Xin-guang, M.S. CM**
Yu Jian-er, M.S. CM   **Liu Jing-feng, Ph. D. CM**
Prof. of Chinese Medicine   Associate Prof. of Chinese Medicine

Liu Dan, M.S. CM   **Yuan Ying, M.S. CM**

Edited by

Bryan McMahon, L. Ac.
Colleen Yvette Robinson, M.S. CM

人民卫生出版社
PEOPLE'S MEDICAL PUBLISHING HOUSE

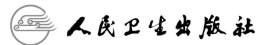

PMPH   PEOPLE'S MEDICAL PUBLISHING HOUSE

http://www.pmph.com

Book Title: Chinese Medicine Study Guide: Fundamentals
中医基础理论图表解

Contact address: No. 19, Pan Jia Yuan Nan Li, Chaoyang District, Beijing 100021, P. R. China, phone: 8610 5978 7340, E-mail: zzg@pmph.com

---

Disclaimer

This book is for educational and reference purposes only. In view of the possibility of human error or changes in medical science, neither the author, editor, publisher nor any other party who has been involved in the preparation or publication of this work guarantees that the information contained herein is in every respect accurate or complete. The medicinal therapy and treatment techniques presented in this book are provided for the purpose of reference only. If readers wish to attempt any of the techniques or utilize any of the medicinal therapies contained in this book, the publisher assumes no responsibility for any such actions.

It is the responsibility of the readers to understand and adhere to local laws and regulations concerning the practice of these techniques and methods. The authors, editors and publishers disclaim all responsibility for any liability, loss, injury, or damage incurred as a consequence, directly or indirectly, of the use and application of any of the contents of this book.

First published: 2007
ISBN: 978-7-117-09240-1/R · 9241

Cataloguing in Publication Data:
A catalog record for this book is available from the CIP-Database China.

Printed in P.R. China

ISBN 978-7-117-09240-1

About the Author

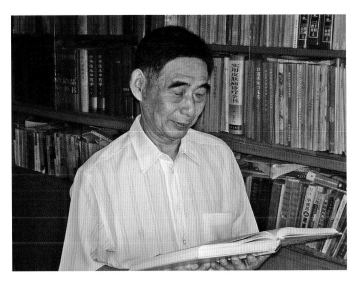

周学胜　教授

Prof. **Zhou Xue-sheng** was born in April, 1940, in Jianhu county, Fujian province, China. He accomplished 6 years of study (1962-1968) at Nanjing University of Chinese Medicine (CM), and practiced as a CM physician in Guannan county, Jiangsu province from 1968 to 1972. After that, he transferred teaching CM basic theory at Xinyi Hospital, Jiangsu province, which led to become a professor at Nanjing University of CM.

Having achieved the titles of instructor, associate professor and professor, Prof. Zhou shoulders the responsibilities of being chief of CM basic theory education and provincial principal of CM basic theory, and associate director of commission of CM basic theory in Jiangsu provincial CM academy.

During past 40 years of working in the education and research department of CM basic theory, Prof. Zhou has lead several projects including Development of Opto-electronic Teaching Aids in CM Basic Theory, supported by Educational Science Research Program of Jiangsu province. He also has lead a research on Figure Illustration in CM Basic Theory, supported by Research Program of CM Higher Education of Jiangsu province, and has accomplished the monograph *Figure Illustration of Basic Theory of CM*. He has also published more than 40 research articles and taken part in editing and publishing 10 CM academic books.

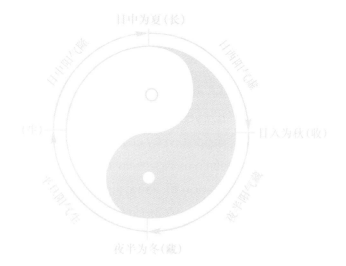

Preface

Chinese Medicine Study Guide: Fundamentals is a companion for the textbook *Basic Theory of Chinese Medicine*. Since its Chinese edition was first published in March 2000, it has gained a lot of popularity among readers because of its comprehensible format and important guideline of Chinese Medicine theory. After revision and translation in English, we bring to you its 2nd edition to facilitate the understanding of TCM around the globe.

In the 2nd Chinese edition, care has been taken to include additional chapters and sections with respect to guidelines of the book by adding organized contents, easy-to-read charts, insightful figures and clear diagrams to help the TCM student and practitioner quickly and efficiently grasp important knowledge. Popular and proper TCM terms were chosen with concise and refined language to express the exact meaning of the text, and facilitate comprehensive.

To avoid confusion of the ancient language used in the classical text, we have chosen to quote them as little as possible and have used modern expressions. We have also cited them altogether after the text to retain the theoretical evidence and to allow different readers to become easily accustomed to the ancient knowledge they provide.

In this new approach to the *Basic Theory of Chinese Medicine* written and designed specifically for students of Chinese medicine, we deliver a more complete and correct theoretical TCM system and a new and innovative way to help the readers understand and memorize the important TCM concept. Last but not the least, we sincerely hope you will point out any possible inadequacy or errors in this book, and share them with us so we can continue to improve and offer you the best final product. Your sincere assistance is always highly appreciated.

Zhou Xue-sheng, Prof. of Chinese Medicine
Nanjing University of Chinese Medicine
August, 2007

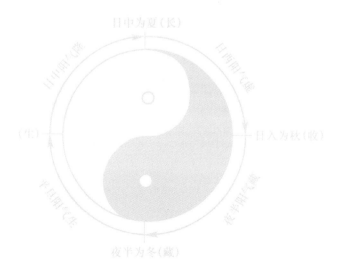

Contents

Chapter 3 Essence, Qi, Blood and Fluid

Chapter 4 Channels and Collaterals

Chapter 5   Body Constitution

Chapter 6   Etiology

Chapter 7   The Onset of Disease

Chapter 8   Pathomechanism

Chapter 9   Principles for Prevention and Treatment

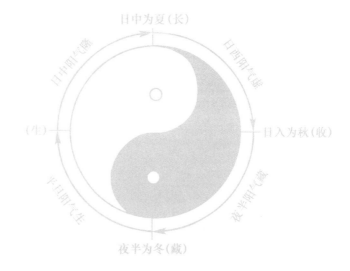

Introduction

The Formation and Development of the Theoretical System of Chinese Medicine

The theoretical system of Chinese medicine is an integration of theory, method, prescriptions and herbs. It is a system of scientific knowledge that includes the basic concepts, rationale and tools of Chinese medicine. This unique system of medical theory is characterized by holism as its dominant underlying principle, with essential qi, yin-yang, and five-phase theory as its philosophical foundation; *zang-fu* organs, channels and collaterals, as well as essential qi, blood and fluid as it's physiological and pathological foundation; and syndrome differentiation and treatment as its diagnostic and healing approach.

① The Formation of the Theoretical System of Chinese Medicine (Fig. Introduction-1)

Chinese medicine originates from the Pre-*Qin* (先秦) era. Its theoretical system was compiled over several centuries from *the Warring States Period* (战国, 475-221 BC) to the *Qin* (秦, 221-207 BC) and *Han* (汉, 206 BC-220AD) Dynasties.

(1) Foundations for the formation of the Chinese medical theoretical system

The theoretical system of Chinese medicine is the resulting combination of accumulated knowledge and theoretical summarization of long-term medical practice together with the traditional culture of China. It is heavily influenced and informed by ancient philosophical concepts.

a. Social and cultural foundations

The appearance of medical science is one result of the evolution of human culture. The climate of Chinese nation states during *the Spring and Autumn Period* (春秋, 770-476 BC), *Qin* and *Han* Dynasties provided favorable socio-cultural conditions for the formation of the theoretical system of Chinese medicine. These factors included drastic social reforms, increases in productivity, and the development of various disciplines such as philosophy, agronomy, astronomy, phenology, botany, mineralogy and smelting etc., as well as academic interaction between various schools of thought.

China is characterized by a long history and a diverse and deep culture. The Chinese medical understanding of biological activity, structure and function of the human body, the etiology and pathology of diseases, as well as the prevention and treatment of diseases has been profoundly influenced by Chinese culture.

b. The accumulation of medical knowledge

The formation of the theoretical system of Chinese medicine was a slow and lengthy process. In the long-term struggle for survival and productivity, as well as in daily life experience and medical practice, the forefathers of the Chinese race battled continually with sickness. This led to a gradual accumulation of raw medical knowledge and a grasp of diagnostic methods and treatment of illness that would later lay the foundation for

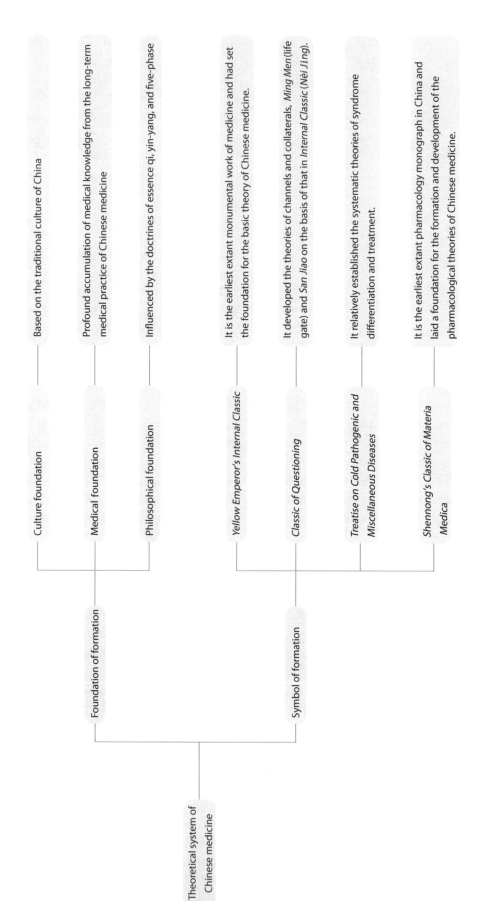

Fig. Introduction-1   Formations and milestones in the formation of the theoretical system of Chinese medicine

the formation of the theoretical system of Chinese medicine.

Medical knowledge required objective organization and summarization in order to develop theories and systems. Socio-cultural development provided favorable condition for this. Under the influence and guidance of ancient philosophical concepts, the earliest extant medical work, *The Yellow Emperor's Internal Classic* (*Huáng Dì Nèi Jīng*, 黄帝内经)*, was written with the combined efforts of numerous physicians.

c. The permeation of ancient philosophical concepts

The formation and development of any discipline of natural science cannot be separated from philosophy, and is necessarily governed and constrained by its philosophical basis. This was especially relevant in ancient societies where philosophy and natural sciences were not clearly separated. The Chinese society of the *Spring and Autumn* and *Warring States* Periods saw revolutionary changes in politics, economy and culture, dramatic increases in productivity, and a flourishing of the natural sciences that resulted in a breakthrough in the worldview of the people of that period. It is only natural then that the physicians of this period utilized these new philosophical and scientific developments to undertake a deep inquisition into the nature of being and the origins of life, health and sickness.

The elements of philosophical thought that have most profoundly influenced the formation of the theoretical system of Chinese medicine are the essential qi, yin-yang and five-phase theories. Using simple theories of materialism and symptom differentiation as guidance, ancient physicians integrated the vast body of medical knowledge with contemporary achievements in the natural sciences, then summarized and systematized these theories. As a result, the theories of Chinese medicine were created and built upon from perceptual to rational knowledge. Chinese medicine uses the concepts and categories of philosophy to observe various phenomena. It is used to shed light on all problems within the field of Chinese medicine and penetrates every aspect of the theoretical system.

The Yellow Emperor's Internal Classic (*Huáng Dì Nèi Jīng*, 黄帝内经), *The Classic of Questioning* (*Nàn Jīng*, 难经), *Treatise on Exogenous Febrile and Miscellaneous Diseases* (*Shāng Hán Zá Bìng Lùn*, 伤寒杂病论), and *Shennong's Classic of Materia Medica* (*Shén Nóng Běn Cǎo Jīng*, 神农本草经) are the four major representative works of Chinese medicine. The completion of these medical classics fundamentally marked the establishment of the theoretical system of Chinese medicine.

The Yellow Emperor's Internal Classic (*Huáng Dì Nèi Jīng*, 黄帝内经) includes two books: *Plain Questions* (*Sù Wèn*, 素问) and *Miraculous Pivot* (*Líng Shū*, 灵枢), usually is called as *The Internal Classic* (*Nèi Jīng*, 内经). It is the earliest extant work of Chinese medicine and a compilation of medical practices and theories of the Pre-Qin and *Western Han* Dynasties. The book comprehensively and systematically discusses the theoretical methods of Chinese medicine, the relationship between mankind and nature, the anatomy, physiology, and pathology of the human body, as well as the diagnosis, prevention and treatment of disease, in other words, the framework for the theoretical system of Chinese medicine. *The Internal Classic* (*Nèi Jīng*, 内经) stresses the importance of holism, stating that, internally, the human body is an organic, interconnected whole and also that externally, mankind is closely tied to its natural and social environment. It systematically introduced ancient philosophical thought into the field of medicine as a way to explain the birth of human life and its processes, the cause, mechanisms, as well as the diagnosis, prevention and treatment of disease. It expounded the physiological functions of *zang-fu* organs, the composition, distribution and actions of the channel system and established the theories of visceral manifestations and channels and collaterals. *The Internal Classic* (*Nèi Jīng*) not only laid the foundation for the theoretical system of Chinese medicine, but is also the basis for all later development of its theories and practice.

Classic of Questioning (*Nàn Jīng*, 难经) is a

medical composition of comparable beauty to *The Internal Classic (Nèi Jīng)*. It utilizes the form of dialogue to discuss the basic theories of *zang-fu* organs, channels and collaterals, pulse reading, pathology and acupuncture methods. This work further developed the theories of channels and collaterals, *Ming Men* (life gate, 命门) and *San Jiao* (三焦) as put forth in *The Internal Classic (Nèi Jīng)*. Like *The Internal Classic (Nèi Jīng)*, *The Classic of Questioning (Nàn Jīng)* has played a central role in giving direction to clinical practice of Chinese medical physicians for generations to come.

Treatise on Exogenous Febrile and Miscellaneous Diseases (Shāng Hán Zá Bìng Lùn, 伤寒杂病论), was penned by Zhang Zhong-jing (张仲景) during the *Eastern Han* Dynasty, and can be divided into two books, *Treatise on Exogenous Febrile Diseases (Shāng Hán Lùn, 伤寒论)* and *Synopsis of Golden Chamber (Jīn Guì Yào Lüè, 金匮要略)*. The former uses the six-channel system to differentiate pathogenic cold diseases; the latter discussed miscellaneous diseases of the *zang-fu* organs. His work outlines the four examinations of Chinese medicine including inspection, smelling and listening, inquiry, palpitation and pulse diagnosis, the eight principles of yin, yang, exterior, interior, cold, hot, deficiency, excess, as well as the eight therapeutic methods of diaphoresis, emetic, purging, warming, clear-heat, harmonizing, resolving (diuresis) and tonifying. This treatise contains theory, method, prescriptions and herbs, established a major theoretical system of syndrome differentiation and treatment, tightly coupled the basic theory and clinical practice of Chinese medicine, and laid a firm foundation for the development of clinical medicine.

Shennong's Classic of Materia Medica (Shén Nóng Běn Cǎo Jīng, 神农本草经) is the earliest extant pharmacological monograph in China. The book collected 365 kinds of herbs, classified into three grades (top, medium and low grades) according to their medical efficacy and toxicity. It records the performance, and indications of these herbs as well as proposed the pharmacological theories of the four natures (cold, hot, warm, cool), five flavors (spicy, sweet, sour, bitter, salty), and seven affects (single

effect, mutual reinforcement, mutual assistance, mutual restraint, mutual inhibition, mutual antagonism, mutual detoxication). In addition to laying the basis for the development of pharmacological theory in China, *Shennong's Classic of Materia Medica (Shén Nóng Běn Cǎo Jīng, 神农本草经)* provided proof for the clinical applications of various herbs and organization for prescriptions.

② The Development of the Theoretical System of Chinese Medicine

The early establishment of the theoretical system of Chinese medicine in turn led to the development of various medical theories and practices. These developments reflect the cultural, scientific and technological standards of subsequent historical periods.

(1) Wei, Jin, Sui and Tang dynasties

The physicians of this period not only inherited and commented on medical classics such as *The Yellow Emperor's Internal Classic (Huáng Dì Nèi Jīng, 黄帝内经)*, and *Treatise on Exogenous Febrile and Miscellaneous Diseases (Shāng Hán Zá Bìng Lùn, 伤寒杂病论)* in order to elucidate their theories, but also compiled clinical experiences, and highlighted the relationship between basic nature and phenomena of disease. Important works include:

Pulse Classic (Mài Jīng, 脉经), by Wang Shu-he (王叔和) of the *Jin* Dynasty (晋, 265-420 AD), is the first monograph on pulse examination. For the first time the book systematically and comprehensively discussed pulse examination from its basic theory to clinical practice. It enriched both the elementary knowledge and the theory of pulse diagnosis.

A-B Classic of Acupuncture and Moxibustion (Zhēn Jiǔ Jiǎ Yǐ Jīng, 针灸甲乙经), by Huang-*fu* Mi (皇甫谧) of the *Jin* Dynasty, is the earliest extant monograph on the science of acupuncture and moxibustion in China.

General Treatise on Causes and Manifestations of All Diseases (Zhū Bìng Yuán Hóu Lùn, 诸病源候论) written by Chao Yuan-fang (巢元方) during the *Sui* Dynasty (隋, 581-618 AD) is the first monograph on etiology, pathogenesis and syndrome differentiation.

Essential Recipes Worth a Thousand Gold Pieces (*Qiān Jīn Yào Fāng*, 千金要方) and *A Supplement to Recipes Worth a Thousand Gold Pieces* (*Qiān Jīn Yì Fāng*, 千金翼方), two medical books written by Sun Si-miao (孙思邈) in the *Tang* Dynasty (唐, 618-907AD), expounded in detail the medical theories, prescriptions, diagnostic techniques, treatment methods, diet and nutrition etc. prior to the *Tang* Dynasty. These two books are often referred to as the first medical encyclopedia of China.

(2) Song, Jin and Yuan dynasties

Drawing upon his clinical experience, Chen Yan (Chen Wu-ze, 陈言 or 陈无择) wrote *The Unified Treatise on Diseases, Patterns, and Remedies According to the Three Causes* (*Sān Yīn Jí Yī Bìng Zhèng Fāng Lùn*, 三因极一病证方论) in the Southern *Song* Dynasty (宋, 960-1279 AD). This work expanded upon the concept of *"The diversity of pathogens may be reduced to no more than three classes."* from Zhang Zhong-jing (张仲景)'s *Han* Dynasty *Synopsis of Golden Chamber* (*Jīn Guì Yào Lüè*, 金匮要略) and Ge Hong (葛洪)'s "Doctrine of the Three Causes" from his *Jin* Dynasty work, *Handbook of Prescriptions for Emergency* (*Zǒu Hòu Bèi Jí Fāng*, 肘后备急方). Chen Yan proposed the *"theory of the three causes of disease"* and systematically detailed it with far-reaching influence on the development and differentiation of etiology of later generations.

During the *Jin* (金, 1115-1234 AD) and *Yuan* (元, 1271-1368 AD) Dynasties, Liu Wan-su (刘完素), Zhang Cong-zheng (张从正), Li Gao (李杲) and Zhu Zhen-heng (朱震亨), often collectively referred to as the "Four Great Physicians of the Jin and Yuan Dynasties, 金元四大家" also contributed greatly to the development of the body of Chinese medical theory.(Table Introduction-1)

Liu Wan-su (nickname Shou-zhen, as founder of the *He Jian* School is also respectfully referred to as Liu He-jian by later generations, 刘河间) advocated *"the theory of fire-heat, 火热论"*. He proposed that "The six climatic factors all originate from fire," and that "excesses of the five emotions produce heat." Believing all diseases originate from fire-heat pathogens, Liu Wan-su often prescribed cool/cold herbs to clear heat. His line of thought therefore became known as "The Cool-Cold School, 寒凉派" (*He Jian* School, 河间派, Representative works include *Exploration of Pathogenesis in Plain Questions* (*Sù Wèn Xuán Jī Yuán Bìng Shì*, 素问玄机原病式) and *Treasury of Pathogenesis and Favorable Qi for Sustaining Life in Plain Questions*(*Sù Wèn Bìng Jī Qì Yí Bǎo Mìng Jí*, 素问病机气宜保命集).

Zhang Cong-zheng (nickname Zi-he, 子和) advocated *"the theory of attacking pathogens, 攻邪论"*.He believed that pathogens are not something that reside within the human body and proposed, "If the pathogen is expelled, the right qi will naturally return to equilibrium." He treated illness by attacking pathogens with aggressive methods of diaphoresis, emetics and purging. Later generations named his approach to treating disease the "Pathogen-Attacking School, 攻邪派". His representative work is *Confucians' Duties to Parents* (*Rú Mén Shì Qīn*, 儒门事亲).

Li Gao (nickname Ming-zhi, title Dong-yuan the Elder, respectively referred to as Li Dong-yuan, 李东垣) created the "Spleen-Stomach theory, 脾胃论". He raised the idea, "Internal damage of the spleen and stomach gives rise to various diseases." He stressed tonifying the spleen and stomach when treating diseases, which lead to the title, "Tonifying Earth School (Spleen-Stomach School), 补土派". His major works are the *Treatise on Spleen and Stomach* (*Pí Wèi Lùn*, 脾胃论), Treatise on Differentiation of Internal and External Impairment (*Nèi Wài Shāng Biàn Huò Lùn*, 内外伤辨惑论).

Zhu Zhen-heng (nickname Yan-xiu, title Dan-xi the Elder, respectively referred to as Zhu Dan-xi, 朱丹溪) created the "theory of ministerial fire, 相火论". He put forward "Yang is always excessive, and yin always insufficient." He treated disease mainly through methods of nourishing yin to temper fire. His followers were therefore referred to as the "Nourishing Yin School, 滋阴派". His representative work is *Further Discourses on the Properties of Things* (*Gé Zhì Yú Lùn*, 格致余论).

Table Introduction-1   Summary of the "Four Great Physicians of the *Jin* and *Yuan* Dynasties"

Representative physician	Main academic view	Academic school	Representative works
Liu Wan-su 刘完素	Advocated the theory of fire-heat; thought that various diseases are caused by fire heat; used cool and cold drugs to clear heat	The Cool-Cold School	*Exploration of Pathogenesis in Plain Questions* (*Sù Wèn Xuán Jī Yuán Bìng Shì*); *Treasury of Pathogenesis and Favorable Qi for Sustaining Life in Plain Questions* (*Sù Wèn Bìng Jī Qì Yí Bǎo Mìng Jí*).
Zhang Cong-zheng 张从正	Advocated the theory of attacking pathogens; thought that pathogens are not a material part of the human body; treated disease with diaphoresis, emetic and purgative methods to attack the pathogen	Pathogen-Attacking School	*Matters of Confucian Filial Piety* (*Rú Mén Shì Qīn*)
Li Gao 李杲	Created the spleen-stomach theory; believed "internal damage of the spleen and stomach gives rise to various kinds of disease"; stressed tonifying the spleen and stomach when treating disease	Tonifying Earth School	*Treatise on Spleen and Stomach* (*Pí Wèi Lùn*), *Treatise on Differentiation of Internal and External Impairment* (*Nèi Wài Shāng Biàn Huò Lùn*)
Zhu Zhen-heng 朱震亨	Created the theory of ministerial fire; put forth "yang is always excessive, and yin always insufficient"; treated disease with methods for nourishing yin to temper fire	Nourishing Yin School	*Further Discourses on the Properties of Things* (*Gé Zhì Yú Lùn*)

(3) Ming and Qing dynasties

During the *Ming* (明, 1368-1644 AD) and *Qing* (清, 1644-1911 AD) Dynasties, practitioners further refined Chinese medical theories and practices, edited large numbers of medical pandects, series and encyclopedias. There were numerous significant medical innovations and inventions, for example, the appearance of *Ming Men* (life gate, 命门) theory in the *Ming* Dynasty provided new material for the theory of visceral manifestations of Chinese medicine. The formation and development of the doctrine of warm diseases in the *Ming* and *Qing* Dynasties was another important theoretical breakthrough of this period.

Wu You-xing (吴有性) of the *Ming* Dynasty and Ye Gui (叶桂), Xue Xue (薛雪), Wu Tang (吴塘), Wang Shi-xiong (王士雄) etc. of the *Qing* Dynasty devoted great effort to the formation and development of the doctrine of warm diseases.

Wu You-xing (nickname You-ke, 吴又可) wrote *On Contagious Warm Diseases* (*Wēn Yì Lùn*, 温疫论), proposing the "pestilent qi theory, 戾气说", a new concept for the etiology of pestilent diseases.

Ye Gui (nickname Tian-shi, 叶天士) wrote *A Piece on Warm-Heat Diseases* (*Wēn Rè Bìng Piān*, 温热病篇), illuminating the patterns in the occurrence and development of warm/heat disease, and established the defensive, qi, nutrition, and blood phase (卫气营血) theory of syndrome differentiation.

Xue Xue (nickname Sheng-bai, 薛生白) wrote *A Piece on Damp-Heat Disease* (*Shī Rè Bìng Piān*, 湿热病篇) pointing out that damp-heat disease is different from pathogenic cold and warm-heat diseases, and expounded the etiology, symptoms, transmission, treatment principles and treatment methods of damp-heat disease.

Wu Tang (nickname Ju-tong, 吴鞠通) wrote *Item by Item Differentiation of Warm-Heat Disease* (*Wēn Rè Tiáo Biàn*, 温热条辨), founding the *San Jiao* (三焦) theory of syndrome differentiation warm-heat disease.

Wang Shi-xiong (nickname Meng-ying, 王孟英) wrote *Longitude and Latitude of Warm-Heat Diseases* (*Wēn Rè Jīng Wěi*, 温热经纬), compiling, editing, and gradually refining and systematizing the doctrine of warm diseases.

(4) Modern and contemporary times

In the modern era (1840-1949 AD) following the Opium War, together with emerging social changes and the introduction of western science, technology and culture, Chinese medical theory reflects a mutual inclusion of both new and old theories, both Chinese and Western. The more traditionally oriented doctors continued compiling and refining the academic achievements of their Chinese predecessors, while others began to integrate Chinese and Biomedicine and develop a school to bring the traditional theories of Chinese medicine into alignment with the biomedical model.

In contemporary times following the establishment of the P.R.C. (1949-present), official Chinese medical policy has been regulated by the central government. The integration of Chinese and biomedicines has been vigorously advocated. The theories of Chinese medicine became more systematized and standardized following large organizational and research projects. Multidisciplinary methods are being applied to study Chinese medicine and its theories continue to be brought under the supervision of modern scientific researchers. Contemporary research on the theoretical system of Chinese medicine continues to produce remarkable new developments.

The Principal Components of the Theoretical System of Chinese Medicine

There are many components of Chinese medicine for understanding the physiological functions and pathological changes of the human body, as well as the diagnosis and treatment of illness. However, they all relate back to two fundamental characteristics, namely, holism and syndrome differentiation and treatment.

① Holism (Fig. Introduction-2)

Holism is the recognition of the integrated, united, and relative nature of things and phenomena. "Holism" in Chinese medicine is twofold: the recognition of the completely integrated nature of the human body and the unity between the human body and its external environment. Holism penetrates the physiology, pathology, diagnostic techniques, syndrome differentiation, health preservation, prevention

and treatment of Chinese medicine and is the most basic guiding theory in its clinical practice.

(1) The human body as an organic whole

a. Structural holism

Each constituent part of the human body is connected via the *zang-fu* organs or communicates through the channel and collateral system to form an interconnected structure that cannot be broken down.

b. Functional holism

The *zang-fu* organs and tissues that constitute the human body have different physiological functions, but combine to form one entity with mutual interaction, promotion and restriction.

Chinese medical holism also stresses that the physical structure of *zang-fu* organs and other structural elements is intimately tied to its individual function and to that of the human body as a whole (five *zang* organs one body view). The physical and spiritual activities of an individual are also dependent upon each other and share an inseparable relationship (holistic view of body and spirit). Essence, qi, blood and fluid are the primary substances that constitute and maintain life activity in the human body. They are also the material foundation for the human physique, physiological activity of the *zang-fu* organs, and sensory functions of the orifices. They serve to further reinforce the unity of function and activity among the *zang-fu* organs and other structural elements.

c. Pathological holism

Chinese medicine utilizes a holistic approach to analyzing the laws of pathology. The illnesses of different viscera can affect each other. An illness of the viscera can affect its corresponding physical structure as well as the relevant orifice, and vise versa. Thereby, local pathological changes are unified into a general pathologic reaction.

d. Diagnostic holism

A given region of the body and the whole are dialectically united. There are also interrelations and interactions among the *zang-fu* organs, channels and collaterals, physical structure and orifices. Thus, when examining a patient, by checking and analyzing the external manifestations of the physique and orifices,

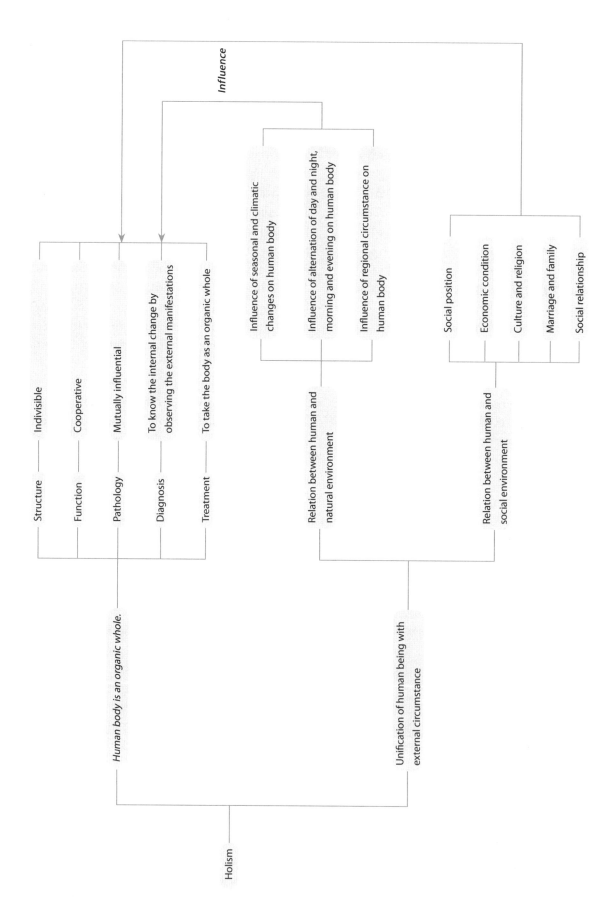

Fig. Introduction-2   Outline of holism

together with color and pulse, the internal pathological changes of the *zang-fu* organs can be surmised. Therefore, acute diagnosis can be made and treatment guidelines can be formulated by the comprehensive analysis of data gained from the four diagnostic methods and careful observation of internal and external changes.

Mencius: Chapter Gaozixia (Mèng Zǐ: Gào Zǐ Xià, 孟子·告子下) states: *"The myriad of internal changes must manifest externally."*

Miraculous Pivot: Chapter The Various Conditions of Internal Organs Relating Different Diseases (Líng Shū: Běn Zàng, 灵枢·本藏) states: *"Observing external manifestations is to know the changes of the internal viscera and thus the patient's illness."*

e. Holism in methods of treatment

Localized symptoms are the reflection of pathological change throughout the whole body. The treatment of such symptoms must start from a holistic perspective and take into account the condition of the entire body. Appropriate treatment principles and methods can be established based on exploring the inner link between local symptoms and the body as a whole.

In short, the five-*zang* viscera compose the central core of the human body, and are organically connected to the six-*fu* viscera, five body constituents, five sense organs, nine orifices, four extremities and bones via the channel and collateral system. It is an intimately unified whole with the interior and the exterior, the upper and the lower in close communication. The various *zang-fu* organs, physical structures and orifices have different composition and functions. They are however, not independent, but interrelated, with mutual promotion and restriction. Therefore, the elements of the human body are indivisible and correlative in construction. They coordinate physiologically and exert a mutual influence upon each other pathologically. In making a diagnosis, one should deduce internal changes by observing external manifestations in accordance with holistic theory. In treatment, these interrelationships must be considered when determining the method of treatment, and only afterward should adjustments be made for

localized pathology.

(2) The unity of human beings and their external environment

The holistic theory of Chinese medicine not only emphasizes the integrated nature of the internal environment of the human body, but also stresses the unity of human beings with their external environment. External environment refers to the world that surrounds the individual, and can be divided into natural and social environments. Environment is the culmination of social and material conditions that human beings rely upon for survival and development.

A. The relationship between human beings and the natural environment

Humans live as part of a natural world that possesses the elements necessary for their survival. *The Internal Classic (Nèi Jīng)* first put forward the view that *"Man and the heavens are mutually dependent"*, meaning that mankind and the natural environment are intimately linked to one another. Environmental factors mainly include seasonal and climatic changes, alternation of day and night, geographic environment etc. They exert a definite influence on the physiological activity of human body, its pathological changes, diagnosis of diseases and treatment.

Miraculous Pivot: Chapter Retention of the Evil Qi (Líng Shū: Xié Kè, 灵枢·邪客) states: *"Man and the heavens are mutually dependent upon one another."*

Miraculous Pivot: Era (Líng Shū: Suì Lù, 灵枢·岁露) states: *"Man mutually interacts with heaven and earth; are mutually respondent to the sun and moon. "*

a. The influence of seasonal and climatic changes on the human body

Each year the four seasons follow the same pattern of change: warm in spring, hot in summer, cool in autumn and cold in winter. Therefore, the physiological activity of the body also follows in accord with these changes: sprouting in spring, growing in summer, harvesting in autumn and storing in winter, maintaining a correlation of the wax and wane of the body's yin and yang energies with that of the seasons and climates. Abnormal season changes often find the human body unable to adapt, thus resulting in outbreaks of seasonal illness and epidemic disease. Therefore, seasonal and climatic factors must be taken into consideration when examining a patient in keeping with the clinical principle to "treat illness according to the season".

Plain Questions: Chapter Discussion on Important Ideas in the Golden Chamber (*Sù Wèn: Jīn Guì Zhēn Yán Lùn*, 素问·金贵真言论) states: "*In spring, one is apt to develop runny nose and nose bleeds. In midsummer, one is apt to contract diseases of the chest cavity. In mid-summer, one is apt to develop cold diseases of the middle burner. In autumn, one is apt to develop wind malaria. In winter, one is apt to develop arthralgia and cold extremities.*"

b. Influence of the changes of night and day upon the human body

The theory that "Man and the heavens are mutually dependent" teaches that not only do seasonal and climatic changes have effects on the human body, but that the 24-hour cycle of morning; day, evening and night does as well. This is evident in the fluctuation of body temperature and varying states of wake and rest. *Plain Questions: Chapter Discussion on the Interrelationship between Life and Nature* (*Sù Wèn: Shēng Qì Tōng Tiān Lùn*, 素问·生气通天论) states that the yang qi in the human body begins to rise to action on the body surface in the morning, becomes most vigorous at noon, gradually wanes in the evening and is completely dormant within the body by midnight. Thus, it is said that the human body changes with the daily cyclical wax and wane of the yin and yang energies of the natural world. (Fig. Introduction-3)

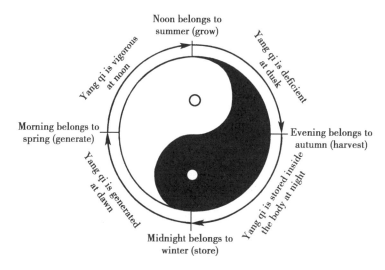

Fig. Introduction-3   Outline of the daily cyclical wax and wane of the body's yang qi

Miraculous Pivot: Chapter The Human Healthy Qi in the Day and Night Corresponds with the Qi of the Four Seasons (*Líng Shū: Shùn Qì Yī Rì Fēn Wéi Sì Shí*, 灵枢·顺气一日分为四时) states: "*The normal cycle of qi is to emerge in spring, grow in summer, harvest in autumn and store in winter. The human body also corresponds to this cycle. If the day is divided into four seasons, morning is equivalent to its spring, noon its summer, evening its autumn and night equivalent to its winter.*"

Plain Questions: Chapter Discussion on the

Interrelationship between Life and Nature (*Sù Wèn: Shēng Qì Tōng Tiān Lùn*, 素问·生气通天论) states: "*Yang qi dominates the exterior of the body during daylight hours. The body's qi emerges at daybreak, flourishes at midday, weakens as the sun falls into the west, closing the qi gate.*"

The alteration of day and night also has a clear influence on illness. In general, symptoms lighten during the day and become more severe at night. The relative flourishing and weakening of the right qi and pathogenic qi during the disease process has a direct influence on the state of illness. In general, if the right qi is victorious, the pathogenic qi will weaken, resulting in a positive change in the patient's condition. On the other hand, if the pathogenic qi is victorious, the right qi will weaken, and the patient's condition will worsen. In accordance with the wax and wane of yin and yang throughout the daily cycle, the yang qi (right qi) of the human body follows the pattern of emerging, growth, harvest and storing according to the four seasons of the day. This also affects the relationship between the rise and fall of right qi and pathogenic qi in the course of an illness. Therefore, symptoms also vary in severity being, "peaceful at daybreak, calm at midday, more severe at dusk and extreme at night". (Table Introduction-2)

Table Introduction-2   The relationship between the daily rise and fall of right or pathogenic qi and patient's condition

	Morning (Daybreak)	Noontime (Midday)	Evening (Dusk)	Night (Midnight)
Human qi (Right qi)	Begins to emerge	Grows	Begins to weaken	Enters into storage
Illness qi (Evil qi)	Weakened	Defeated (Right qi overcomes pathogenic qi.)	Begins to emerge	Reigns unchecked in the body
Patient's Condition	Peaceful	Calm	More severe	Extreme

Note: The above table generalizes the patient's condition in accordance with the alternation of morning, day, evening and night. In clinical practice, the patient's status should be analyzed according to the concrete nature of their illness.

Miraculous Pivot: Chapter The Human Healthy Qi in the Day and Night Corresponds with the Qi of the Four Seasons (Líng Shū: Shùn Qì Yī Rì Fēn Wéi Sì Shí, 灵枢·顺气一日分为四时) states: "'Why are most illnesses peaceful at daybreak, calm at midday, more severe at dusk and extreme at night?' Qi Bo (岐伯) replies, 'It is the qi of the four seasons that make it so…At daybreak, the body's qi begins to emerge and the pathogenic qi is weakened, thus symptoms are at rest. At midday, the body's qi grows and the increased qi can thus overcome the pathogenic qi, so symptoms remain calm. In the evening, the body's qi begins to decline and the pathogenic qi begins to emerge, so symptoms increase. At night, the body's qi is stored internally, and the pathogenic qi reigns unchecked within the body, so symptoms become severe.'"

Jing-yue's Complete Works: Section Yin and Yang, Chapter Chuan Zhong Lu, (Jǐng Yuè Quán Shū: Chuán Zhōng Lù, Yīn Yáng Piān, 景岳全书·传忠录·阴阳篇) states: "The Classic of the Central Viscera (Zhōng Zàng Jīng, 中藏经) observes: 'If the patient suffers from yang illness, symptoms will quiet at daybreak; yin illness, symptoms will be quiet during the night. If yang is deficient there will be disorder in the evening; yin deficiency and there is struggle in the morning. This is because yang deficiency benefits from the help of yang energy, so symptoms are light in the morning and severe in the evening. Yin deficiency benefits from the help of yin energy, so symptoms are severe in the morning and light in the evening. This explains the deficiency of yin and yang. If the illness suffers one of excess pathogen, conditions will be opposite. All diseases of excessive yang pathogens will be severe in the morning and light in the evening. Diseases of excessive yin pathogens will be light in the morning and severe in the evening. In summary, yang invigorates yang, and yin strengthens yin.'"

Key Link of Medicine: Chapter Discussion Yin and Yang (Yī Guàn: Yīn Yáng Lùn, 医贯·阴阳论) states: "If the patient suffers from yang illness, symptoms will be severe during the day and light at night. This is because the yang qi and pathogenic qi congeal. If the patient suffers from yin illness, symptoms will be light during the daytime and severe at night. That's because the yin qi and pathogenic qi are vigorous alternatively. Illnesses of yang deficiency are light during the daytime; illnesses of yin deficiency are light at night because yin and yang tend to return to their respective phases."

c. The influence of the regional environment factors on the human body

Regional environmental factors are one of the fundamentals surrounding human life. Differences in terrain, climate, water, soil, produce, culture, living habits and customs exert a varying degree of influence on the human body, and in turn lead to the development of different characteristic physiological functions and constitutions of the human body. For example, the terrain of southeastern China is located close to sea-level, the climate is warm and humid, making the striae and interstitial space of its inhabitants relatively porous. In contrast, the northwestern area of China is a high plateau, the climate is cold and dry, and therefore the striae and interstitial space of local residents is tightly sealed. Thus, long-term residents of a given region often feel uncomfortable upon relocating to a new environment. This is also known as "unsuitable water and earth". The occurrence of many endemic diseases is closely related to the environmental characteristics of a given region. Therefore, regional differences may directly influence the occurrence, development, and nature of disease. Chinese medical practitioners must adhere to the principle of "adjusting treatment to fit local conditions" when making a diagnosis and providing treatment. In *The Internal Classic (Nèi Jīng)* the practice of "treating patients of different regions accordingly" is expounded in detail.

Plain Questions: Chapter Discussion on Different Therapeutic Methods for Different Diseases (Sù Wèn: Yì Fǎ Fāng Yí Lùn, 素问·异法方宜论*)* states: *"The east is near the sea and rich in fish and salt. People there prefer fish and salty flavors… Fish leads to heat retain in the middle jiao and excessive salt intake impairs blood. Therefore, the local people are dark-skinned with porous striae and interstices, and often suffer from carbuncles and ulcers that can be cured by stone-needles…The western region is rich in metal, jade, sand and stone…The people eat fresh and rich food, which makes them heavy and strong. As a result, pathogens cannot attack their body. Their illnesses are usually endogenous and best treated with herbs…The North is nature's place of storage and closure…The people there roam the outdoors and consume dairy, so their viscera easily contract cold and develop illnesses of fullness. Their illnesses are best treated with moxibustion…The South is a nurturing region of growth, plentiful in yang qi… The people prefer sour flavors and fermented food. Their skin is therefore compact and reddish. They often suffer cramps best treated with acupuncture…."* (Table Introduction-3)

Table Introduction-3   Effects of different regions on human body, sickness and treatment

Region	Environment, habits and customs	Constitution	Common Illness	Treatment
East	Close proximity to the sea, rich in fish and salt; the people prefer fish and salty flavors	Black striae	Carbuncles and furuncles	Suitable to use stone needles
West	Rich in metal, jade, sand and stone; the people eat fresh and rich foods that make them heavy and strong	Relatively strong (qi pathogens can not hurt the body)	Tend suffer endogenous illness	Suitable for herbal treatment
North	A place of natural storage and closure; the people there live outside and consume dairy	Relatively strong	Viscera easily contract cold and develop diseases of abdominal fullness	Suitable for treatment with moxibustion
South	A place of natural growth, plentiful in yang qi; the people prefer sour flavors and fermented food	Striae is compact and skin reddish	Cramps and arthritic pain	Suitable for treatment with thin needles

Medical Ladder (Yī Xué Jiē Tī, 医学阶梯*)* states: *"Therefore, those who are good at treating illness must first differentiate region and terrain. Region and terrain are differentiated in terms of far, close, high and low. The strength and weakness of the individual and the wax or wane of their disease conforms to it."*

Treatise on the Headstream of Medicine: Chapter On Five Orientations and Different Treatment (Yī Xué Yuán Liú Lùn: Wǔ Fāng Yì Zhì Lùn, 医学源流论·五方异治论) states: *"Humans are created through the fusion of the qi of heaven and earth. The body's qi is therefore different in respect to region and terrain. The qi of the people of the northwest region is deep and thick. If attacked by wind-cold pathogens, it is difficult to expel. Therefore, a powerful dispersing formula should be used. The qi of the people of the southeast region is floating and thin. If attacked by wind-cold pathogens, it is easy to expel. So, a light dispersing formula should be used."*

B. The relationship between humans and their social environment

Humans possess both natural and social attributes. The life activities of a person are not only influenced by various natural environmental factors, but are also constrained by various social factors, including political, economic, cultural, religious, legal, marital, and interpersonal etc. These social factors can both directly and indirectly influence the physical and mental health of an individual, their physiological functions and psychological mood, and in turn the onset of disease and its treatment. Chinese medicine attaches great importance to social and mental factors, especially emotional ones. *"Internal damage from the seven emotions"* is considered in detail in Chinese medical etiology, and is recognized as a key pathogenic factor in the appearance of internal disease.

② Syndrome Differentiation and Treatment (Fig. Introduction-4)

(1) The concept of disease, syndrome and symptoms

Chinese medical diagnosis and treatment emphasizes "treatment based on syndrome differentiation, 辨证论治", not "treatment based on disease differentiation" where one herb or one prescription directly corresponds to one illness. It also does not advocate the treatment of concrete symptoms, or "treatment of symptoms". The concepts of disease, syndrome and symptom therefore need some differentiation.

Disease (病), or illness, is a complex course of pathological changes within the body with certain manifestations and a definite pattern of illness caused by pathogenic factors under the right conditions.

Syndrome (证), or pattern, is the summary of a given phase of pathological development of the body.

Symptoms (症), or manifestations, are specific phenomena that emerge in the course of illness and are the patient's subjective perception of abnormality.

In terms of their reflection of the nature of disease, disease reflect the nature of the overall course of the pathological changes; syndrome reflects the nature of a certain phase of pathological changes; and symptoms are the specific external phenomena of disease, but do not necessarily accurately reflect the true nature of the disease.

Disease, syndrome and symptoms are related in that they all stem from the foundation of pathological change in the human body. Disease includes the whole course of pathological change in terms of both syndrome and symptom. Syndrome is a summation of symptoms that reflects the nature of illness at a given point in time, while symptoms are the basic elements of disease and syndrome; in other words, both disease and syndrome are composed of symptoms. With these differences between the concept of disease, syndrome and symptoms, Chinese medicine emphasizes syndrome differentiation, because a syndrome represents a pathological summary of a given phase of disease. Syndrome includes the etiology, location, nature of the disease, relationship between the wax and wane of right qi and pathogen, as well as the pattern of pathological change. It also reflects the nature of pathological change during a given phase in the course of disease development. In keeping with the principle of "seeking the root cause in treating illness", syndrome reveals the nature of pathological change more completely and deeper than that of symptoms, and reflects the nature of the present phase of pathological change more concretely and more precisely than disease. Therefore, treatment based on syndrome differentiation should be more feasible

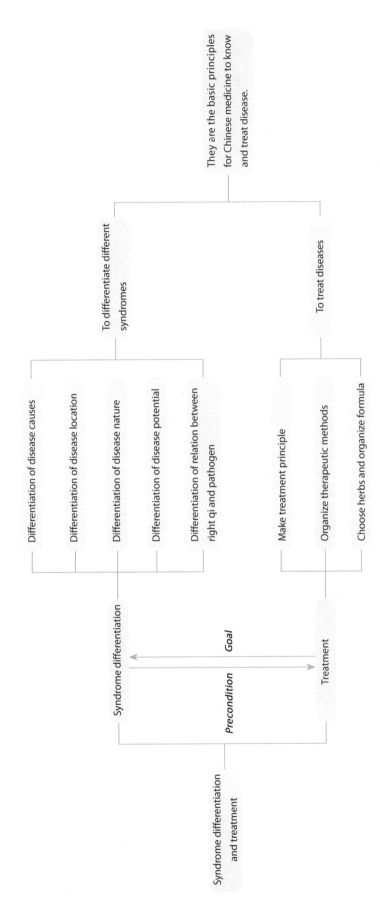

Fig. Introduction-4   Sketch of syndrome differentiation and treatment

and effective. Chinese medicine emphasizes syndrome differentiation and treatment, neither treatment based on disease differentiation nor direct treatment of concrete symptoms.

Note: Regarding the usage of the character 证 "Zheng (syndrome or pattern)" and 症"Zheng (symptom)", Zhang Zhong-jing of the Eastern *Han* Dynasty first classified diseases according to "Mai (Pulse) and Zheng (syndrome)" and divided them into their respective chapters. He proposed the theory of syndrome differentiation and treatment "To observe the pulse and syndrome of a patient to know what the patient suffers from and to then treat the illness according to syndrome." There was no Chinese character "Zheng (symptom)" in the medical works preceeding *Song* Dynasty. In the *Ming* and *Qing* Dynasties, the character was widely used, and in some medical books, the Chinese characters "Zheng (syndrome) and Zheng (symptom)" were used together, often it difficult to distinguish their meanings. *Large Dictionary of Chinese Characters (Zhōng Huá Dà Zì Diǎn)* states that zheng (symptom) is a commonly used form derived from Zheng (syndrome). *The Source of Words (Cí Yuán)* states that Zheng (syndrome) is the archaic character of Zheng (symptom). It is important to note the difference in meaning between syndrome and symptom in modern Chinese medical theory and not to confuse them.

(2) Concept of syndrome differentiation and treatment

Syndrome differentiation and treatment, also called treatment based on syndrome differentiation, is the primary Chinese medical principle in the recognition and treatment of disease. It can be divided into two phases, syndrome differentiation and treatment.

Syndrome differentiation, or distinguishing syndromes, is to amass the information collected through the four examinations (observing, smelling and listening, questioning, and palpation and pulse reading, 望, 闻, 问, 切), including symptoms and signs, and analyze it according to the theories of Chinese medicine; This analysis should result in a clear differentiation of the nature of the syndrome, the cause, location, properties, tendency of pathological change of the disease, as well as the relationship between the wax and wane of right qi and pathogen.

Etiological Differentiation: To deduce the primary cause of illness according to the etiological theory of the analysis of symptoms and physical signs and to treat an illness based on its etiology, namely, "To distinguish symptoms and signs to identify etiology, and to treat disease according to its cause."

Differentiation of Disease Location: Different pathogenic factors invade different regions of the human body and cause different disease syndromes. Differentiation of disease location is to pinpoint the location of a disease based upon external manifestations of pathological change and in turn, provide appropriate treatment.

Differentiation of the Nature of Disease: To determine the nature of a syndrome in terms of yin, yang, exterior, interior, cold, heat, deficiency and excess according to the manifestations of the pathological change.

Differentiation of Disease Potential: All diseases have certain laws of development and transmission. Differentiation of disease potential is to predict its tendency to change and provide an accurate disease prognosis.

Differentiation of the Relationship between Right Qi and Pathogen: In the development and evolution of a disease, its wax and wane is a reflection of the constant battle between right qi and pathogen. The relationship of the wax and wane of right qi and pathogen is also responsible for the deficiency or excess property of a syndrome, as well as the determination of disease potential. This is the basis for the practice of the treatment principle "strengthen right qi to eliminate the pathogenic factor".

Treatment, or treating disease, is to the result of syndrome differentiation, to establish relevant clinical treatment and methodology, to select appropriate therapeutic methods and techniques, as well as to choose proper prescriptions and herbs in accordance with the patient's syndrome. Syndrome differentiation and treatment are two interrelated and indivisible elements in the diagnostic and treatment process. Syndrome differentiation is the precondition and foundation for determining treatment and treatment is the aim of syndrome differentiation, confirming the accuracy of syndrome differentiation. Therefore, syndrome differentiation and treatment, is the process of recognizing and resolving disease.

(3) The relationship between syndrome differentiation and disease differentiation

Both syndrome differentiation and disease differentiation are part of the larger analytical process of recognizing disease, providing instruction for treatment based upon the clinical manifestations of the patient. As practitioners continue to raise the level of the practice of methods unique to Chinese medical syndrome differentiation and treatment, they must also take advantages of the advancements in diagnostic techniques of biomedical science and technology. Over the course of a patient's illness, syndrome differentiation and disease differentiation must be equally stressed, with emphasis on the principle of syndrome differentiation and treatment.

(4) Treatment of the same disease with different methods and treatment of different diseases with the same method

Treating the same disease with different methods and treating different diseases with the same methods are a concrete embodiment of the principle of syndrome differentiation and treatment in the clinical process of diagnosing and treating a disease.

Treating the same disease with different methods refers to the different treatment of one disease in multiple patients with different syndromes, the result of discrepancies in time of occurrence, terrain, phase of a disease, or constitution of the patient. Treating different diseases with the same methods refers to the use of the same treatment for several different diseases in patients who have the same or approximately the same pathological changes that in turn manifests as the same or approximately the same syndrome.

As a result, it can be said that Chinese medicine treats disease not with an eye to the similarities and differences of "Bing (disease, 病)", but rather to the differentiation of "Zheng (syndrome, 证)". The same syndrome is treated with fundamentally the same clinical methods and different syndromes with different clinical methods. This is "To treat the same syndrome with same treatment; to treat different syndromes with different treatments". The principle of resolving conflicts of discrepancy in the process of illness development through the use of different methods is the essence of syndrome differentiation and treatment.

Plain Questions: Chapter Major Discussion on the Administration of Five-Motions (Sù Wèn: Wǔ Cháng Zhèng Dà Lùn, 素问·五常政大论) states: "The weather in the northwest is cold, so one must disperse the external cold and clear away internal heat; the weather in the southwest is warm and hot, one must collect and restrain the excreted yang energy and warm internal coldness. This is treating the same disease with different methods."

Chapter 1
Chinese Medicine and Ancient Philosophy

The scientific theories of the natural sciences cannot evolve or develop without a strong philosophical grounding and are guided and bounded by philosophical thought. During the course of the evolution and development of the theoretical system of Chinese medicine, it is inevitable that ancient philosophical thought would exert a strong influence. Amidst this influence, the doctrines of essence and qi, yin-yang and the five phases have exerted the most profound influence on Chinese medicine.

These three doctrines are philosophical theories of ancient China that represent the perspectives and methodology for the ancients to cognize the world and explain its changes. When Chinese medical theory was being formed, sages utilized these ancient philosophies to explain the vital phenomena of the human body, with far-reaching influence on all fields of Chinese medicine to expound physiological functions and pathological changes, as well as to diagnose and treat disease. Therefore, the doctrines of essential qi, yin-yang and the five phases are not only the guiding principles in the evolution and development of Chinese medical theory, but also a fundamental part of its theoretical system.

Section 1　Doctrine of Essential Qi

Concept of Essential Qi (Fig. 1-1)

①Philosophical Meaning of Essential Qi

The doctrine of essential qi is an ancient philosophy prevailing in the period prior to the *Qin* and *Han* Dynasties that utilizes essential qi to explain the origin and creation of all things in the universe, their development and changes. It holds that everything in the universe consists of essence and qi and that their development and changes are produced by its function.

Yi Zhuan: Chapter Xicishang (Yì Zhuàn: Xì Cí Shàng, 易传·系辞上) states: "*Essential qi creates everything.*"

Lun Heng: Chapter Nature (Lùn Héng: Zì Rán, 论衡·自然) states: "*The qi of heaven and earth combine, naturally giving rise to the myriad of forms.*"

Plain Questions: Chapter Major Discussion on the Law of Motions and Changes in Nature (Sù Wèn: Tiān Yuán Jì Dà Lùn, 素问·天元纪大论) states: "*It is manifested as qi in the heavens and takes form on earth. The interplay of qi and form produces all.*"

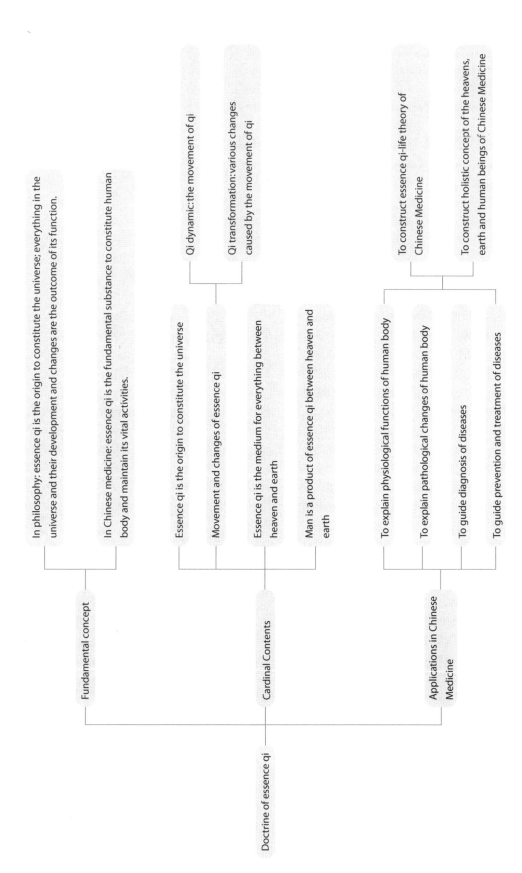

Fig. 1-1   Outline of the doctrine of essential qi

② Concept of Essential Qi in Chinese Medicine

The theoretical system of Chinese medicine took shape primarily during the *Qin* and *Han* Dynasties, thus the contemporary prevailing doctrine of essential qi would exert a profound influence on its formation. Medical experts at that time introduced this theory into Chinese Medicine to expound vital phenomena of the human body. It is considered that the essential qi is the fundamental substance that constitutes the human body and maintains its vital activities.

Huai Nan Zi: *Chapter Explanation of the Universe* (*Huái Nán Zǐ: Tiān Wén Xùn*, 淮南子·天文训) states: "*Essential qi forms the human body.*"

Zhuang Zi: *Chapter Zhi Traveling to the North* (*Zhuāng Zǐ: Zhì Běi Yóu*, 庄子·知北游) says: "*Human life is a gathering of qi. As qi gathers there is life, when it scatters, death.*"

Lun Heng: *Chapter Discussion of Death* (*Lùn Héng: Lùn Sǐ*, 论衡·论死) says: "*Man is alive is because of essential qi. When a man dies, the essence and qi perish.*"

③ Various Meanings of Essence and Qi as Applied in Chinese Medicine

In ancient philosophy, in regard to the origin of all the things in the universe, such expressions as essence, qi, essential qi, and original qi are used simultaneously. This phenomenon had a certain degree of influence on Chinese medicine as well. Generally speaking, essence, qi, essential qi or original qi all refer to the fundamental substance that constitutes the human body, maintains its vital activities, and provides a substantial basis for the functional activities of all viscera and bowels, tissues and organs. For this reason, essence and qi are of the same meaning in some respects in the Chinese medical application and can be used as substitutes for each other. For instance, essence from water and food, qi from water and food, essential qi from water and food can often be used interchangeably, as can Kidney qi, essential qi of the Kidneys, and original qi of the Kidneys.

However, in some regards, essence and qi are different in Chinese medicine. It is believed that essence and qi are two different kinds of substances that emerge from vital activities. Essence is the condensed and static state of qi, and qi is the diffused and mobile state of essence. Thus, it is said that essence can transform into qi and qi can transform into essence. Sometimes "essence" is used to modify qi. Essential qi is the refined, extracted part of qi. For example, qi from Water and food can be classified into essential qi from water and food, and vigorous qi from water and food. Therefore, the different applications of essence, qi, essential qi and original qi in Chinese medicine depend on the situation, and the implications will have corresponding distinctions.

Basic Contents of the Doctrine of Essential Qi (Fig. 1–1)

① Essential Qi: The Structural Origin of the Universe

It is held that everything in the universe, including mankind, is composed of essential qi, the primordial matter of all things between heaven and earth. The formation, development and changes of the universe are all the result of the motion of essential qi, namely, the interaction of the qi of heaven and earth (yin and yang), the root cause of all phenomena.

Concerning its states of existence, the ancients have divided essential qi into "form" and "formless" through their direct observation. The formless indicates essential qi in a diffuse and mobile state that fills the vast universal space and is invisible, hence the name. That with form indicates essential qi in a condensed and comparatively static state that has formed a visible and tangible entity. Therefore, the diffuse and formless is usually called qi, and the formed and comparatively static is called form. The formless qi can condense into physical form, and form can transform into formless qi. Therefore, the formed and formless are in a constant state of transformation. The mutual transformation of essence and qi is an embodiment of this principle.

Yi Zhuan: *Chapter Xicixia* (*Yì Zhuàn: Xì Cí Xià*, 易传·系辞下) states: "*Heaven and earth enshrouded*

in mist, bring all things to fruition. The intercourse of the male and females essence results in the growth of all the things."

Lun Heng: Chapter Yandu (Lùn Héng: Yán Dú, 论衡·言毒) says: *"The emergence of the ten thousand forms all depends on original qi."*

② Movement and Changes of Essential Qi

Essential qi is a refined substance full of vitality in constant motion. The movement and change of everything in nature is the result of that of essential qi. The movement and change of essential qi are called qi dynamics and qi transformation.

Qi dynamics refers to the movement of qi. Its patterns vary and are summarized by *Internal Classic (Nèi Jīng, 内经)* into the four basic forms of ascending, descending, entering and exiting. The movement of qi is one of its intrinsic features and a universal law. It is the movement of qi that promotes the decline and disappearance of old forms, and the formation and growth of new things. Thus, the balance of the cycle of nature is maintained.

Qi transformation points to the various changes caused by the movement of qi. Its process is very complicated. All modes of change throughout the universe such as those in form, function and manifest pattern are the outcome of qi transformation.

Plain Questions: Chapter Major Discussion on the Abstruseness of the Six Kinds of Qi (Sù Wèn: Liù Wēi Zhǐ Dà Lùn, 素问·六微旨大论) says: *"The ascent and descent of qi is the alternating action of heaven and earth…Qi descends after ascending, the descending is the qi of heaven; qi ascends after descending, the ascending is the qi of earth. The qi of heaven descends and flows upon the earth, while the qi of earth ascends and evaporates into the heavens. Therefore, high and low mutually welcome one another, ascending and descending rely upon one another. Thus, change occurs…the generation of things depends on transformation, and the extremity of things is known as change. Interaction of transformation and change is the basis of formation and destruction…Formation and destruction are engendered from movement, and endless movement leads to change."*

③ Essential Qi: The Medium for All Between Heaven and Earth

Medium embodies the indirect connection of different things or different factors of the same thing. It is the intermediary link between the transformation and development of objective things.

Heaven, earth, and all things between them are, relatively speaking, independent matter. However, they are not independent of each other and, on the contrary, are filled with formless qi by which they are connected into a seamless entity. Formless qi can also penetrate form, playing the role of communicating and connecting, bringing all things into interaction and harmony.

The Book of Changes: Section Xian (Xián), Chapter Xiajing, (Zhōu Yì: Xià Jīng, Xián, 周易·下经·咸) states: *"The interaction of heaven and earth gives rise to the ten thousand forms."*

Plain Questions: Chapter Major Discussion on the Law of Motions and Changes in Nature (Sù Wèn: Tiān Yuán Jì Dà Lùn, 素问·天元纪大论) states: *"It manifests as qi in the heavens and form on earth. The interaction of qi and form produces everything."*

④ Man as the Product of the Interaction of the Essential Qi of Heaven and Earth

Ancient philosophers believed that man is produced through the combination of the essential qi of heaven and earth, the original structural matter of the human body. Human beings are different from other living things in the universe due to the possession of conscious mental functions above and beyond simple life instincts. Man is engendered from a refined portion of ethereal qi (called "essential qi" in *Huai Nan Zi*). The birth and death of human life is the process of the gathering and scattering of qi.

Guanzi: Chapter Nei Ye (Guǎn Zǐ: Nèi Yè, 管子·内业) states: *"Human life is the combination of essence endowed by the heavens and substance endowed by the earth."*

Plain Questions: Chapter Discussion on Preserving Health and Protecting Life (Sù Wèn: Bǎo Mìng Quán Xíng Lùn, 素问·宝命全形论) states: *"A man is generated by the qi of heaven and earth and*

grows according to the law of the four seasons." "The combination of the qi of heaven and earth is animated and called man."

Miraculous Pivot: Chapter On Channels (Líng Shū: Jīng Mài, 灵枢·经脉) states: *"The start of human life is the formation of essence."*

Lun Heng: Chapter Discussion of Death (Lùn Héng: Lùn Sǐ, 论衡·论死) states: *"Essential qi is the means by which man is born." "The course of qi generating man is just like Water becoming ice. The solidification of Water is ice, and that of qi is man."*

Huai Nan Zi: Chapter Explanation of the Universe (Huái Nán Zǐ: Tiān Wén Xùn, 淮南子·天文训) states: *"Disrupted qi forms worms while essential qi forms man."*

Zhuangzi: Chapter Zhi Traveling to the North (Zhuāng Zǐ: Zhì Běi Yóu, 庄子·知北游) states: *"Human life is a gathering of qi. As qi gathers there is life, when it scatters there is death."*

The Application of the Doctrine of Essential Qi in Chinese Medicine (Fig. 1-1)

① Theoretical System of Chinese Medicine

A. Used to create the essential qi-life theory of Chinese medicine

It is believed that essential qi is the origin of human life, i.e. man is produced by essential qi. At the same time, essential qi is also the most fundamental substance that maintains the vital activities of the human body. Therefore, Chinese medicine utilizes it to expound reproduction and growth of the body as well as to explain the physiological functions and pathological changes of the viscera and bowels, tissues and organs.

B. Used to create the holistic concept of heaven, earth and human beings in Chinese medicine

Chinese medical theory holds that all things between heaven and earth (including mankind) are composed of essential qi. Heaven, earth and human beings (three *cai*, 三才) are integrated through essential qi. Its natural environment will therefore inevitably influence the phenomena of human life. The physiological functions and pathological changes of the human body as well as the prevention and treatment of disease are all closely related to the natural and social environments. Thus, the integrity of three *cai* was formed. This is the view that *"Man mutually interacts with heaven and earth"* as stated in *Internal Classic (Nèi Jīng, 内经).*

② Concrete Contents of Chinese Medicine

The dotrine of essential qi runs through every aspect of Chinese medicine, which is used to explain the physiological functions and pathological changes of the body, to guide diagnosis, prevention and treatment of disease (see related chapters for details).

Section 2　Doctrine of Yin-Yang

The doctrine of yin-yang is a materialistic and dialectic world view and methodology of the ancients to understand nature and explain its changes. It considers the world to be a materially integrated whole, the product of the opposition and unity of yin and yang. Everything in the world emerges, develops and changes through the interaction of yin qi and yang qi.

Chinese medicine adopted the doctrine of yin-yang to consider many medical questions. As a result, Chinese medicine combined with the doctrine of yin-yang to form the Chinese medical yin-yang theory. It penetrates every aspect of Chinese medicine to explain the vital activities of the human body, occurrence of disease and its pathological changes, as well as to guide diagnosis and prevention. It has become an indispensable foundation of the theoretical system of Chinese medicine.

Yi Zhuan: Chapter Xicishang (Yì Zhuàn: Xì Cí Shàng, 易传·系辞上) states: *"One yin, one yang, this is called Dao (道)."*

Plain Questions: Chapter Major Discussion on the Theory of Yin and Yang and the Corresponding Relationships Among All the Things in Nature (Sù Wèn: Yīn Yáng Yìng Xiàng Dà Lùn, 素问·阴阳应象大论) states: *"Yin-yang is the Dao (道) of heaven and earth, the guiding principle of all things, the origin of change, the root of life and death, and the residence of the brilliant spirit."*

Fundamental Concept of Yin–Yang

1 Definition of Yin-Yang

Yin-yang is a general underlying notion of ancient Chinese philosophy that can be summarized as the opposing aspects of correlative things or phenomena in the universe. The original meaning of yin-yang is rather simple, meaning the sunny or shadowy side of an object. The side exposed to the sun may be characterized as yang, the shadowy side, yin. Together with the constantly growing range of subjects for observation, the application of yin-yang gradually enlarged. For example, daytime can be characterized as yang and night yin, warm as yang while cold yin, etc. Thus, almost all things and phenomena in nature can be delineated according to yin and yang. Yin-yang has come to represent an abstract concept to summarize two complimentary attributes of things or phenomena in nature.

Classic of Poetry: Chapter Gong Liu, volume Daya, (Shī Jīng: Dà Yǎ, Gōng Liú, 诗经·大雅·公刘) states: "Look out over the scenery and the mountain ridges, observe its yin and yang, and watch its running springs."

Explanation of Chinese Characters (Shūo Wén, 说文) explains the meaning of yin and yang: "Yin means dark, indicating southern banks of rivers and northern slopes of mountains." "Yang means high and bright."

Laozi: Chapter 42nd (Lǎo Zǐ, 老子) states: "All things inwardly bear yin and outwardly embrace yang."

Miraculous Pivot: Chapter The Yin and Yang of Human Body Relate to Sun and Moon (Líng Shū: Yīn Yáng Xì Rì Yuè, 灵枢·阴阳系日月) states: "Yin-yang is a term without shape."

Classified Classic: Chapter Category of Yin-Yang (Lèi Jīng: Yīn Yáng Lèi, 类经·阴阳类) says: "Yin-yang is the one divided into two."

2 Attributes of Things According to Yin-Yang

It is believed that the opposing aspects in corresponding things and phenomena have two contrary natures, which can be symbolized by yin and yang, known as their yin-yang attribute. In other words, yin-yang is a summarization of the attributes of opposing, dualistic things and phenomena in nature.

A. The categorization of things according to yin-yang

How should opposing, dualistic things and phenomena be categorized according to their yin-yang attributes? Water and Fire are used as the basic symbols of yin and yang in *Plain Questions: Chapter Major Discussion on the Theory of Yin and Yang and the Corresponding Relationships Among All the Things in Nature (Sù Wèn: Yīn Yáng Yìng Xiàng Dà Lùn, 素问·阴阳应象大论)*. Yin-yang is abstract while Water and Fire are concrete, so *Internal Classic (Nèi Jīng)* uses them as a basis for categorization, i.e., "Water and Fire are signs of yin and yang", "Water is characterized as yin and Fire as yang." Water is cool, downward flowing and relatively still, thus, it embodies yin. Fire is hot, upward flaring and comparatively active, thus representing yang.

Therefore, in general, anything that has the characteristics of activeness, directed upward or outward, formlessness, warmth and heat, brightness, excitement, strength, etc, belongs to yang; whereas anything that has the characteristics of stillness, directed downward or inward, coldness and coolness, darkness, inhibiting, weakness, etc, belongs to yin (Table 1-1). These are also called the basic properties of yin-yang.

Plain Questions: Chapter Major Discussion on the Theory of Yin and Yang and the Corresponding Relationships Among All the Things in Nature (Sù Wèn: Yīn Yáng Yìng Xiàng Dà Lùn, 素问·阴阳应象大论) states: "Yin is still while yang is active… yang generates qi and yin takes form…Water belongs to yin while Fire belongs to yang. Qi is attributed to yang and taste to yin…Medicines with acrid, sweet tastes and lifting functions belong to yang, while those with sour, bitter tastes that promote emesis and purging belong to yin. Yin and yang are the male-female properties of blood and qi. Left and right are the routes of yin-yang movement. Water and Fire are the embodiment of yin-yang."

Table 1-1   Categorization of yin-yang Attributes (Examples)

Attributes	Yang	Yin
Position (Space)	Up	Down
	Outside	Inside
	Left	Right
	South	North
	Sky	Earth
Time	Day	Night
Seasons	Spring and summer	Autumn and winter
Temperature	Warm	Cold
Humidity	Dry	Moist
Brightness	Bright	Dark
Substance or Function	Function	Substance
State of Movement	Ascending	Descending
	Motion	Stillness
	Rapid	Slow
Functional State	Excitement	Inhibition
	Hyperactivity	Hypoactivity
	Transforms qi	Takes form
Others	—	—

Key Link of Medicine: Chapter Discussion Yin and Yang (Yī Guàn: Yīn Yáng Lùn, 医贯·阴阳论) says: *"Yin-yang is just an empty name; Water and Fire are the concrete embodiments."*

B. Relativity of yin-yang attributes

It is held that the yin or yang attribute of any given phenomena are by no means absolute and unchangeable, but relative and variable. This is the relativity of yin-yang attributes. In other words, with the passing of time, differences in the scale in question, or changes in the features of an object or its relative opposite, its yin-yang attribute will change accordingly.

The relativity of yin-yang mainly manifests as follows:

Firstly, an object's yin-yang attribute is determined by comparison. The yin-yang attribute of an object or phenomena is classified by comparison. Once the object of comparison changed, the yin- yang attributes will change in accordance.

Secondly, yin and yang can transform into each other. Under certain conditions, an object may exhibit, also changing their yin-yang attributes. Yin can transform into yang, and yang into yin.

Thirdly, there exists yin and yang within yin or yang. Things are infinitely divisible, as is the yin-yang classification used to conceptualize them. That is to say, any aspect of yin or yang can also be divided into yin and yang. Day and night are used as an example to explain the unlimited divisibility of yin-yang in *Plain Questions: Chapter Discussion on Important Ideas in the Golden Chamber (Sù Wèn: Jīn Guì Zhēn Yán Lùn*, 素问·金匮真言论). Day is characterized as yang and night as yin. Day may be further divided, with morning as yang within yang, and afternoon as yin within yang; for night, the first half may be conceptualized as yin within yin, and the latter half, yang within yin (Fig. 1-2). Hence, yin and yang within yin and yang embodies the unlimited divisibility of things.

In Chinese medicine, according to the categorization of yin-yang attributes, substance is attributed to yin and function to yang. According to the relativity of yin-yang, yin substances and functions are those that possess condensing,

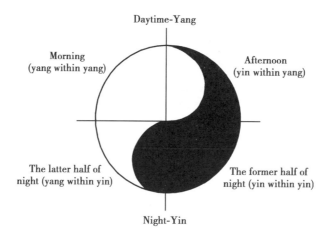

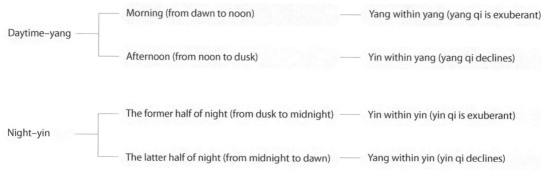

Fig. 1-2 Subdivision of the yin and yang of day and night

moistening and inhibiting properties, while generating, warming and exciting substances and functions are yang.

Plain Questions: Chapter Discussion on Important Ideas in the Golden Chamber (Sù Wèn: Jīn Guì Zhēn Yán Lùn, 素问·金匮真言论) states: *"There is yin within yin and yang within yang. The period from dawn to noon, the yang of the heavens, is yang within yang. That from noon till dusk, the yang of the heavens, is yin within yang. The period from dusk to midnight, the yin of the heavens, is yin within yin, and the period from midnight to dawn, the yin of the heavens, is yang within yin."*

Elaboration of Bureau Prescriptions (Jú Fāng Fā Huī, 局方发挥) states: *"The implication of yin-yang is relative, and its indication is not fixed."*

③ Universal Nature of Yin-Yang

The mutual opposition and interconnection of two aspects of things or phenomena in nature is universal and infinite. Yin-yang summarizes not only two opposite aspects of correlative objects or phenomena, but also two internal opposite attributes of the same thing. In other words, each individual object or phenomenon embraces yin and yang and can be sub-divided into two aspects. Therefore, the application of yin-yang theory is universal.

Plain Questions: Chapter Major Discussion on the Theory of Yin and Yang and the Corresponding Relationships Among All the Things in Nature (Sù Wèn: Yīn Yáng Yìng Xiàng Dà Lùn, 素问·阴阳应象大论) states: *"Yin-yang is the Dao of heaven and earth."*

Plain Questions: Chapter Separation and Combination of Yin and Yang (Sù Wèn: Yīn Yáng Lí Hé Lùn, 素问·阴阳离合论) states: *"The applications of yin-yang can be enumerated as high as ten, expanded to as high as one hundred, enumerated as high as one thousand, expanded to as high as ten thousand, even on to infinity, but in the end, there must still exist the unity of one."*

Basic Contents of the Doctrine of Yin–Yang

① Opposition of Yin and Yang (Fig. 1-3)

Opposition refers to the mutual repulsion and antagonism of two contradictory aspects within a single body. The opposition of yin and yang is used to explain the dualistic repelling, antagonistic and restricting relationship between two opposite natures of objects and phenomena.

The two opposite aspects of yin and yang exist within all things and phenomena of the natural world, making the opposition of yin and yang absolute.

The two opposites of yin and yang are also interconnected, interacting and mutually restraining, or mutually restrictive. The mutual opposition of yin and yang mainly manifests in their mutual antagonism and restriction. Antagonism is the root cause of change and development in all things; there would be no changes or development without this antagonism. Restriction implies that the existence and change of one thing takes as a condition the existence and change of another. Things maintain a relative balance between themselves through restriction, without which the balance would be upset. Therefore, the antagonism and restriction of yin and yang maintain the unity of things. In conclusion, the two aspects of yin and yang are both opposite as well as integrated in nature, that is, their unity is the result of their opposition.

In Chinese medicine, the opposing restriction theory of yin and yang is used to explain the physiological state of human body. The opposing forces of yin and yang within the human body are in a constant state of mutual antagonism and restriction that allows for the maintenance of a dynamic balance, i.e. *"yin calms and yang steadies, 阴平阳秘"* If this relationship of opposing restriction is broken, preventing yin and yang from maintaining a balanced state, an imbalance of yin and yang results and disease occurs.

Yi Zhuan: Chapter Xicishang (Yì Zhuàn: Xì Cí Shàng, 易传·系辞上) states: *"One yin, one yang, this is known as Dao (道)."*

Classified Classic: Chapter Category of Yin-Yang (Lèi Jīng: Yīn Yáng Lèi, 类经·阴阳类) states: *"Yin-yang is the one divided into two."*

Supplementary to the Classified Classic: Chapter Medicine and Changes (Lèi Jīng Fù Yì: Yī Yì, 类经附翼·医易) states: *"Extreme motion must be calmed with stillness; hyperactivity of yin must be pacified by yang."*

Plain Questions: Chapter Major Discussion on the Theory of Yin and Yang and the Corresponding Relationships Among All the Things in Nature (Sù Wèn: Yīn Yáng Yìng Xiàng Dà Lùn, 素问·阴阳应象大论) states: *"Overly dominant yin leads to disorders of yang, and overly dominant yang leads to disorders of yin. Yang dominance leads to heat, and yin dominance leads to cold."*

② Interdependence of Yin and Yang (Fig. 1-4)

Interdependence can be defined as being the mutual basis for each other, which is the source of the existence, development and movements of objects and phenomena in mutual opposition. The interdependence of yin and yang is to use yin-yang to explain that the two mutually opposing aspects of a given object or phenomena take each other as the precondition of their own existence and that any single aspect cannot exist without the other. Their relationship is one mutual utilization, mutual nourishment, and mutual replenishment.

Interdependence shows the inseparability of the two opposing aspects of yin and yang. The main manifestations are as follows:

Firstly, yin and yang take each other as their basis in categorizing the yin-yang attributes of objects and phenomena. The two aspects of yin and yang are opposite as well as interdependent. Therefore, when analyzing the yin-yang attributes of something, it is crucial to first grasp its fundamental properties. At the same time, one must pay attention to the correlation of things. Only when these two aspects exist unified within a single body, can it be analyzed by yin-yang, i.e. *"if there is yin, so must there also be yang; if there is yang, so must there also be yin."*

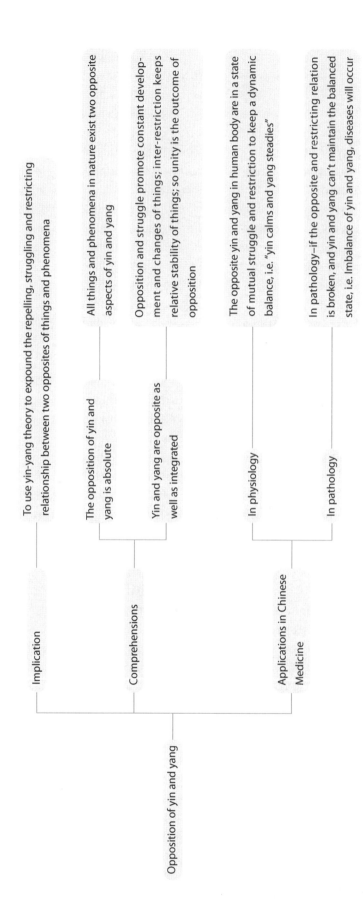

Fig. 1-3   Summary of the opposition of yin and yang

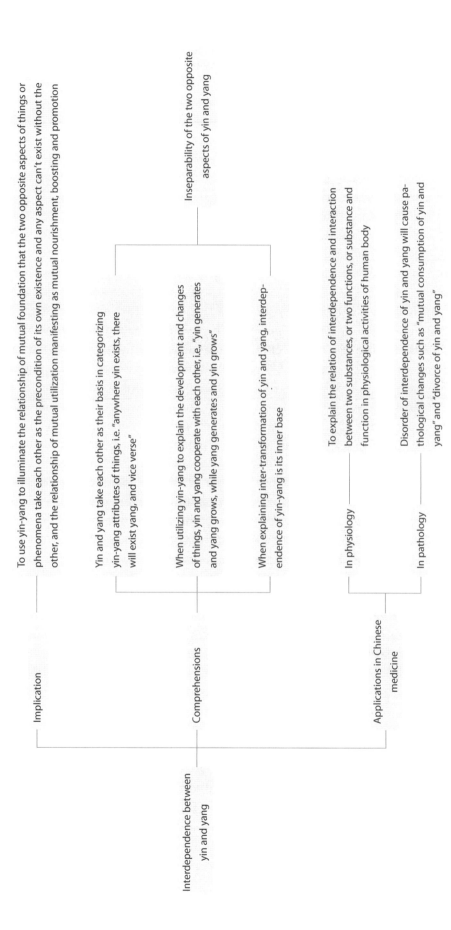

Fig. 1-4   Summary of the interdependence of yin and yang

Interdependence between yin and yang

Implication — To use yin-yang to illuminate the relationship of mutual foundation that the two opposite aspects of things or phenomena take each other as the precondition of its own existence and any aspect can't exist without the other, and the relationship of mutual utilization manifesting as mutual nourishment, boosting and promotion

Comprehensions

— Yin and yang take each other as their basis in categorizing yin-yang attributes of things, i.e. "anywhere yin exists, there will exist yang, and vice verse"

— When utilizing yin-yang to explain the development and changes of things, yin and yang cooperate with each other, i.e., "yin generates and yang grows, while yang generates and yin grows"

— When explaining inter-transformation of yin and yang, interdependence of yin-yang is its inner base

Inseparability of the two opposite aspects of yin and yang

Applications in Chinese medicine

In physiology — To explain the relation of interdependence and interaction between two substances, or two functions, or substance and function in physiological activities of human body

In pathology — Disorder of interdependence of yin and yang will cause pathological changes such as "mutual consumption of yin and yang" and "divorce of yin and yang"

Secondly, the interdependence of yin and yang is the source of development and change for all things. When utilizing yin-yang to explain the development and change of things, yin and yang exist in cooperation with each other, i.e., "*Yin is generated and yang grows; yang is generated and yin grows.*"

Thirdly, the interdependence of yin-yang is an inner foundation for the mutual transformation of yin and yang. The mutual transformation of yin and yang under certain conditions is based upon their interdependence. If there is no relationship of interconnection and interdependence, this transformation into its opposite can not occur.

In Chinese medicine, the theory of interdependence and interaction of yin and yang can be used to explain the nature of a relationship between two substances, or two functions, or substance and function in the physiological activities of the human body. In pathology, disorder of the interdependence of yin and yang could lead to pathological changes, such as the "mutual consumption of yin and yang" and the "separation of yin and yang".

Notation of *Plain Questions: Chapter Major Discussion of Regulation of Spirit According to the Changes of the Four Seasons (Sù Wèn: Sì Qì Tiáo Shén Dà Lùn,* 素问·四气调神大论) by Wang Bing (王冰, *Tang* Dynasty) states: "*Yang qi is rooted in yin and yin qi rooted in yang. Yang can not generate without yin and yin can not transform without yang.*"

Key Link of Medicine: Chapter Discussion Yin and Yang (Yī Guàn: Yīn Yáng Lùn, 医贯·阴阳论) states: "*Yin and yang are the sources of each other. Yang is rooted in yin and yin in yang. Yin can not generate without yang and yang can not transform without yin.*"

Plain Questions: Chapter Major Discussion on the Theory of Yin and Yang and the Corresponding Relationships Among All The Things in Nature (Sù Wèn: Yīn Yáng Yìng Xiàng Dà Lùn, 素问·阴阳应象大论) states: "*Yin remains inside, the guardian of yang, while yang remains outside, the envoy for yin.*"

Plain Questions: Chapter Discussion on the Interrelationship between Life and Nature (Sù Wèn: Shēng Qì Tōng Tiān Lùn, 素问·生气通天论) says:

"*If yin calms and yang steadies, the essence and spirit will function normally; if yin and yang separate, the essential qi will be exhausted.*"

Supplementary to the Classified Classic: Chapter Seeking the Right Way (Lèi Jīng Fù Yì: Qiú Zhèng Lù, 类经附翼·求正录) states: "*Yin can not exist without yang because there would be nothing from which to generate form; yang can not exist without yin because there would be no form to carry qi.*"

③ Wax and Wane of Yin and Yang (Fig. 1-5)

Wax and wane, increase and decrease, or flow and ebb. The wax and wane of yin and yang is to use yin-yang theory to clarify that the opposing aspects are not in a state of stillness but in a state of constant motion of waxing and waning change. The dynamic balance of the waxing and waning change between yin and yang has a defined limit, within which normal development and changes of things is maintained.

The two opposing aspects of correlative objects or phenomena in nature are moving and changing constantly, so the waxing and waning of yin and yang is a fund amental law of movement and change in all things. It includes a process of "quantitative change".

The factors that cause waxing and waning are twofold. Firstly, the mutual opposition and antagonism between the opposing natures of yin and yang inevitably bring about a situation that one should increase while the other decreases, or one grows while the other declines, i.e. one waxes while the other wanes, or one wanes while the other waxes. Secondly, the interdependence and interaction of yin and yang lead to a state of simultaneous waxing and waning, i.e. one wanes and the other wanes, or one waxes and the other waxes.

The forms of yin-yang's waning and waxing movement caused by their mutual restriction and antagonism of each other leads to decreasing and increasing changes of yin and yang. The first is that one waxes while the other wanes, including yin waxes while yang wanes and yang waxes while yin wanes; the second is one wanes while the other waxes, including yin wanes while yang waxes and yang wanes while yin

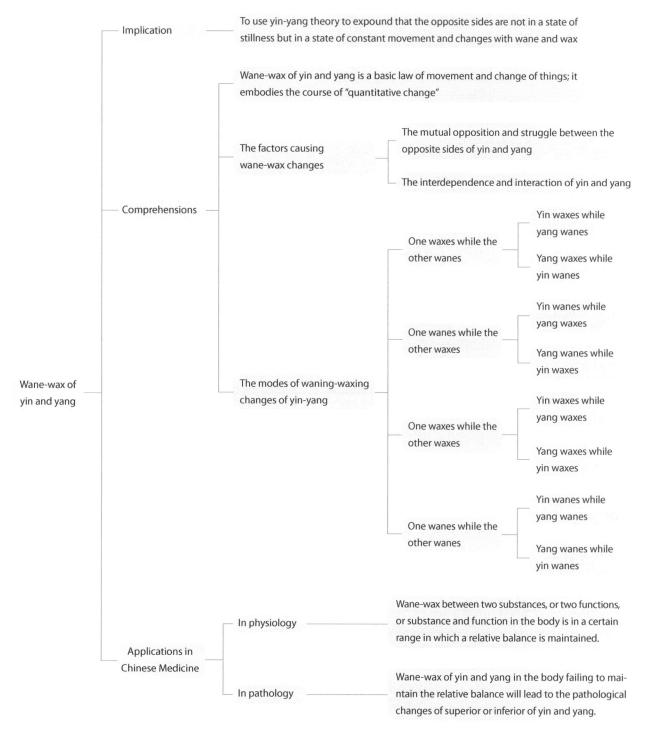

Fig. 1-5   Summary of the waxing and waning of yin and yang

waxes. The forms caused by interdependence and interactions of each other lead to simultaneous decreasing or increasing. The first form is one waxes while the other waxes including yin waxes while yang waxes and yang waxes while yin waxes; the second is one wanes while the other wanes including yin wanes while yang wanes and yang wanes while yin wanes. (Fig. 1-6)

The waxing and waning theory of yin and yang in Chinese medicine can be taken both to clarify human physiological changes and to analyze pathological changes. However, there

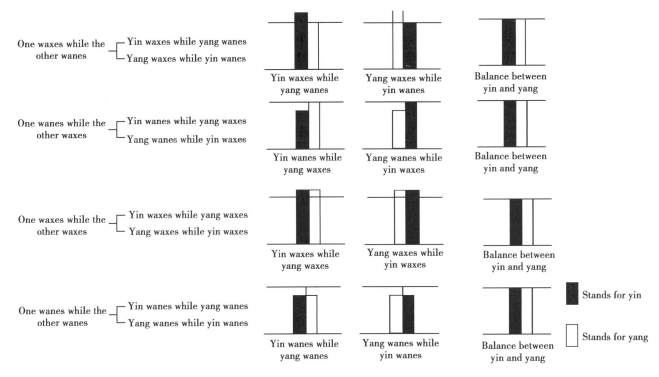

One waxes while the ⌐ Yin waxes while yang wanes
other wanes   └ Yang waxes while yin wanes

One wanes while the ⌐ Yin wanes while yang waxes
other waxes   └ Yang wanes while yin waxes

One waxes while the ⌐ Yin waxes while yang waxes
other waxes   └ Yang waxes while yin waxes

One wanes while the ⌐ Yin wanes while yang wanes
other wanes   └ Yang wanes while yin wanes

Yin waxes while yang wanes · Yang waxes while yin wanes · Balance between yin and yang

Yin wanes while yang waxes · Yang wanes while yin waxes · Balance between yin and yang

Yin waxes while yang waxes · Yang waxes while yin waxes · Balance between yin and yang

Yin wanes while yang wanes · Yang wanes while yin wanes · Balance between yin and yang

■ Stands for yin
□ Stands for yang

Fig. 1-6   Waxing and waning forms of yin and yang

are differences between their nature and degree. Physiological changes of waxing and waning yin and yang are within a certain range in which a relative balance is maintained. Pathological changes are beyond that certain limit where the relative balance is upset leading to superiority or inferiority of yin and yang.

Plain Questions: Chapter Discussion on the Essentials of Pulse (Sù Wèn: Mài Yào Jīng Wēi Lùn, 素问·脉要精微论) states: "*On the forty-fifth day after the winter solstice, yang qi ascends slightly while yin qi descends slightly. On the forty-fifth day after the Summer Solstice, yin qi rises mildly and yang qi falls mildly.*"

Plain Questions: Chapter Discussion on Jue Syndrome (Sù Wèn: Jué Lùn, 素问·厥论) states: "*There is more yang qi than yin qi in spring and summer, while yin qi becomes predominant while yang qi decreases in autumn and winter.*"

Plain Questions: Chapter Major Discussion on the Theory of Yin and Yang and the Corresponding Relationships Among All the Things in Nature (Sù Wèn: Yīn Yáng Yìng Xiàng Dà Lùn, 素问·阴阳应象大论) states: "*Overly dominant yin leads to yang disorder, and overly dominant yang leads to yin disorder.*"

④ Transformation of Yin and Yang (Fig. 1-7)

Transformation, namely transition and change, indicates that under certain conditions, opposing aspects transform themselves into their opposites through antagonism. Transformation of yin and yang is to utilize yin-yang to explain how the two opposite aspects of things or phenomena are able to transform into their opposite under certain conditions, i.e., yin can transform into yang and yang can transform into yin.

The transformation of yin and yang is one of the fundamental laws of the movement of all things. The development of phenomena manifests as the inter-transformation course from quantitative change to qualitative change and then from qualitative change to quantitative change. Using waxing and waning and transformation of yin and yang to explain the process of development of all things includes the processes of quantitative and qualitative change. If the waxing and waning of yin and yang is considered as a process of quantitative change, then the transformation of yin and yang should be considered a process of qualitative change. The waxing and waning (quantitative change)

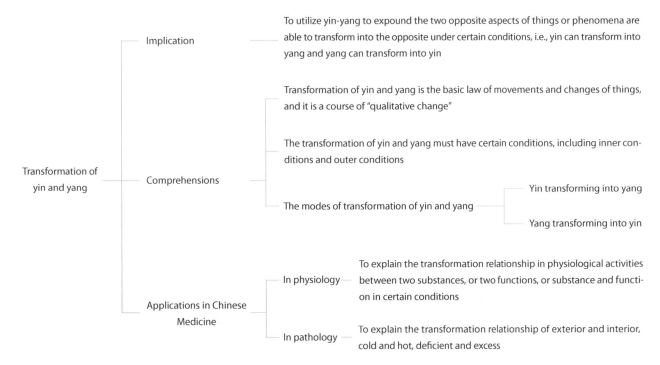

Fig. 1-7   Summary of the transformation of yin and yang

and transformation (qualitative change) are two inseparable phases of the whole course of development of all things. Waxing and waning of yin and yang is a precondition of transformation, and transformation is the inevitable result of waxing and waning.

The transformation of yin and yang must be provided for with certain conditions. One is constant motion. There exist factors in each aspect of the transformation into its opposite, and this is the internal foundation for transformation. On the other hand, there must also be certain external conditions for transformation. The transformation will not occur without the internal foundation and suitable external conditions. In Chinese Medicine, such words as "extreme", "utmost" and "excess" are used to reflect conditions necessary for transformation. The necessary internal and external conditions for generating transformation vary according to specific situations.

There are two forms of transformation of yin and yang: yin transforming into yang and yang transforming into yin.

The mutual transformation theory of yin and yang, in Chinese medicine, can be taken to explain the transformative relationship in

physiological activities between two substances, or two functions, or substance and function under certain conditions, as well as the transformative relationship of exterior and interior, cold and hot, deficient and excess, etc, in the disease process.

Plain Questions: Chapter Major Discussion on the Abstruseness of the Six Kinds of Qi (Sù Wèn: Liù Wēi Zhǐ Dà Lùn, 素问·六微旨大论) states: "The generation of things depends on transformation, and the extremity of things leads to change. The interaction of transformation and change is the cause of formation and destruction…Formation and destruction are engendered by movement, and constant movement leads to change."

Plain Questions: Chapter Major Discussion on the Theory of Yin and Yang and the Corresponding Relationships Among All the Things in Nature (Sù Wèn: Yīn Yáng Yìng Xiàng Dà Lùn, 素问·阴阳应象大论) states: "Extreme yang turns into yin, and extreme yin turns into yang." "Cold in its extreme will give rise to heat, and heat in its extreme will give rise to cold."

Miraculous Pivot: Chapter To Determine the Disease by Inspecting the Skin of the Anterolateral Side of the Forearm (Líng Shū: Lùn Jí Zhěn Chǐ, 灵枢·论疾诊尺) states: "The changes of the four seasons are caused by the alternating superiority of cold and heat. Extreme yang turns into yin, and extreme yin turns into yang. Therefore, yin dominates cold and yang dominates heat. Excessive cold turns into heat and excessive heat turns into cold. So it is said that cold can generate heat and heat can generate cold. This is the transformation of yin and yang."

Applications of the Yin–Yang Doctrine in Chinese Medicine

① To Explain the Organizational Structure of the Human Body

The human body is an organic whole. The yin-yang attributes of every organizational part of the body can be determined according the theory of opposition and interdependence of yin and yang.

The attributes of yin or yang of viscera, channels, body constituents and tissues can be classified according to this theory. With regard to general regions of the human body, the upper half is characterized as yang and the lower half as yin; the superficial as yang and the internal as yin. The back is attributed to yang while the abdomen to yin; the lateral surface of the limbs to yang, and the medial surface to yin. As for the viscera, five *zang* organs are considered to be yang, and six *fu* organs, yin; within the five *zang* organs, the Heart and Lungs, located in the chest are classified as yang, while the Liver, Spleen and Kidney, located in the abdomen, as yin. As for the twelve channels, the channels circulating on the lateral surface are labeled as yang, while those on the medial surface as yin. (Fig. 1-8)

There are two justifying principles for categorizing the yin-yang attributes of the organizational structure of the human body. The first is *"Water and Fire are the embodiment of yin and yang"*; the other is the relativity of yin-yang attributes, i.e. the subdivision of yin and yang. It can therefore be concluded that the categorization of the yin-yang attributes of the human body is also relative.

Plain Questions: Chapter Discussion on Preserving Health and Protecting Life (Sù Wèn: Bǎo Mìng Quán Xíng Lùn, 素问·宝命全形论) states:

"Man is born with a form that cannot be separated from yin and yang."

Plain Questions: Chapter Discussion on Important Ideas in the Golden Chamber(Sù Wèn: Jīn Guì Zhēn Yán Lùn, 素问·金匮真言论) states: *"As for the yin and yang of mankind, the external is characterized as yang, while the internal as yin. As for the yin and yang of the body, the back is yang, while the abdomen is yin. As for the yin and yang of the viscera, zang organs are yang, while fu organs are yin. The Liver, Heart, Spleen, Lung and Kidney, or five zang organs, all belong to yang, while the Gallbladder, Stomach, Large Intestine, Small Intestine, urinary Bladder and San Jiao, or six fu organs, all to yin…The back is attributed to yang, so the Heart is yang within yang, and the Lungs yin within yang. The abdomen is characterized as yin, so the Kidneys are yin within yin, the Liver is yang within yin, and the Spleen is extreme yin within yin."*

② To Explain Physiological Functions of the Human Body

Yin-yang doctrine regards normal activities and on-going physiological functions of the human body as the result of a harmonious balance of yin and yang. This balance depends upon their opposition and restriction, interdependence and interaction, waxing and waning and transformation.

In the relationship between substance and function in human vital activities, the material foundation is called yin essence (bodily yin, 体阴), while functional activity is referred to as yang qi (functional yang, 用阳). Human physiological activity (yang) is based on substance (yin). Yang qi can't be generated without yin essence, while physiological activity constantly replenishes the yin-essence. Thus, substance and function (bodily yin and functional yang) are together in a unity of mutual opposition, dependence, waxing and waning and transformation, maintaining a dynamic balance, which guarantees the normal processes of vital activity.

③ To Expound Pathological Changes of the Human Body

Pathology includes the mechanisms of onset,

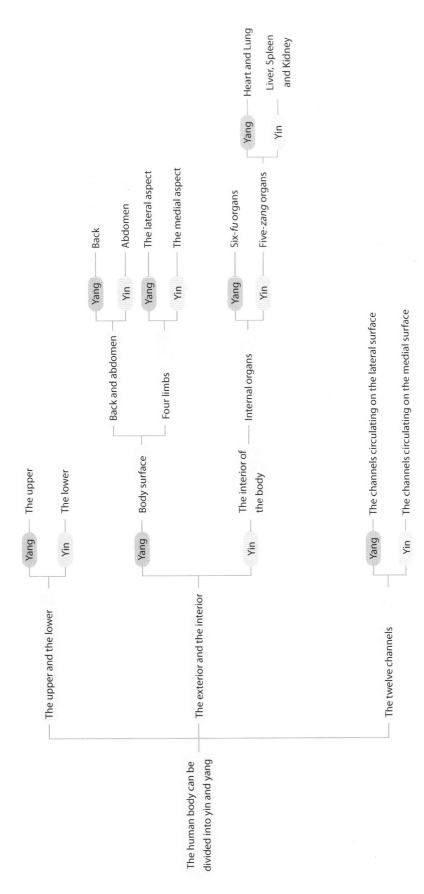

Fig. 1-8 Summary of the yin and yang of the human organizational structure (Example)

the development and changes of disease. The doctrine of yin-yang asserts that amidst all the complicated physiological activity of the human body, maintaining a balanced and coordinated relationship between opposition, interdependence, waxing and waning and transformation of yin and yang, i.e. yin calms while yang steadies, is the prerequisite condition for the continuation of normal vital activities. Whenever this relationship is destroyed, it leads to an imbalance of yin and yang, and disease ensues. Therefore, imbalance of yin and yang is the basis for onset, development and changes of disease. The occurrence of disease is related to two aspects, the vital qi and the evil qi. The struggle between the right and the evil qi leads to an imbalance of yin and yang and consequently the occurrence of disease (this will be discussed in pathogenesis). Though they are complicated, pathological changes generally fall into the two categories, which include relative superiority of yin or yang and relative inferiority of yin or yang.

A. Relative superiority of yin or yang (Fig. 1-9)
Superiority indicates that the evil qi is overly dominant. Relative superiority of yin or yang means yin or yang evil is relatively dominant, and has reached a pathological state where yin or yang is above the normal level. "*Dominant evil qi results in excessive syndromes*", mean that the relative superiority of yin or yang results in excess syndromes. In the pathological course of the relative superiority of yin or yang, superiority (dominance) of evil qi will inevitably restrict or impair the right qi of the human body. As a result, it is often complicated with symptoms of deficiency.

a. Relative superiority of yin
This represents predominant yin evil with pathological changes that manifest as excess cold syndrome, i.e., "superiority of yin leads to cold syndrome". Excess yin can also impair yang qi of the human body leading to yang deficiency. Hence, excess cold syndrome caused by superiority of yin usually is complicated by yang deficiency, i.e., "*superiority of yin leads to yang illness*".

b. Relative superiority of yang

This represents predominant yang evil with pathological changes that manifest as excess heat syndrome, i.e., "superiority of yang leads to heat syndrome". Excess yang can also impair yin fluid of the human body leading to yin deficiency. Hence, excess heat syndrome caused by superiority of yang is usually complicated by yin deficiency, i.e., "*superiority of yang leads to yin illness*".

B. Relative inferiority of yin or yang (Fig. 1-9)
Inferiority indicates that the right qi is weak. It includes relative inferiority of yin and relative inferiority of yang, a pathological state where yin fluid or yang qi is depressed below the normal level. "Loss of essence qi results in deficiency", means that relative inferiority of yin or yang leads to a deficient syndrome.

a. Relative inferiority of yin
This represents an insufficiency of yin fluid in pathological course that leads to deficient yin failing to restrict yang, thus yang is relatively superior accompanied with heat symptoms. This kind of heat is caused by yin deficiency, as a deficient heat it may be summarized as "inferiority of yin results in heat syndrome".

b. Relative inferiority of yang
This points to insufficient yang qi in a pathological course that leads to deficient yang failing to restrict yin, thus yin is relatively superior accompanied with cold symptoms. This kind of cold is caused by yang deficiency, as a deficient cold; it may be summarized as "inferiority of yang results in cold syndrome".

c. Mutual consumption of yin and yang
Due to the interdependence and interaction between yin and yang, there occur such pathological changes as the impairment of yin affecting yang, impairment of yang affecting yin and impairment of both yin and yang. When yin is deficient to a certain degree, it fails to generate yang and bring on yang deficiency. This is called "*impairment of yin affecting yang*". When yang is deficient to a certain degree, it fails to generate yin and then it will occur deficiency of yin. This is called "*impairment of yang affecting yin*". The impairment of yin affecting yang and the impairment of yang affecting yin will

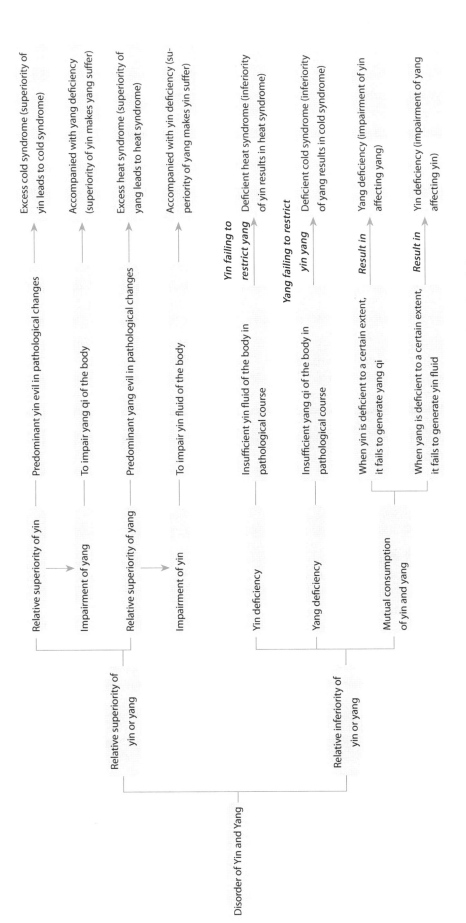

Fig. 1-9 Summary of the relationship between relative superiority or inferiority of yin or yang and nature of syndrome

eventually lead to the pathological state of the deficiency of both yin and yang.

In addition, the pathological changes of yin and yang also include the transformation of yin and yang, yin and yang repulsion and depletion of yin or yang, which will be discussed under pathological mechanisms.

Plain Questions: Chapter General Discussion on Deficiency and Excess (Sù Wèn: Tōng Píng Xū Shí Lùn, 素问·通评虚实论) says: "Dominance of evil qi results in excess syndromes, and loss of essential qi results in deficient syndromes."

Plain Questions: Chapter Major Discussion on the Theory of Yin and Yang and the Corresponding Relationships Among All the Things in Nature (Sù Wèn: Yīn Yáng Yìng Xiàng Dà Lùn, 素问·阴阳应象大论) says: "Superiority of yin leads to yang illness, and superiority of yang leads to yin illness.

Superiority of yang leads to heat syndromes, and superiority of yin leads to cold syndromes."

Plain Questions: Chapter Discussion on the Regulation of Channels (Sù Wèn: Tiáo Jīng Lùn, 素问·调经论) says: "Deficiency of yang leads to exterior cold, and deficiency of yin leads to interior heat."

④ Application to the Diagnosis of Disease

The diagnostic process in Chinese medicine includes two main aspects, or diagnostic methods and syndrome differentiation. There are two main applications of the yin-yang doctrine to diagnosis of diseases: to analyze the yin-yang attributes of symptoms and signs collected through the four examinations and differentiate yin-yang attributes of syndromes.

A. Analyzing data collected from the four examinations (Table 1-2)

Table 1-2　Yin-yang attributions of symptoms and signs

Four Examinations		Yang Attribute	Yin Attribute
Observing	Complexion	Bright	Dark and dull
Listening and Smelling	Voice	A piercing voice with a high tone, rambling speech accompanied with restlessness	A feeble voice with a low tone, silence, accompanied with quiet body language
	Breath	Forceful, loud and coarse	Faint, low and timid
Questioning	Preference or Aversion to Cold and Heat	Fever, aversion to heat with preference for cold	Chills, aversion to cold with preference to heat
	Thirst	Dry mouth with thirst	Moist mouth without thirst
Palpating (Pulse Diagnosis)	Position	*Cun*	*Chi*
	Trend	Arriving (rising)	Leaving (falling)
	Frequency	Rapid	Slow
	Shape	Floating, rapid, surging and slippery	Deep, slow, thready and rough

Yin-yang theory can be used to analyze the yin-yang attributes of concrete symptoms and signs collected from the four examinations of observing, listening and smelling, questioning, and palpating. In observing complexion, a bright color is indicative of yang and a dark or dull color of yin. When listening and smelling, a piercing voice with a high tone is characteristic of yang, while a feeble voice with a low tone of yin. In questioning favor or aversion to heat and cold, aversion to heat with preference for cold is reflective of yang, and aversion to cold with

preference for heat of yin. When reading the pulse, floating, rapid, surging and slippery pulses pertain to yang; deep, slow, thready and rough pulses pertain to yin. Distinguishing yin-yang attributes of symptoms and signs provide the foundation for syndrome differentiation.

B. Differentiating syndromes of disease

Disease syndromes can be quite complex. Syndrome differentiation according to yin-yang theory is mainly to distinguish yin or yang attributes of syndromes. For instance, among the eight principles of syndrome differentiation, yin-yang is the fundamental principle; the exterior, excess and heat belong to yang, while interior, deficient and cold to yin. As another example, in external inflammatory diseases, local manifestations of red, swollen, hot and painful symptoms belong to yang, while pale, flat or collapsed, absence of heat and mild, dull pain symptoms to yin. Distinguishing yin-yang attributes of syndromes is of great value in recognizing the nature of diseases and provides a foundation for treatment.

Plain Questions: Chapter Major Discussion on the Theory of Yin and Yang and the Corresponding Relationships Among All the Things in Nature (Sù Wèn: Yīn Yáng Yìng Xiàng Dà Lùn, 素问·阴阳应象大论) states: "*One who is good at diagnosis always first distinguishes yin or yang when observing color and feeling pulse.*"

Plain Questions: Chapter Discussion on the Essentials of Pulse (Sù Wèn: Mài Yào Jīng Wēi Lùn, 素问·脉要精微论) states: "*Feeling the pulse is a perceptive and subtle technique that one must study carefully. There is a guiding principle in this study which begins with distinguishing yin and yang.*"

Plain Questions: Chapter Separate Discussion On Yin and Yang (Sù Wèn: Yīn Yáng Bié Lùn Piān, 素问·阴阳别论篇) states: "*As far as yin and yang are concerned, leaving pertains to yin and arriving to yang; stillness pertains to yin and movement to yang; slowness pertains to yin and rapidness to yang.*"

Jing-yue's Complete Works: Section Yin and Yang, Chapter Chuan Zhong Lu, (Jǐng Yuè Quán Shū: Chuán Zhōng Lù, Yīn Yáng Piān, 景岳全书·传忠录·阴阳篇) says: "*When diagnosing and treating disease, one must first distinguish yin and yang. This is the general principle of medicine. If yin and yang are clearly differentiated, how can mistakes occur in treatment? Though the way of medicine is complicated, to sum it up in one word, there is only yin and yang. Therefore, there is yin and yang in syndromes, pulses and herbs. In syndromes, the exterior belongs to yang while the interior to yin; heat belongs to yang and cold to yin; the upper belongs to yang while the lower to yin; qi belongs to yang while blood to yin; activeness to yang while stillness to yin; rambling speech belongs to yang while quiet to yin; preference for light belongs to yang while preference for darkness to yin; patients with feeble yang find it difficult to exhale, and those with feeble yin find it difficult to inhale; patients with yang disease can't prostrate, and those with yin disease can't lie on their back. In pulse, floating, large, slippery and rapid pulses all pertain to yang, while deep, faint, thready and rough pulses all to yin…Though the way of medicine is profound, if a doctor clearly grasps yin-yang theory, he has already traveled beyond the halfway point.*"

⑤ Application to the Prevention and Treatment of Disease

A. To guide health maintenance and disease prevention

Health maintenance is to preserve and nurture life and good health. The purpose of health maintenance is to strengthen the body, prevent disease and prolong lifespan. Yin-yang doctrine holds that, if the changes of yin and yang of the human body are in accordance with the natural cycle of the four seasons, immunity to disease and longevity will be attained. It is advocated that one must comply with natural law to preserve heath and be sure to nurture yang in spring and summer, yin in autumn and winter, conserve the essence and spirit internally, keep a proper diet, keep regular sleeping and waking hours, follow the law of yin-yang, and thus maintain the body's internal balance as well as a harmony with the external environments so as to achieve the purpose of furthering health and preventing disease.

According to the principle of "*nurturing yang in spring and summer, nurturing yin in autumn and winter*", for an individual with a constitution of deficient yang and predominant yin who is "able to endure summer but not winter", herbs with warm and hot natures should be used to reinforce yang preemptively, thus disease will not easily occur in winter; for one with a constitution of deficient yin and predominant yang who is "able to endure winter but not summer", herbs with cool and moist natures should be adopted to nourish yin preemptively, thus disease will not easily occur in summer. This is what is called "treating illnesses of winter in summer" and "healing illnesses of summer in winter".

Plain Questions: Chapter Major Discussion of Regulation of Spirit According to the Changes of the Four Seasons (Sù Wèn: Sì Qì Tiáo Shén Dà Lùn, 素问·四气调神大论*)* says: *"Yin and yang of the four seasons are the root of all things. Therefore the saint, complies with this principle and nurtures yang in spring and summer, and yin in autumn and winter in order to adjust to the basic changes of the four seasons. If people go against principle, they will injure their root and spoil their origin. Therefore yin and yang of the four seasons is the start and end of all things, and the ultimate source of death and birth. Violating this principle, disasters will occur; obeying it, diseases will not happen. This is called understanding Dao."*

B.To guide treatment of disease

Guidance of yin-yang theory for the treatment of disease includes the two main aspects of determining treatment principles and categorizing the natures of herbs.

a. To determine treatment principles (Fig. 1-10)

Since the imbalance of yin and yang is the fundamental pathological cause of disease, application of yin-yang doctrine in treatment is to determine treatment principles mainly according to this fundamental pathological change, i.e., regulating relative superiority or inferiority of yin and yang in order to restore their harmonious balance. Therefore, regulating imbalance of yin and yang is the fundamental principle of treating disease.

Treatment principles for relative superiority of yin or yang: Relative superiority of yin or yang is an excess syndrome in which the evil qi dominates, and the principle of "eliminating the excess (expelling evil)" should be applied. For an excess cold syndrome caused by the relative superiority of yin, herbs with a hot nature should be applied, known as "heating what is cold" in *Internal Classic (Nèi Jīng)*. When overly dominant yin impairs yang, resulting in accompanying symptoms of yang deficiency, herbs to replenish yang should be carefully added in order to take this deficiency into account. For an excess heat syndrome caused by relative superiority of yang, herbs with cold nature should be applied, referred to as "cooling what is hot" in *Internal Classic (Nèi Jīng)*. When overly dominant

yang damages yin, resulting in accompanying symptoms of yin deficiency, herbs to nourish yin should be added to the prescription in order to take this deficiency into account.

Treatment principles for relative inferiority of yin or yang: Relative inferiority of yin or yang results in deficient syndromes where the right qi is insufficient, where the principle "supplementing what is insufficient (strengthening the right)" should be used. For a deficient heat syndrome caused by yin deficiency failing to restrict yang where yang is relatively dominant, herbs to tonify yin should be applied to nourish yin and bring yang into check. This therapeutic method of "nourishing the origin of Water (Kidney yin) in order to control the light of yang" is called "treating yin for yang illnesses" in *Internal Classic (Nèi Jīng)*. In a deficient cold syndrome caused by yang deficiency failing to restrict yin where yin is relatively dominant, herbs to tonify yang should be applied to replenish yang and bring yin into check, This therapeutic method of "supplementing the source of Fire (Kidney yang) in order to expel the yin fog" is also called *treating yang for yin illnesses* in *Internal Classic (Nèi Jīng)*.

Treatment principles for mutual consumption of yin and yang: Mutual consumption of yin and yang will lead to the deficiency of both. Treatment should therefore tonify both yin and yang. According to the interdependence and interaction of yin and yang, for syndromes of mutual deficiency caused by impairment of yin affecting yang, which manifest mainly as yin deficiency, treatment should focus on tonifying yin, therefore tonifying yang as well. As for those caused by impairment of yang affecting yin, manifest mainly as yang deficiency, treatment should focus on strengthening yang, in order to nourish yin.

Plain Questions: Chapter Discussion on the Most Important and Abstruse Theory (Sù Wèn: Zhì Zhèn Yào Dà Lùn, 素问·至真要大论*)* states: *"Observe the yin-yang of a disease and harmonize them with balance as the end goal." "Purge that which is excessive, tonify that which is deficient." "Heat that which is cold; cool that which is hot."*

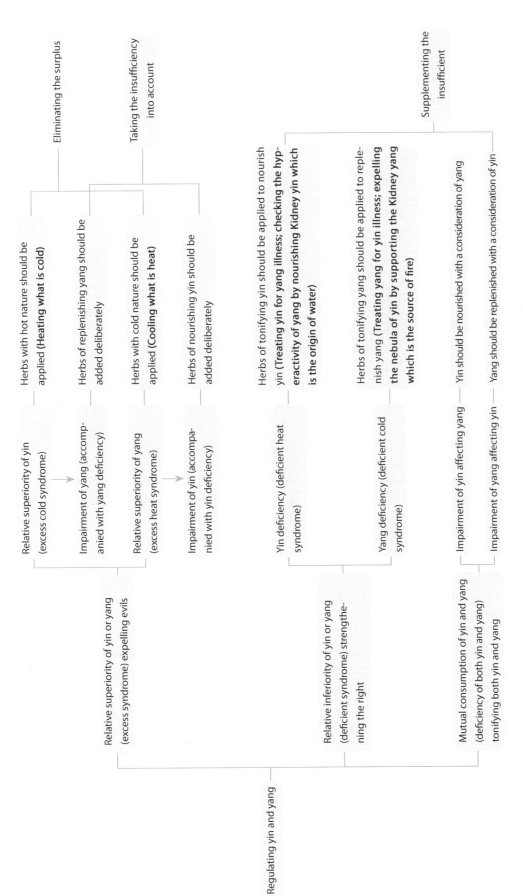

Fig. 1-10 Summary for regulating the imbalance of yin and yang

Miraculous Pivot: Chapter Retention of the Evil Qi (Líng Shū: Xié Kè, 灵枢·邪客) states: "*Supplement the body's deficiencies and eliminate its excesses.*"

Plain Questions: Chapter Major Discussion on the Theory of Yin and Yang and the Corresponding Relationships Among All the Things in Nature (Sù Wèn: Yīn Yáng Yìng Xiàng Dà Lùn, 素问·阴阳应象大论) states: "*Treat yin for yang illnesses, and treat yang for yin illnesses.*"

Notation of *Plain Questions: Chapter Discussion on the Most Important and Abstruse Theory (Sù Wèn: Zhì Zhèn Yào Dà Lùn, 素问·至真要大论)* by Wang Bing (王冰) states: "*Supplement the source of Fire (Kidney yang) in order to expel the yin fog; nourish the origin of Water (Kidney yin) in order to control the light of yang.*"

b. To categorize the properties of herbs (Table 1-3)

Table 1-3 Categorization of yin-yang attributes of herbal properties

Herbal Properties	Yin	Yang
Natures (Four qi)	Cold, cool	Warm, hot
Five Flavors	Sour, bitter, salty	Acrid, sweet (bland)
Lifting, Lowering, Floating and Sinking	Falling, sinking	Rising, floating

Yin-yang can be used to analyze and categorize natures, flavors and functions of herbs and serves as the basis for guiding their clinical administration. The properties of Chinese herbs include its nature, flavor, and its rising, falling, floating or sinking action, which can be categorized and explained by yin-yang theory.

The nature of herbs includes hot, cold, warm and cool, known as the "four qi, 四气". Among them, herbs of cold and cool natures can clear heat and purge Fire, and alleviate or eliminate heat symptoms. Thus, they are categorized as yin and are often used to treat yang and heat syndromes. Herbs of hot and warm natures can expel cold and warm the interior, and alleviate or eliminate cold symptoms. They are categorized as yang and are often used in treatment of yin and cold syndromes.

The five flavors include acrid, sweet, sour, bitter and salty. Among them, the acrid has the function of dispersing and the sweet is tonifying. They belong to the category of yang herbs. The sour has an astringent function, the bitter purges Fire and the salty softens hardness. They are classified as yin.

The concept of rising, falling, floating and sinking outlines the acting tendencies of herbs on the body. Among them, herbs with rising and floating tendencies are recognized as yang, while those with falling and sinking tendencies as yin.

Plain Questions: Chapter Discussion on the Most Important and Abstruse Theory (Sù Wèn: Zhì Zhèn Yào Dà Lùn, 素问·至真要大论) says: "*The acrid and sweet disperse and are of yang; the sour and bitter with emetic and purging functions are of yin; the salty with emetic and purging functions also belongs to yin; the bland with its seeping function is classified as yang.*"

Key Link of Medicine: Chapter Discussion Yin and Yang (Yī Guàn: Yīn Yáng Lùn, 医贯·阴阳论) states: "*Shennong (神农) tasted herbs, and according to yin and yang, he classified them into cold, hot, warm, cool, acrid, sweet, sour, bitter and salty. The acrid and the sweet belong to yang, as do the warm and hot; the cold and the cool belong to yin, as do the sour, bitter and salty.*"

Jing-yue's Complete Works: Section Yin and Yang, Chapter Chuan Zhong Lu, (Jǐng Yuè Quán Shū: Chuán Zhōng Lù, Yīn Yáng, 景岳全书·传忠录·阴阳篇) states: "*To speak of herbs, those with rising and dispersing functions belong to yang; those with astringent and falling to yin; the acrid and the hot belong to yang, the bitter and the cold to yin; those that circulate qi are labeled as yang, and those that circulate blood as yin; those with an active and moving nature belong to yang, and those with a still and guarding natures to yin.*"

Section 3   Doctrine of the Five Phases

The doctrine of the five phases is a materialistic and dialectic category of ancient China. It postulates that the universe is composed of the five elements, or phases, of Wood, Fire, Earth, Metal and Water. The development and changes of various objects and phenomena in nature are the outcome of the constant motion and interaction of these five elements.

In applying this doctrine of the five phases to medicine, Chinese medical theory draws upon it to explain the organic connections among parts of the body, a part and the whole body, the superficial and viscera as well as the unity of the human body and its external environment. The doctrine of five phases runs throughout every aspect of the theoretical system of Chinese Medicine to explain human physiological functions and pathological changes and to guide diagnosis and treatment of disease, making it a fundamental component of Chinese medical theory.

Fundamental Concept of Five Phases

① Definition of the Five Phases

Five phases refers to the five materials of Wood, Fire, Earth, Metal and Water, their movement and their transformations.

The five phases were initially called the "five elements". Over a long period of experience in living and agricultural production, ancient Chinese people gradually came to understand that these five materials of Wood, Fire, Earth, Metal and Water are the most common, indispensable and fundamental substances of everyday life.

Afterwards, the original meaning of these five concrete materials underwent abstraction and its scope of application was widened to accommodate the world view that all concrete forms and intangible phenomena are generated from the movement and change amongst these materials. The theory of generation and restriction was conceived of upon this foundation to explain the mutual relationships amongst these various forms and phenomena, thus forming the doctrine of the five phases.

Zuo's Commentaries on the Spring and Autumn: Chapter the 27th Year of Xianggong (Zuǒ Zhuàn: Xiāng Gōng Èr Shí Qī Nián, 左传·襄公二十七年) says: "*The heavens produced the five elements to be used by mankind. Man cannot be without any of them.*"

Guoyu: Chapter Zhengyu (Guó Yǔ: Zhèng Yǔ, 国语·郑语) says: "*The emperors of ancient times mixed Earth with Metal, Wood, Water and Fire to give form to the myriad things.*"

② Properties of the Five Phases

The properties of the five phases refer to each individual's inherent characteristics. They are theoretical ideas taken by the ancients from everyday life experience, abstracted and gradually developed based upon a simple understanding and intuitional observation of the nature of the five elements of Wood, Fire, Earth, Metal and Water. The properties of five phases are as follows:

"*Wood bends and straightens*, 木曰曲直" meaning that trees have the ability to both bend and straighten. By extension anything that has the properties of growing, rising, extending and unfolding is attributed to Wood.

"*Fire burns and flares*, 火曰炎上" meaning that Fire has the properties of ascending heat. By extension anything that has the properties of warmth or heat, rising, and brightness is attributed to Fire.

"*Earth provides for sewing and reaping*, 土爰稼穑" meaning that Earth can be sewed and reaped. By extension anything that has the properties of generating, holding and receiving is attributed to Earth.

"*Metal complies and transforms*, 金曰从革" meaning that Metal has the properties of compliance and change. By extension anything that has the properties of cold lifelessness, astringing and sinking is attributed to Metal.

"*Water moistens and descends*, 水曰润下"

which means that Water has the properties of moistening and tending to flow downwards. By extension anything that has the properties of moistening, descending, storing and is cool or cold is attributed to Water.

Shang Shu: Chapter Hong Fan (Shàng Shū: Hóng Fàn, 尚书·洪范) states: "*Wood bends and straightens, Fire burns and flares, Earth provides for sewing and reaping, Metal complies and transforms, and Water moistens and descends.*"

③ The Categorization of Attributes of Things According to the Five Phases (Table 1-4)

A. Categorizing method

The various phenomena of the natural world are attributed to one of the five phases through a combination of analogical connection with a specific elemental image and deductive reasoning based upon an association with one of the five phases.

Table 1-4　Association of things with the five phases

		Jiao角	Zhi徵	Gong宫	Shang商	Yu羽
Nature	Five Sounds					
	Five Flavors	Sour	Bitter	Sweet	Acrid	Salty
	Five Colors	Green	Red	Yellow	White	Black
	Five Transformations	Germination	Growth	Transformation	Reaping	Storing
	Five Climatic Agent	Wind	Summer-heat	Damp	Dryness	Cold
	Five Orientations	East	South	Middle	West	North
	Five Seasons	Spring	Summer	Late summer	Autumn	Winter
Five Phases		Wood	Fire	Earth	Metal	Water
Human Body	Five *zang* Organs	Liver	Heart	Spleen	Lung	Kidney
	Five *fu* Organs	Gall bladder	Small intestine	Stomach	Large intestine	Urinary Bladder
	Five Body Constituents	Tendons	Pulse	Muscles	Skin	Bones
	Five Sense Organs	Eyes	Tongue	Mouth	Nose	Ears
	Five Emotions	Anger	Joy	Contemplation	Sadness	Fear
	Five Voices	Shouting	Laughing	Singing	Crying	Moaning
	Five Changes	Grasping	Worrying	Hiccup	Cough	Trembling
	Five Pulses	Wiry	Surging	Moderate	Floating	Deep
	Five Liquids	Tears	Sweat	Saliva	Mucus	Spittle

a. Analogical connection with the elemental image

Forming a connection with the image means to search for specific characteristics in the image of something (including shapes, functions and properties) that reflects its true essence. A category indicates a collection of individuals of the same characteristics. Analogy is to compare sorts of things, has the meaning of attribution and categorization. Attribution of things to five phases by this method is to compare the unique characteristics of things with the abstract properties of the five phases in order to determine their association to one of them. For instance, if the unique characteristics of something are similar with the properties of Wood, it can be attributed to Wood. The same goes for each of the other five phases as well.

b. Deduction

This is to deduce and categorize the associations of related things based upon something that has already been attributed to one of the five phases. For instance, it is already known that the Liver is related to Wood, and the Gallbladder, tendons and eyes are closely related to the Liver, therefore it can be deduced that they also pertain to Wood. The same can be applied to the other elements as well.

B. Opinions on association with the five phases

Association with the five phases is a method

of the ancients used to categorize things and phenomena and to set forth their philosophical meaning. It is convenient for analyzing and explaining the close relationships among the same class of things (horizontal row in the next table) and things of the same association with the five phases (vertically column in the next table).

In Chinese medicine, association with the five phases, connects the human vital activities with things and phenomena in nature in order to expound the unity of the human body and the holistic nature of the human body and the environment.

The basis for association with the five phases is that things and phenomena must be five in number. This is difficult to accord with actual conditions of reality. Moreover, sometimes it is also difficult to accept the practice of using the theories of mutual generation and restriction of the five phases to explain the relationship among things strictly on the basis of association.

Plain Questions: Chapter Major Discussion on the Theory of Yin and Yang and the Corresponding Relationships Among All the Things in Nature (Sù Wèn: Yīn Yáng Yìng Xiàng Dà Lùn, 素问·阴阳应象大论*)* states: *"The east generates wind…it manifests as wind in the sky, Wood on the ground, tendons in the body, the Liver as a viscera, green as a color, jiao as a sound, shouting as a voice; in change it becomes a grasp, the eyes as an orifice, sour as a flavor, and anger as an emotion."*

"The south generates heat…it manifests as heat in the sky, Fire on the ground, the pulse in the body, the Heart as a viscera, red as a color, zhi as a sound, laughter as a voice; in change it becomes worry, the tongue as an orifices, bitter as a flavor, and joy as an emotion."

"The middle generates damp…it manifests as damp in the sky, earth on the ground, muscles in the body, the Spleen as a viscera, yellow as a color, gong

as a sound, singing as a voice; in change it becomes a hiccup, the mouth as an orifice, sweet as a flavor, and contemplation as an emotion."

"The west generates dryness…it manifests as dryness in the sky, Metal on the ground, skin and hair on the body, the Lungs as a viscera, white as a color, shang as a sound, crying as a voice; in change it becomes a cough, the nose as an orifice, acrid as a flavor, and sadness as an emotion."

"The north generates cold…it manifests as cold in the sky, Water on the ground, bones in the body, the Kidneys as a viscera, black as a color, yu as a sound, moaning as a voice; in change it becomes trembling, the ears as an orifice, salty as a flavor, and fear as an emotion."

Fundamental Contents of the Doctrine of Five Phases

① Mutual Generation, Restraint and Interaction of the Five Phases (Appendix: Dominance and Recovery of the Five Phases)

A. Mutual generation of the five phases

Mutual generation means mutual production, multiplication and promotion. Mutual generation of the five phases indicates that there exists a productive, promotional relationship among Wood, Fire, Earth, Metal and Water respectively.

The sequence of the mutual generation of the five phases is: Wood generates Fire, Fire generates Earth, Earth generates Metal, Metal generates Water, and Water generates Wood. (Fig. 1-11)

Classic of the Central Viscera: Chapter 3, Discussion on Generation (Zhōng Zàng Jīng:Shēng Chéng Lùn Dì Sān, 中藏经·生成论第三*)* states: *"Metal generates Water, Water generates Wood, Wood generates Fire, Fire generates Earth, and Earth generates Metal. Thus, creation circulates endlessly."*

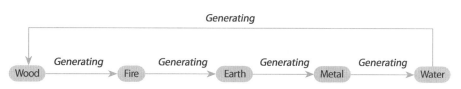

Fig. 1-11   Sequence of inter-generation of five phases

Within this relationship of mutual generation, each phase has two aspects: "generating" and "generated", likened to "a mother and child" in the *Classic of Questioning* (*Nàn Jīng*, 难经). The "generating" phase represents the mother, and the "generated" phase the child. Take Fire as an example, because Wood generates Fire, Wood is the mother of Fire (generating); because Fire generates Earth, Earth is the child of Fire (generated). (Fig. 1-12)

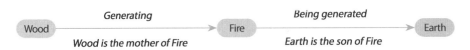

Fig. 1-12   Mother-child relationship of the five phases (Example)

B. Mutual restraint of the five phases
Mutual restraint includes the functions of reciprocal restriction and suppression. Mutual restraint of the five phases indicates that there exists a restrictive and suppressive relationship among Wood, Fire, Earth, Metal and Water respectively.

The sequence of mutual restraint of the five phases is: Wood restrains Earth, Earth restrains Water, Water restrains Fire, Fire restrains Metal, and Metal restrains Wood. (Fig. 1-13)

Plain Questions: Chapter Discussion on

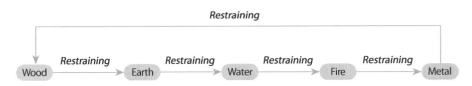

Fig. 1-13   Sequence of the mutual restraint of the five phases

Preserving Health and Protecting Life (Sù Wèn: Bǎo Mìng Quán Xíng Lùn, 素问·宝命全形论) states: "*Wood is felled by Metal, Fire is snuffed out by Water, Earth is burrowed through by Wood, Metal is melted by Fire, and Water is separated by Earth. Everything conforms to this law.*"

Within this relationship of mutual restraint, each phase has two aspects: "restraining" and "restrained", also termed the "inferior" and "superior" in *Internal Classic* (*Nèi Jīng*). The "restraining" phase is the superior, while the "restrained" phase is the inferior. To use Fire as an example, Water restrains Fire, making Water superior to Fire (restraining); Fire restrains Metal, making Metal inferior to Fire (restrained). (Fig. 1-14)

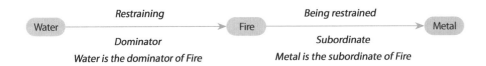

Fig. 1-14   Superior-inferior relationships of the five phases

C. Interaction of the five phases
Interaction means the two complimentary functions of generation and restriction. Interaction of the five phases is a combination of mutual generation and mutual restraint. Any one phase is generated, as well as, restrained by the others (Fig. 1-15), maintaining a relationship of restriction within generation

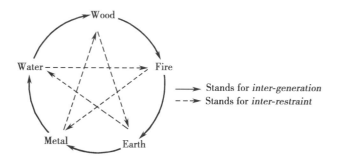

Fig. 1-15　Mutual generation and mutual restraint of the five phases

and generation within restriction. That is to say, mutual generation and mutual restraint are two inseparable processes. There would be no birth and development without generation; without restraint, development would lead to excess and result in disaster. Therefore, a relative balance and coordination among the forces of nature can only exist under the conditions of restraint within generation and generation within restraint.

Plain Questions: Chapter Major Discussion on the Abstruseness of the Six Kinds of Qi (Sù Wèn: Liù Wēi Zhǐ Dà Lùn, 素问·六微旨大论) states: "*Excess brings about harm, while restraint leads to order. With restraint, things flourish and decline according to the natural order; when harmed, things fall into chaos and the natural order is destroyed.*"

Illustrated Supplementary to the Classified Classic: Chapter the Upper Part of Five Circuit Phases and Six Climatic Factors (Lèi Jīng Tú Yì: Yùn Qì Shàng, 类经图翼·运气上) states: "*The processes of nature can not be without either generation or restriction. Without generation, there would be no birth and development; without restriction, excessive growth would result in harm.*"

The law of interaction of five phase is: Wood generates Fire, Fire generates Earth, and Wood restrains Earth; Fire generates Earth, Earth generates Metal, and Fire restrains Metal; Earth generates Metal, Metal generates Water, and Earth restrains Water; Metal generates Water, Water generates Wood, and Metal restrains Wood; Water generates Wood, Wood generates Fire, and Water restrains Fire. Take the relationships shared by Wood, Fire and Earth as an example. Wood can generate Fire, and Fire generates Earth, thus Earth will be too excessive; but Wood restrains

Earth to prevent it from becoming excessive (Fig. 1-16). Hence, there exists mutual restraint within generation, and mutual generation within restraint.

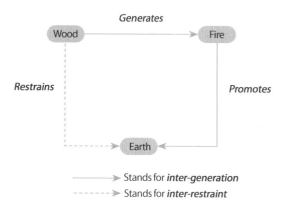

Fig. 1-16　Interaction of the five phases (Example)

Appendix: Dominance and Recovery of the Five Phases

A. Concept of dominance and recovery of the five phases

Dominance and recovery involves a dominant qi and a recovery qi. Among the five phases, when one phase is hyperactive and overly restrains its subordinate, it becomes the dominant qi, causing retaliatory suppression by its superior. The phase that retaliates against the dominant phase is called the recovery qi. In *Plain Questions: Chapter Discussion on the Most Important and Abstruse Theory (Sù Wèn: Zhì Zhèn Yào Dà Lùn*, 素问·至真要大论), this system is used to discuss the changes of the six climatic agents and the onset of disease.

B. Relation between dominant qi and recovery qi

The appearance of the dominant qi is caused by hyperactivity of one phase (including absolute hyperactivity and relative hyperactivity) and the appearance of recovery qi is a reaction to it, meaning the dominant qi appears first leading to the appearance of the recovery qi. Their relationship is that the recovery qi is the superior of the dominant qi, such that if the dominant qi is Wood then the recovery qi would be Metal; if the dominant qi is Fire then the recovery agent would be Water; if the dominant qi is Wood then the recovery agent would be Metal; if the dominant qi is Metal then the recovery agent would be Fire; if the dominant qi is Water then the recovery agent would be Earth. (Table 1-5)

Table 1-5   Relationship between the dominant qi and the recovery qi

Dominant Qi	Recovery Qi	Relationship: The recovery qi is the superior of the dominant qi
Wood	Metal	Metal is the superior of Wood
Fire	Water	Water is the superior of Fire
Earth	Wood	Wood is the superior of Earth
Metal	Fire	Fire is the superior of Metal
Water	Earth	Earth is the superior of Water

Plain Questions: Chapter Discussion on the Most Important and Abstruse Theory (Sù Wèn: Zhì Zhèn Yào Dà Lùn, 素问·至真要大论*)* says: *"If there is a dominant qi, there is a recovery qi; if there is no dominant qi, there is no recovery qi." "Where there is dominant qi, there will be recovery qi."*

C. Regulating principle of dominant qi and recovery qi

The dominant qi and the recovery qi of the five phases are automatically regulated according to the law of mutual restraint. Take the hyperactivity of Wood as an example. Hyperactivity of Wood (appearance of the dominant qi) restrains Earth, leading to its weakening. Weakened Earth fails to restrict Water, leading in turn to the hyperactivity of Water. Hyperactive Water restrains Fire, causing it to weaken. Weakened Fire fails to restrict Metal, causing the hyperactivity of Metal. Hyperactive Metal (emergence of the recovery qi) restrains Wood leading to the suppression of the hyperactivity of Wood. (Fig. 1-17) Each of the other four phases proceeds in the same manner.

② Extreme Restraint and Counter Restraint of the Five Phases

A. Extreme restraint of the five phases

Extreme restraint means to torment, suggesting an encroachment on that which is weak. Extreme restraint of the five phases is an abnormal condition of mutual restraint where any one of the five phases suppresses its inferior to an excessive degree.

The sequence of extreme restraint of the five phases is the same for that of mutual restraint,

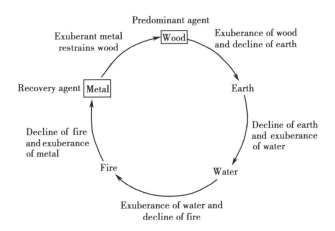

Fig. 1-17   Regulating principle of the dominant qi and the recovery qi

i.e. Wood overly restrains Earth, Earth overly restrains Water, Water overly restrains Fire, Fire overly restrains Metal, and Metal overly restrains Wood. (Fig. 1-18)

There are two causes that result in extreme restraint among the five phases, "excess" and "insufficiency".

If one phase is excessively active, it will overly restrain its inferior (its "restrained" element).

If one phase is insufficient, it will be overly restrained by its superior (its "restraining" element).

Take Wood as an example: if Wood is excessive, it will overly restrain Earth; if Wood is insufficient, Metal will overly restrain it. (Fig. 1-19)

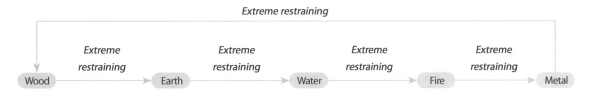

Fig. 1-18   Extreme restraint of the five phases

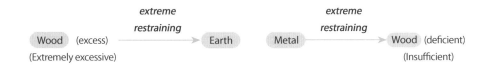

Fig. 1-19   Excess and insufficiency resulting in extreme restraint of the five phases (Example)

Although mutual restraint and extreme restraint follow the same sequence, they are different in nature. Mutual restraint is the restrictive relationship among the five phases under normal conditions, while extreme restraint represents a deviation from them. In terms of the human body, mutual restraint is a physiological phenomenon, while extreme restraint is a pathological one.

B. Counter restraint of the five phases

Counter restraint also refers to a process of torment or insult. Counter restraint among the five phases is an abnormal phenomenon of mutual restraint where one of the five phases conversely restrains its superior.

The sequence of counter restraint is opposite to that of mutual restraint, i.e. Wood counter restrains Metal, Metal counter restrains Fire, Fire counter restrains Water, Water counter restrains Earth, and Earth counter restrains Wood. (Fig. 1-20)

The two factors leading to counter restraint among the five phases are also "excess" and "insufficiency".

If one phase is excessively active, it will counter restrain its superior (its "restraining" element).

If one phase is insufficient, it will be counter restrained by its inferior (its "restrained" element).

Take Wood as an example: if Wood is excessive, it will counter restrain Metal; if Wood is insufficient, Earth will counter restrain it. (Fig. 1-21)

Plain Questions: Chapter Discussion on the Changes of Five-Motions (Sù Wèn: Wǔ Yùn Xíng Dà Lùn, 素问·五运行大论) states: "*As qi becomes excessive, it will restrict its inferior and counter*

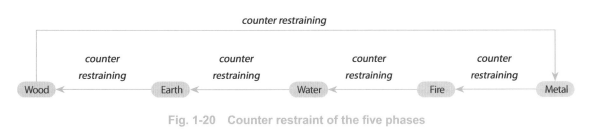

Fig. 1-20   Counter restraint of the five phases

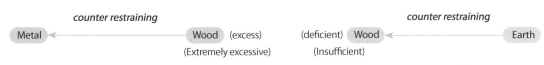

Fig. 1-21   Excess and insufficiency resulting in counter restraint of the five phases (Example)

restrain its superior; as qi becomes deficient, its superior will overly restrain it and its inferior will counter restrain it." (See Fig. 1-22 for explanation with Wood as an example)

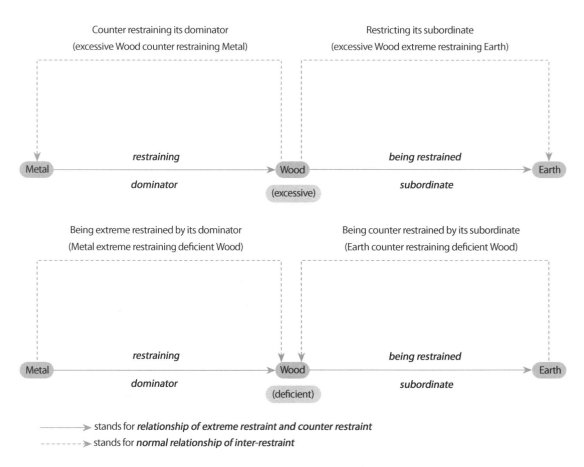

Fig. 1-22   Reasons and principles of extreme restraint and counter restraint (Example)

C. Involvement between mother and child of the five phases

Extension, also known as reaching or arriving, means to be entangled or to exert reciprocal influence. The extension of mother and child within the five phases, also known as affliction of mother and child, is an abnormal phenomenon of mutual generation caused by a break down in the conventional relationship among the five phases. This includes extension of mother to child (affliction of the child by its mother's illness) and extension of child to mother (affliction of the mother by its child's illness).

The sequence of extension from mother to child is in keeping with that of mutual generation, while the sequence of extension from child to mother is opposite to that of mutual generation. To use Wood as an example, abnormality of Wood affects Fire, which is in accordance with the sequence of mutual generation, known as extension from mother to child; Wood also affects Water, which is opposite to the sequence of mutual generation, and represents extension of illness from child to mother. (Fig. 1-23)

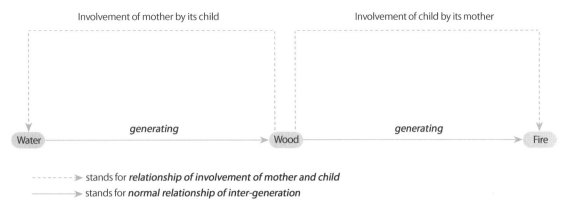

Fig. 1-23   Extension of mother and child (Example)

Application of the Doctrine of Five Phases in Chinese Medicine

① To Expound the Physiological Function of the Five *Zang* Organs and Their Relationships

(1) To expound the physiological function of the five zang organs

The doctrine of five phases associates the five *zang* organs of the human body with the five phases and endows the physiological functions of five *zang* organs with the properties of the five phases. For example, Wood has the properties of extending and rising. The Liver likes to expand and branch out while it loathes suppression, and has the function of smoothing and discharging. The warmth and heat of Fire rises, and the Heart yang has the function of warming the body. Earth has the properties of receiving and generating, while the Spleen has the functions of transporting and transforming Water and food and generating qi and blood. Metal has the properties of cold lifelessness and astringency, while the Lungs have the functions of purification and lowering. Water has the properties of moistening and descending, while the Kidneys have the functions of managing Water and storing essence.

(2) To expound mutual relationships among the five zang organs

A. To explain the reciprocal generating relationships among the five *zang* organs with the mutual generation of the five phases

The five *zang* organs are paired with the five phases to account for the mutually beneficial relationships between physiological functions of the human body. For instance, the blood of the Liver nourishing the Heart corresponds with Wood generating Fire; Heart yang warming the Spleen corresponds with Fire generating Earth; Spleen qi transporting essential substances to the Lung corresponds with Earth generating Metal; Lung qi lowering Water to the Kidneys corresponds with Metal generating Water; Kidney essence nourishing the blood of the Liver corresponds with Water generating Wood. (Fig. 1-24)

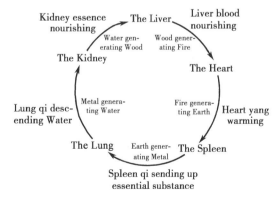

Fig. 1-24   Mutual generating relationships among the five *zang* organs as explained by the five phases theory

B. To expound mutually restrictive relationships among five *zang* organs with mutual restraint of five phases

The aspect of mutual restraint between the five

phases can be used to explain the physiological functions of mutually restrictive relationships among the five *zang* organs. For instance, expansion of the Liver qi discharging stagnation of the Spleen corresponds with Wood restraining Earth; the Spleen transporting and transforming Water preventing overflow in the Kidneys corresponds with Earth restraining Water; Kidney yin (Water) restricting excessive Fire in the Heart corresponds with Water restraining Fire; Heart yang warmth restricting excessive descent of Lung qi corresponds with Fire restraining Metal; descent of Lung qi restricting excessive rising of Liver qi corresponds with Metal restraining Wood. (Fig. 1-25)

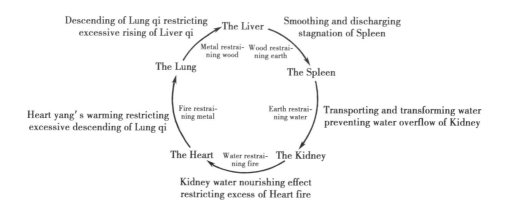

Fig. 1-25 **Mutually restrictive relationships among the five *zang* organs as explained by the five phases theory**

Plain Questions: Chapter Discussion on Various Relationships Concerning the Five Zang-Organs (Sù Wèn: Wǔ Zàng Shēng Chéng Piān, 素问·五脏生成篇*)* states: *"The Heart's superior is the Kidney." "The Lung's superior is the Heart." "The Liver's superior is the Lung." "The Spleen's superior is the Liver." "The Kidney's superior is the Spleen."* (Superior refers to the restraining viscera)

② To Explain Mutual Pathological Affliction among the Five *Zang* Organs

Mutual pathological affliction among five *zang* organs means simply that an illness of any one organ may adversely affect one or more others, and conversely the illnesses of one or more other organs may adversely affect the organ in sequence. This kind of mutual pathological affliction is called "transmission". Transmission is classified according to the mutual generation and mutual restraint relationships of the five phases to explain its existence among the five *zang* organs. (Fig. 1-26) The Liver can be used as an example to clarify the relationship of pathological transmission between the Liver and the four other organs.

A. Transmission following relationships of mutual generation

This includes the two aspects of "disorder of the mother extends to the child" and "disorder of child extends to the mother".

a. Disorder of the mother extending to the child indicates pathological transmission from mother-organ to its child-organ

For instance, disease of the Liver transmitted to the Heart or disease of the Kidneys transmitted to the Liver. (Fig. 1-26)

b. Disorder of child extending to the mother indicates pathological transmission from child-organ to its mother-organ

For instance, disease of the Liver transmitted to the Kidneys or disease of the Heart transmitted to the Liver. (Fig. 1-26)

B. Transmission following relationships mutual restraint

This includes the two aspects of "transmission of extreme restraint" and "transmission of counter

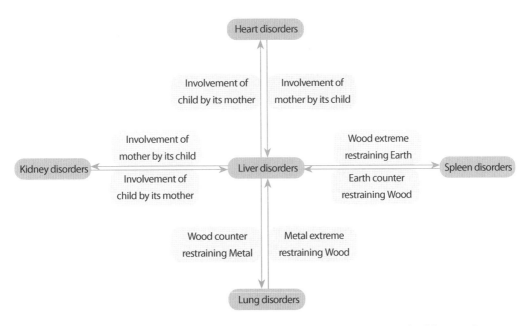

Fig. 1-26   Relationship of pathological transmission between the Liver and
the other four organs

restraint".

a. Extreme restraint indicates over restriction leading to the occurrence of disease

It includes two conditions: extreme restraint caused by excess of a *zang* organ and extreme restraint caused by deficiency of a *zang* organ.

An excessive *zang* organ overly restrains its inferior *zang* organ. For example, excess of the Liver overly restrains the Spleen. (Fig. 1-27)

A deficient *zang* organ is overly restrained by its superior *zang* organ. For example, deficient Spleen is over restrained by the Liver. (Fig. 1-27)

b. Counter restraint indicates the normal restraining order is reversed, thus leading to the occurrence of disease

It includes two conditions: counter restraint caused by excess of a *zang* organ and counter restraint caused by deficiency of a *zang* organ.

An excessive *zang* organ conversely restrains its superior *zang* organ. For example, excess of the Liver counter restrains the Lungs. (Fig. 1-28)

A deficient *zang* organ is conversely restrained by its inferior *zang* organ. For instance, deficiency of the Lungs is counter restrained by the Liver. (Fig. 1-28)

(3) Application to the Diagnosis of Disease

The human body is an organic whole. When the viscera is struck by disease, it is be reflected in

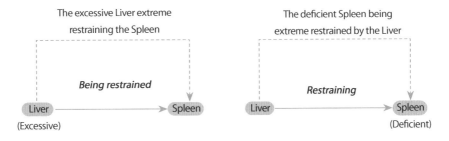

Fig. 1-27   Excessive Liver extreme restraining the Spleen and deficient Spleen extreme
restrained by the Liver

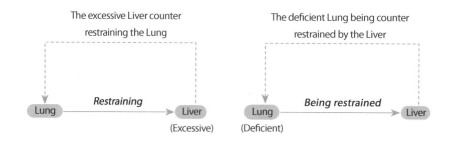

Fig. 1-28 Excessive Liver counter restraining the Lungs and deficient Lung counter restrained by the Liver

corresponding external tissues and organs on the surface of the body, appearing as abnormal changes in complexion, pulse and flavor, etc. Association with the five phases and the law of mutual generation, mutual restraint, extreme restraint and counter restraint can be used to diagnose disease and infer its status through symptoms and signs obtained through the four examinations.

A. To diagnose disease

Pathological changes of the five *zang* organs can be diagnosed through changes in corresponding color, pulse and flavor. For instance, a patient with a blue-green complexion, a preference for sour food and a wiry pulse can be diagnosed with Liver trouble. A reddish complexion accompanied by a bitter taste in the mouth and a surging pulse can be diagnosed with hyperactivity of the Heart Fire. A patient with Spleen deficiency displaying a blue-green complexion and a wiry pulse can be diagnosed with Liver illness that has spread to the Spleen (Wood overly restraining Earth).

B. To infer the status of disease

The prognosis of a disease can be inferred from the relationships of mutual generation and mutual restraint between complexion and pulse. The doctrine of five phases holds that when a *zang* organ is afflicted by disease, if complexion is in accordance with its corresponding pulse, this indicates the expected course of illness. In situations where the complexion does not match with its corresponding pulse, if the pulse restrains the complexion, it indicates an unfavorable prognosis; if the pulse generates the complexion, it indicates a favorable prognosis. For instance, a patient with Liver trouble has a blue-green complexion and a wiry pulse. This is in keeping with the five phases, meaning complexion matches with pulse. If this same patient's pulse is not wiry, but instead floating, this is a restraining pulse, or a pulse of the restraining color (Metal restrains Wood), making the prognosis unfavorable. If the patient has a deep pulse, this is a pulse of the generating color (Water generates Wood), indicating a good prognosis. (Table 1-6)

Mencius: Chapter Gaozixia (Mèng Zǐ: Gào Zǐ Xià, 孟子·告子下) states: "*Where there are internal changes, there are external symptoms.*"

Miraculous Pivot: Chapter the Various

Table 1-6 Mutual generation and mutual restraint relationships between complexion and pulse of Liver disease and its prognosis

	Complexion	Pulse	Relationship between Complexion and Pulse	Prognosis
Liver Trouble	Blue-green	Wiry	Concurrent	Normal
	Blue-green	Floating	Pulse restraining color	Death (unfavorable)
	Blue-green	Deep	Pulse generating color	Recovery (favorable)

Note: The prognosis of disease should be inferred by analyzing the data gathered from the four examinations comprehensively, and not confined only to the mutual generation and mutual restraint relationship between complexion and pulse.

Conditions of Internal Organs Relating Different Diseases (Líng Shū: Běn Zàng, 灵枢·本藏) states: *"Observe the external response to understand the internal viscera, and thus know the nature of the disease."*

Classic of Questioning: The Sixty-first Question (Nàn Jīng: Liù Shí Yī Nàn, 难经·六十一难) states: *"Understanding through observation is to recognize disease by studying the five colors. Understanding through listening is to recognize disease by analyzing the five sounds. Understanding through questioning is to recognize disease by inquiring of the desire for the five flavors. Understanding through palpating is to recognize the diseased zang or fu organs by reading the Cun Kou (寸口) pulse and determine excess or deficiency."*

Plain Questions: Chapter Discussion on Various Relationships Concerning the Five Zang-Organs (Sù Wèn: Wǔ Zàng Shēng Chéng Piān, 素问·五脏生成篇) states: *"To diagnose disease by combining complexion and pulse is to be complete."*

Miraculous Pivot: Chapter the Visceral Diseases Caused by Evil Qi (Líng Shū: Xié Qì Zàng Fǔ Bìng Xíng, 灵枢·邪气脏腑病形) states: *"A complexion without its corresponding pulse, accompanied instead by its restraining pulse indicates that the patient will die; if accompanied instead by the generating pulse, they will recover."*

Golden Mirror of Medicine: Chapter the Inmost Methods of Four Examinations (Yī Zōng Jīn Jiàn:Sì Zhěn Xīn Fǎ, 医宗金鉴·四诊心法) states: *"When the complexion matches with the pulse, blue-green complexion with a wiry pulse, red with surging, yellow with moderate, white with floating, and dark with deep, there is no cause for great concern. When a complexion appears without its corresponding pulse, if the pulse restrains the color, the patient will die; if the pulse generates the color, the patient will survive."*

④ Application to the Treatment of Disease

(1) To check the transmission of disease

The patterns of development for diseases of the five *zang* organs can be inferred by the mutual generating, mutual restraining, extreme restraining and counter restraining laws of the five phases. If one *zang* organ is diseased, it can affect the other four *zang* organs, while diseases of the

other *zang* organs can also affect the original *zang* organ in question. Therefore, transmission can be checked in treatment by harmonizing excess and the deficiency according to these laws. Take the Liver as an example. Excessive Liver qi will inevitably overly restrain the Spleen; if the Spleen is strengthened in advance, it will prevent Liver illness from spreading to the Spleen. Whether the disease is transmitted or not depends mainly on the functional state of five *zang* organs, meaning it is more prone to transmit if the five *zang* organs are relatively deficient and not transmit if they are excessive.

Classic of Questioning: The Seventy-seventh Question (Nàn Jīng: Qī Shí Qī Nàn, 难经·七十七难) states: *"When a disease of the Liver appears, it should be recognized that it may be transmitted to the Spleen, so the Spleen qi should be strengthened in advance in order to prevent the Spleen from contracting the evil qi of the Liver. This is referred to as treating disease before it occurs."*

(2) To determine principles and methods of treatment

A. To determine principles and methods of treatment according to the law of mutual generation of the five phases (Fig. 1-29)

The treatment principles according to the law of mutual generation of the five phases is "tonifying the mother and purging the child".

Tonifying the mother element, namely to "tonify the mother of that which is deficient", is to treat deficiency syndromes of the *zang* organs in accordance with the mother-child relationship by tonifying the mother of the deficient *zang* organ. For instance, deficiency of Liver yin can be treated by nourishing the yin of the Kidneys.

Purging the child, namely "purging the child of that which is excessive", is to treat excessive syndromes of the *zang* organs in accordance with mother-child relationship by purging the child of the excessive *zang* organ. For instance, excess of Liver Fire can be treated by purging Heart Fire.

The commonly used methods of treatment determined according to the law of mutual generation of the five phases include replenishing Water to nourish Wood, aiding Fire to strengthen Earth, reinforcing Earth to strengthen Metal and mutually generating Metal and Water.

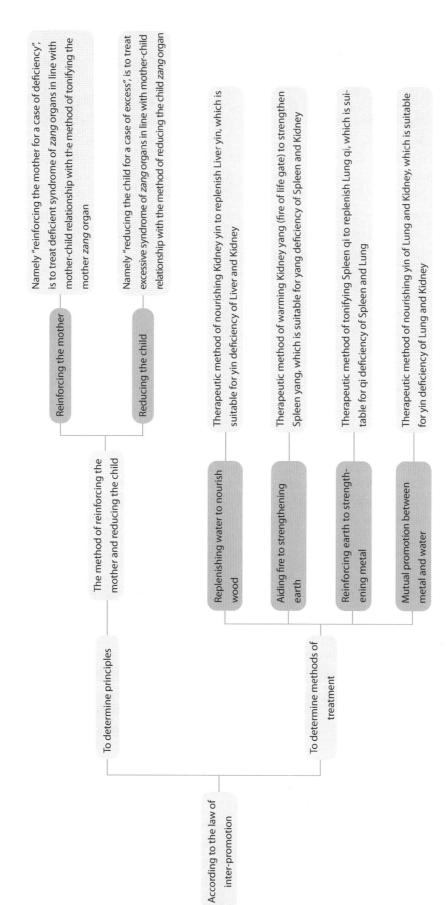

Fig. 1-29 Summary of determining principles and methods of treatment according to the law of mutual generation of the five phases

Classic of Questioning: The Sixty-nineth Question (Nàn Jīng: Liù Shí Jiǔ Nàn, 难经·六十九难) says: *"Tonify the mother of that which is deficient, and purge the child of that which is excessive."*

B. To determine principles and methods of treatment according to the law of mutual restraint of the five phases (Fig. 1-30)

The treatment principle according to the law of mutual restraint of the five phases is to "inhibit the strong and support the weak".

When the relationship of mutual restraint among the five phases is abnormal, the pathological changes of extreme restraint and counter restraint will inevitably occur, the cause of which is nothing more than simple excess and deficiency. Excess is characteristic of the strong and manifests as hyperactivity; deficiency is characteristic of the weak and manifests as hypoactivity. As a result, the principle of inhibiting the strong and supporting the weak can be adopted in treatment to facilitate recovery.

Inhibiting the strong means to reduce the strength of that which is excessive, this is suitable for extreme restraint and counter restraint caused by excessive restricting. For instance, if the Liver qi is excessive and conversely invades the Spleen, leading to disharmony between the Liver and the Spleen, it is called Liver-Wood over restrains Spleen-Earth, and should be treated mainly by soothing and pacifying the Liver. Another example, stagnation of Spleen-Earth with accumulating damp brings about disharmony of the Liver and the Spleen, known as Spleen-Earth counter restraining Liver-Wood and should be treated by activating the Spleen and resolving the damp. If the strong is inhibited, the function of the weak is apt to recover.

Supporting the weak means to improve the weakened condition of that which is deficient, this is suitable for extreme restraint and counter restraint caused by a lack of restriction. For instance, if the Spleen qi is deficient and the Liver qi invades the Spleen, leading to disharmony between the Liver and the Spleen, it is called invasion of the Liver due to deficiency of the Spleen, and should be treated mainly by strengthening the Spleen and replenishing qi. Another example, deficiency of Spleen qi failing to control Water flow leading to the syndrome of overflowing Water and dampness, known as counter restraint of Water due to deficiency of the Spleen, and should be treated by strengthening the Spleen and purging excess Water. Supporting the weak can aid in its recovery of normal functions.

The commonly used treating methods determined by the law of mutual restraint include inhibiting Wood to assist Earth, amassing Earth to control Water, assisting Metal to check Wood and reducing the south while reinforcing the north.

(3) To guide administration of herbs in accordance with the zang-fu organs

Different Chinese herbal medicinals are of different colors and flavors. Classified by color, they possess the "five colors, 五色" of green, red, yellow, white and black. Differentiated by flavor, they have the "five flavors, 五味" of sour, bitter, sweet, acrid and salty. According to association with the five phases, five colors, five flavors and five *zang* organs have their own selective nature, i.e. blue-green and sour enter the Liver, red and bitter enter the Heart, yellow and sweet enter the Spleen, white and acrid enter the Lungs, and black and salty enter the Kidneys. The association of colors and flavors of medicine to the five *zang* organs is the referential basis for the selective administration to visceral pathological changes.

Plain Questions: Chapter Discussion on the Most Important and Abstruse Theory (Sù Wèn: Zhì Zhèn Yào Dà Lùn, 素问·至真要大论) states: *"The five flavors tend towards the organ of which they are fond of after entering the Stomach. Therefore, sour enters the Liver first, bitter enters the Heart first, sweet enters the Spleen first, acrid enters the Lungs first, and salty enters the Kidneys first."*

In addition, the doctrine of five phases is of certain guiding value in acupuncture and moxibustion therapy as well as in the treatment of emotional diseases.

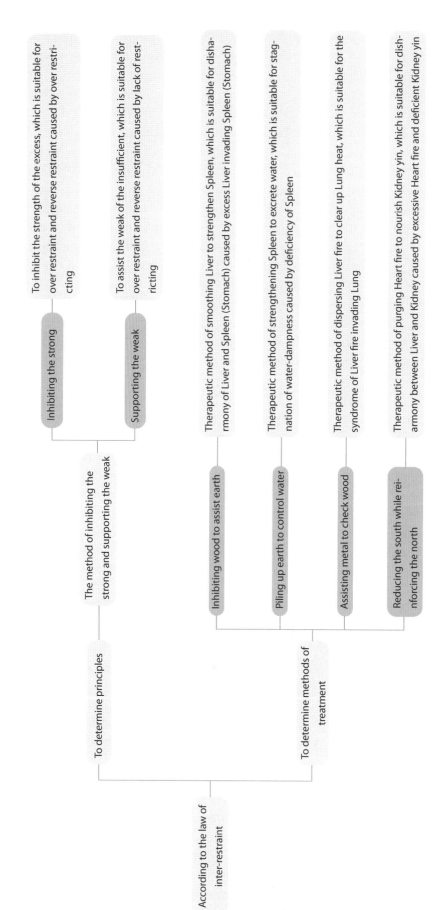

Fig. 1-30 Summary of determining principles and methods of treatment according to the law of mutual restraint of the five phases

Chapter 2
Visceral Manifestations

Introduction

(1) Basic Definition of Visceral Manifestations

(1) The meaning of visceral manifestations (Fig. 2-1)

The two Chinese characters *Zang Xiang* (visceral manifestations) were first seen in *Plain Questions: Discussion on Six-Plus-Six System and the Manifestations of the Viscera (Sù Wèn: Liù Jié Zàng Xiàng Lùn,* 素问·六节藏象论). This chapter takes visceral manifestations as its name and expounds upon the physiological functions of the five *zang* organs and six *fu* organs, as well as the relationship between *zang-fu* organs and the natural environment.

The meaning of "*Zang*藏" is the same as that of "*Zang*脏", and refers to the organs that hide deep inside the body, including the five *zang* organs, six *fu* organs and the extraordinary *fu* organs together known as the *zang-fu* organs (脏腑).

"*Xiang*象" has many meanings: a. It refers to figure, namely the anatomical shape of the *zang-fu* organs, and is the morphological foundation for the physiological functions of viscera; b. It refers to sign, namely the physiological and pathological phenomena of *zang-fu* organs manifesting externally; c. It refers to respondent image, namely the physiological and pathological images of *zang-fu* organs that respond to the yin and yang of the four seasons. Generally speaking, visceral manifestations refer to the viscera that hide in the human body and the physiological and pathological phenomena of the viscera that manifest externally.

"*Zang* (藏 viscera)" is the inbeing of image or manifestation, "Xiang (象 image or manifestation)" is the external reflection of viscera, and a combination of the two characters is called "*Zang* Xiang (Visceral manifestations)". Chinese medicine primarily studies the physiological activities and pathological changes of viscera through the transmutation of "Xiang (象 manifestation)" externally. Namely it is what is called "to examine the viscera by manifestations".

(2) Definition of the theory of visceral manifestations

The theory of visceral manifestations is a theoretical discussion of the morphological structures, physiological functions, pathological changes and their correlations among the *zang-fu* organs, body constituents, sense organs and orifices. Therefore, the contents of the theory of visceral manifestations primarily analyzes the physiological function of the five *zang* organs, six *fu* organs and extraordinary *fu* organs and the relationship between different *zang-fu* organs, as well as the physiological function of the body constituents, sense organs and orifices and their relation to the viscera.

Plain Questions: Discussion on Six-Plus-Six

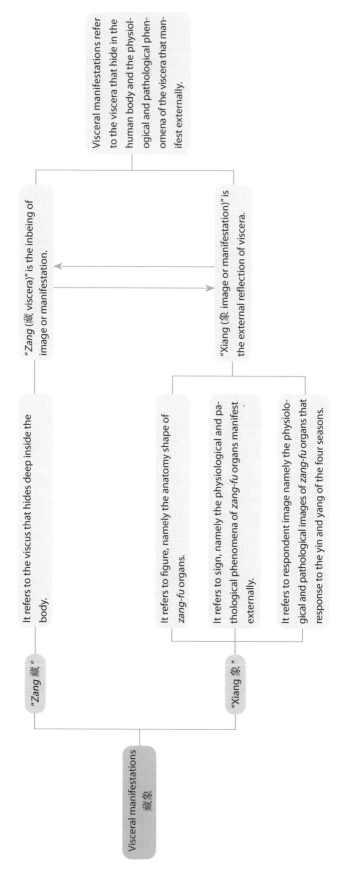

Fig. 2-1　Chart for the meaning of visceral manifestations

System and the Manifestations of the Viscera (*Sù Wèn: Liù Jié Zàng Xiàng Lùn*, 素问·六节藏象论) says: "Yellow Emperor (黄帝) *said: How about the visceral manifestations? Qi Bo* (岐伯) *said: The Lung is the root of qi, where the inferior spirit is located; its quintessence appears in the fine hair of the body, and its function is to nourish skin. The Lung belongs to greater yin within yang, so its qi communicates with autumn. The Kidney manages closure and is the root of storage and the place where the essence is housed; its quintessence appears in the hair, and its function is to nourish bone. The Kidney is shaoyin within yin, so its qi communicates with winter. The Liver is the root of the four limbs, it is the place where the soul lies, its quintessence appears on the nails, its function is to nourish tendons and produce blood, its taste is sour and its color is green. The Liver belongs to shaoyang within yang and communicates with spring qi. The Spleen, Stomach, Large Intestine, Small Intestine, San Jiao, and the Bladder are the root of the granary where the nutrient qi resides and are called the containers. They can store food, transform draff and manage the transformation, absorption and the discharge of the flavors. The Spleen demonstrates its quintessence on the lips, nourishing the muscles, and associating with sweet tastes and yellow color. The Spleen belongs to zhiyin within yin and communicates with earth qi.*"

The note by Wang Bing (王冰)"*Xiang* (象 *manifestation*) *refers to what manifests outside and can be seen.*"

Variorum of Plain Questions of The Yellow Emperor's Internal Classic (*Huáng Dì Nèi Jīng Sù Wèn Jí Zhù*, 黄帝内经素问集注) says: "*Xiang* (象 *manifestation*) *refers to Xiang* (像 *image*). *It is to discuss the image of the zang-fu organs in response to the yin and yang of heaven and earth.*"

Classified Classic: Chapter Class of Visceral Manifestations (*Lèi Jīng: Zàng Xiàng Lèi*, 类经·藏象类) says: "*Xiang* (象) *refers to figure. Zang organs reside internally, with their figure manifesting externally, so this is called visceral manifestation.*"

Miraculous Pivot: Chapter The Various Conditions of Internal Organs Relating Different Diseases (*Líng Shū: Běn Zàng*, 灵枢·本藏) says: "*The inner viscera can be known by observing their external manifestations.*"

② The Concept and Classifcation of *Zang-Fu* Organs (Fig. 2-2)

Zang-fu organs are the general name for all internal viscera, and the basis of the theory of visceral manifestations. The names of the *zang-fu* organs in Chinese medicine are the same as the biomedical terms, but the connotations are different. The internal organs of contemporary biomedicine are a morphologic concept based on anatomy. *Zang-fu* organs of Chinese medicine are a collective concept based on functions that include anatomy, physiology and pathology, serving as an integrative functional unit.

Zang-fu organs are classified into three types according to their physiological functional features in terms of the five *zang* organs (Liver, Heart, Spleen, Lung, Kidney), six *fu* organs (Gallbladder, Stomach, Small Intestine, Large Intestine, Bladder, *San Jiao*) and extraordinary *fu* organs (brain, marrow, bone, vessel, Gallbladder, uterus).

The common physiological features of the five *zang* organs are to transform, generate and store essence qi.

The physiological features of the six *fu* organs are to receive, contain, transport and absorb food and water.

Plain Questions: Chapter Different Discussion on the Five Zang-Organs (*Sù Wèn: Wǔ Zàng Bié Lùn*, 素问·五脏别论) says: The five *zang* organs "*store up essence qi*", and "*are substantial but not filled*", and the six *fu* organs "*transport, digest and absorb water and food*", and "*are filled but not substantial*". "Substantial" refers to the state of being full of essence qi; "filled" refers to the state of being filled up with water and food. The physiological features of the five *zang* organs and six *fu* organs differ, which has certain significance in directing the clinical syndrome differentiation and treatment. Generally, most diseases of *zang* organs are deficiency syndromes; for *fu* organs, they are excess syndromes. Thereby, *zang* disease should be supplemented and *fu* diseases should be reduced.

Morphologically, most extraordinary *fu*-organs are hollow and similar to the six *fu* organs;

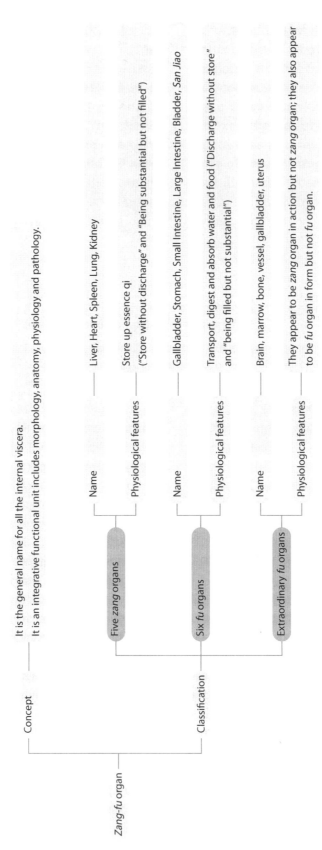

Zang-fu organ

Concept
- It is the general name for all the internal viscera.
- It is an integrative functional unit includes morphology, anatomy, physiology and pathology.

Classification

Five zang organs
- Name —— Liver, Heart, Spleen, Lung, Kidney
- Physiological features —— Store up essence qi ("Store without discharge" and "Being substantial but not filled")

Six fu organs
- Name —— Gallbladder, Stomach, Small Intestine, Large Intestine, Bladder, San Jiao
- Physiological features —— Transport, digest and absorb water and food ("Discharge without store" and "being filled but not substantial")

Extraordinary fu organs
- Name —— Brain, marrow, bone, vessel, gallbladder, uterus
- Physiological features —— They appear to be zang organ in action but not zang organ; they also appear to be fu organ in form but not fu organ.

Fig. 2-2   The conclusion of the contents, classification and concept of zang-fu organs

functionally, they are the same as the five *zang* organs and store essence qi. They appear to be *zang* organs but not *zang* organs; they also appear to be *fu* organs but not *fu* organs, so they are called the extraordinary *fu* organs.

Plain Questions: Chapter Discussion on Important Ideas in the Golden Chamber (Sù Wèn: Jīn Guì Zhēn Yán Lùn, 素问·金匮真言论) says: "The Five zang organs, the Liver, Heart, Spleen, Lung and Kidney belong to yin; the six fu organs, Gallbladder, Bladder and San Jiao belong to yang."

Plain Questions: Chapter Different Discussion on the Five Zang-Organs (Sù Wèn: Wǔ Zàng Bié Lùn, 素问·五脏别论) says: "All of the six organs, brain marrow, bone, vessels, Gallbladder and uterus are generated in accordance with the earth qi and store yin like the earth that contains everything. Therefore they store and don't discharge and are called the extraordinary fu organs. The Stomach, Large Intestine, Small Intestine, San Jiao and Bladder discharge but do not store, and the five organs are generated in accordance with heaven qi, so they function like the heavens, and they discharge without storing up. These so called five zang organs store without discharge, therefore, are substantial but not filled. The six fu organs digest and transport food and drink without storing essence, and so are filled but not substantial."

The notes to *Plain Questions: Chapter Different Discussion on the Five Zang-Organs (Sù Wèn: Wǔ Zàng Bié Lùn, 素问·五脏别论)* by Wang Bing (王冰) record: (Regarding the five *zang* organs) "*Being substantial refers to the essence qi, being filled refers to the water and food, but they only store up essence qi, therefore they are substantial but not filled.*" (Regarding the six *fu* organs) "*They don't store up essence qi, but receive water and food.*"

Classified Classic: Chapter Class of Visceral Manifestations (Lèi Jīng: Zàng Xiàng Lèi, 类经·藏象类) says that extraordinary *fu* organs "*store up and accumulate yin essence.*" "*Qi (奇, extraordinary) means special. Heng (恒, permanent) means constant.*"

Guide to Clinical Practice with Medical Records: Chapter Spleen and Stomach (Lín Zhèng Zhǐ Nán Yī Àn: Pí Wèi, 临证指南医案·脾胃) says: "*Zang organs are suitable to store up and fu organs are suitable to dredge, that's because the forms and*

functions of them are different respectively."

Treatment of Different Kinds of Diseases: Chapter Summarization of Internal Images (Lèi Zhèng Zhì Cái: Nèi Jīng Zōng Yào, 类证治裁·内景综要) says: "*The six fu organs transport but do not store up; they are filled but not substantial, so using elimination as treatment is a form of tonification for them.*"

③ Formation of the Theory of Visceral Manifestations

The theory of visceral manifestations was basically formed in *Internal Classic (Nèi Jīng)*. The chief formative foundations are as follows:

a. Ancient anatomical knowledge: there have been records of anatomical knowledge in the medical work *Internal Classic (Nèi Jīng, 内经)* and *Classic of Questioning (Nàn Jīng, 难经)*. This knowledge laid a morphological foundation for the formation of the theory of visceral manifestations.

b. Observations of physiological and pathological phenomena of the human body: based on anatomical knowledge in ancient times, people understood the physiological and pathological laws of the human body via holistic observation of phenomena of the human body, which provided basis for the formation of the theory of visceral manifestation.

c. The accumulation of experience of long-term medical practice: The physiological functions of *zang-fu* organs were discovered through pathological phenomena and curative effect after long-term medical practice, which is the practical foundation for the theoretical formation of visceral manifestations.

④ Features of Theory of Visceral Manifestations

The basic characteristic of the theory of visceral manifestations is the holism that takes the five-*zang* viscera as its center. The theory of visceral manifestations thinks that the constituents of the human body are structurally indivisible, functionally interactive, and pathologically and mutually infective and constitute an intricate organic whole. The organic whole takes the five *zang* organs as its center, namely it lais special stress on the core actions of the five *zang* organs. It is thought that the five *zang* organs are the core of the life activity of the human body. The six-*fu* organs, body constituents, sense organs and orifices, four-extremity and bones, as well as spirit, passion and emotion are categorized into the five-*zang*-organ system respectively. This forms five large systems with the five *zang* organs as their center, namely the five *zang* organ system. (Fig. 2-3)

Another feature of the theory of visceral manifestation indicates that *zang-fu* organs are not only a morphological concept, but also a collective concept including anatomy, physiology and pathology, i.e. a concept of a functional unit.

Miraculous Pivot: Chapter On Acupoints (*Líng Shū: Běn Shū*, 灵枢·本输) says: "*The Heart connects with the Small Intestine*", "*the Lung connects with the Large Intestine*", "*the Liver connects with the Gallbladder*", "*the Spleen connects with the Stomach*" and "*the Kidney connects with the Bladder.*"

Plain Questions: Chapter Discussion on the Elucidation of Five-Qi (*Sù Wèn: Xuān Míng Wǔ Qì Piān*, 素问·宣明五气篇) says: "*The five secretions derived from the five zang organs are sweating from the Heart, nasal discharge from the Lung, tears from the Liver, saliva from the Spleen and spit from the Kidneys, which are called the five fluids.*"

"*The storage of the five zang organs is: the Heart stores the spirit, the Lung stores inferior spirit, the Liver stores the soul, the Spleen stores ideas, and the Kidneys stores will, together called the storage of the five zang organs.*"

"*Dominances of five zang organs: the Heart dominates vessels, the Lung dominates skin, the Liver dominates tendons, the Spleen dominates muscles, and the Kidneys dominates bone, together called the five dominances.*"

"*The respondent images of the five zang organs: the pulse of the Liver is string-like, the pulse of the Heart is hook-like, the pulse of the Spleen is slow, the pulse of the Lung is floating, and the pulse of the Kidney is deep, together called the five pulses of the five zang organs.*"

Plain Questions: Chapter Discussion on Important Ideas in the Golden Chamber (*Sù Wèn: Jīn Guì Zhēn Yán Lùn*, 素问·金匮真言论) says: "*The Heart opens at the ears*", "*the Liver opens at the eyes*",

"*the Spleen opens at the mouth*", and "*the Kidney opens at the two lower orifices*".

Plain Questions: Chapter Major Discussion on the Theory of Yin and Yang and the Corresponding Relationships Among All the Things in Nature (*Sù Wèn: Yīn Yáng Yìng Xiàng Dà Lùn*, 素问·阴阳应象大论) says: The Heart "*opens at the tongue*"; the Kidney "*opens at the ears*".

Miraculous Pivot: Chapter Determining the Conditions of the Five Viscera by Examining the Five Sense Organs (*Líng Shū: Wǔ Yuè Wǔ Shǐ*, 灵枢·五阅五使) says: "*The nose belongs to the Lung, and takes charge of respiration; the eyes belong to the Liver, they take charge of vision; the mouth belongs to the Spleen, it takes charge of receiving water and food; the tongue belongs to the Heart, it takes charge of distinguishing tastes; the ears belong to the Kidney, they take charge of hearing.*"

Plain Questions: Discussion on Six-Plus-Six System and the Manifestations of the Viscera (*Sù Wèn: Liù Jié Zàng Xiàng Lùn*, 素问·六节藏象论) says of the Heart: "*Its quintessence appears on the face*"; of the Liver, "*its quintessence appears on the nails*"; of the Spleen "*its quintessence appears on the lips*", of the Lung "*its quintessence appears on the fine hair*", and of the Kidney "*its quintessence appears on the hair*".

Plain Questions: Chapter Major Discussion on the Theory of Yin and Yang and the Corresponding Relationships Among All the Things in Nature (*Sù Wèn: Yīn Yáng Yìng Xiàng Dà Lùn*, 素问·阴阳应象大论) says: Of the Liver "*Its mind is anger*"; Of the Heart "*its mind is happy*"; of the Spleen "*its mind is thinking*"; of the Lung "*its mind is sorrow*", and of the Kidney "*its mind is fear*".

Miraculous Pivot: Chapter The Twenty-Five Kinds of People in Different Characteristics of Yin and Yang (*Líng Shū: Yīn Yáng Èr Shí Wǔ Rén*, 灵枢·阴阳二十五人) says: "*In all of heaven and earth, in every direction and with everything, all things are a part of the five elements. People are the same.*"

⑤ Regarding the Problems of Qi, Blood, Yin and Yang of the Five *Zang* Organs

Chinese medicine thinks that the morphological structure of viscera is the material basis for their function and activities. Different viscera have

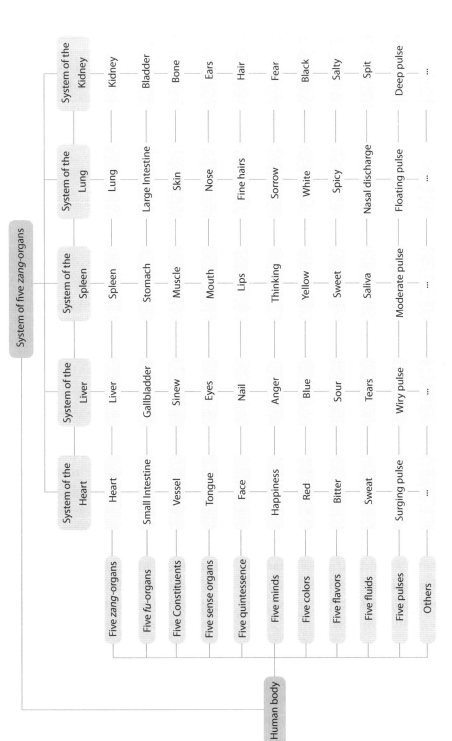

Fig. 2-3 Systematic organization of the patterns of the five *zang* organs

dissimilar morphological structures, and thus have different physiological functions. However, the recognition of the visceral shapes of Chinese medicine is comparatively simple. Chinese medicine expounds the function and activities of viscera with qi, blood, yin and yang, which are considered the material basis of the functions and activities of the viscera.

Chinese medicine understands the qi, blood, yin and yang of the five *zang* organs by the action features of them. Qi, blood, yin and yang are the basic substances maintaining the function and activities of the five *zang* organs. Comparatively speaking, both qi and yang have the actions of warming, pushing and consolidating. Qi is primarily responsible for the functions of pushing and consolidating, and yang for warming. Both blood and yin have the actions of nourishing and moistening. Blood primarily has the action of nourishing, and yin moistening. Since each organ emphasizes qi, blood, yin or yang respectively, they have different physiological functions. The pathological changes engendered by the disorders of the physiological functions of the five *zang* organs always manifests as the imbalance of qi, blood, yin and yang.

The concept of the yin and yang of the five *zang* organs is different from that in the yin-yang theory. The yin and yang of the five *zang* organs is a specific concept and the material basis for maintaining the functions and activities of the five *zang* organs. With physiological activities, substances with the actions of nourishing and moistening belong to the yin of the five *zang* organs; the ones with warming and pushing actions belong to the yang of the five *zang* organs. The yin and yang in the yin-yang theory are abstract concepts and the generalization of the attributes of both sides of the associated items or phenomena in the natural world.

Section 1 Five *Zang* Organs

This section mainly discusses the physiological functions of the five *zang* organs in terms of the Heart, Liver, Spleen, Lung and Kidney, the functions of the body constituents, sense organs and orifices, and emotions and five humors, as well as their relationship to the five *zang* organs, and the physiological properties of the five *zang* organs.

The Heart (Appendix: Pericardium)

The Heart (心) is located in the chest, between the two lungs and above the diaphragm. It is similar in shape to an inverted lotus bud and is guarded by the Pericardium.

The main physiological functions of the Heart are dominating the blood vessels and housing the spirit. In the ancient literature of Chinese medicine, the Heart had different connotations in terms of the Heart of flesh and blood and the Heart of mental activity. The Heart of flesh and blood refers to the substantial Heart that controls the impulses of blood circulation; the Heart of mental activity refers to the conscious, thinking and emotional functions of the Heart that controls the spirit and mind.

The Heart connects with the Small Intestine among the *fu* organs and dominates vessels among the body constituents. Its quintessence appears on the face, it opens onto the tongue, its mind is happiness, and its fluid is sweat.

① Physiological Functions of the Heart (Table 2-1)

(1) The Heart governs blood and vessels

The Heart governing blood and vessels refers to the function of the Heart that controls the blood circulating inside the vessels.

Blood circulates inside the vessels, and the vessels connect with Heart directly. The Heart, blood and vessels constitute one relatively independent Heart-blood-vessel system (the cardiovascular system). The Heart plays a leading role in the system, which is called "the Heart governs blood and vessels".

Normal blood circulation depends on the combined actions of the Heart, blood and vessels, namely, that only abundant Heart yang qi can activate and warm the blood to circulate; only

Table 2-1 Physiologicals of the Heart

Actions	Heart governs blood and vessels	The Heart stores the spirit
Meaning	It refers to the function of the Heart causing blood to circulate inside the vessels.	The Heart dominates the life activity of the whole body and the functions of spirit, consciousness and thinking of humans.
Physiological actions	The necessities for normal blood circulation are abundant yang qi, sufficient yin blood, and free vessel passage. If the blood circulation is normal, the whole body can be nourished. Chief manifestations: normal Heart beat, reddish and lustrous complexion, light red tongue with moist body, moderate and forceful pulse. The Heart governs the blood circulation and also generates the blood.	Normal mental activities manifest as good spirit, clear consciousness, prompt thinking, and rapid response. It dominates the physiological activities of the zang-fu organs, body constituents, sense organs, and orifices, and balances the physiological activities of the whole body.
Chief pathological changes	Insufficient Heart qi & Heart blood deficiency: palpitation, pale complexion, pale tongue body, small and weak pulse. Heart blood stagnation, unsmooth vessel passage: precordial pain, dark complexion, cyanotic lips and tongue, thready uneven pulse or knotted or intermittent pulse.	Imbalance of Heart spirit: insomnia and dreamful sleep, delirium, lags in response, even coma or unconsciousness, disorders of the zang-fu organs, dysfunction of body constituents, sense organs and orifices.

filled Heart yin blood can moisten and nourish the Heart vessel; only free vessels can control and keep free blood circulation. These are the postulates of normal blood circulation.

The physiological action of the Heart governing blood and vessels is to guarantee normal blood circulation. On one hand, it maintains the actions of the Heart itself, i.e. maintaining a regular Heart beat to keep a normal Heart force, rhythm and Heart rate. On the other hand, the Heart transports blood all over the body and exerts blood's function of nourishing the five zang organs and six fu organs, the body constituents, sense organs and orifices, the four extremities, the bones etc., which maintains normal life activities.

In addition, the Heart governs blood also has the meaning of generating blood. It means that water and food, the refined nutritious substances, are transformed into red blood by the action of Heart-fire (Heart yang). (This will be discussed in the contents of the generation of blood.)

Determining whether the function of the Heart governing blood and vessels is normal or not can be determined by the chest (Heart beat), the complexion, tongue body and pulse manifestation etc. The action of the Heart governing blood and vessels is normal, and then the Heart beats normally, the complexion is reddish and lustrous, the tongue body is reddish and moistened, and the pulse manifestation is moderate and forceful. If the action of the Heart governing blood and vessels is abnormal, if the Heart qi is insufficient and the Heart blood is deficient, symptoms of palpitation, pale complexion, a pale tongue body, and a small and weak pulse will occur. If the Heart blood is stagnated and the vessel passages are not free, symptoms of Heart pain, dark complexion, cyanotic lips and tongue body, and uneven pulse occur. (Table 2-1)

Plain Questions: *Chapter Discussion on Flaccidity* (Sù Wèn: Wěi Lùn, 素问·痿论) says: "*The Heart dominates the blood and vessels of the body.*"

Plain Questions: *Discussion on Six-Plus-Six System and the Manifestations of the Viscera* (Sù Wèn: Liù Jié Zàng Xiàng Lùn, 素问·六节藏象论) says: The function of the Heart "*is to fill the vessels*".

Plain Questions: *Chapter Discussion on Various Relationships Concerning the Five Zang-Organs* (Sù Wèn: Wǔ Zàng Shēng Chéng Piān, 素问·五脏生成篇) says: "*All the diseases of blood belong to the Heart.*"

Plain Questions: *Chapter Discussion on the Essentials of Pulse* (Sù Wèn: Mài Yào Jīng Wēi Lùn, 素问·脉要精微论) says: "*Vessels are the house of blood."*

Essay of Reading Medical Works: Chapter Patient becomes Conscious after Maculation of Warm-Heat Disease (Dú Yī Suí Bǐ: Wēn Rè Fā Bān Qí Rén Fǎn Qīng, 读医随笔·温热发斑其人反清) says: "All the blood in the vessels of the whole body originates from the Heart, returns to the Heart and cycles endlessly."

Miraculous Pivot: Chapter On Channels (Líng Shū: Jīng Mài, 灵枢·经脉) says: "If the qi of the hand shaoyin channel is exhausted, the vessels will be obstructed, and the blood will not circulate, and the hair will not be lustrous, therefore the complexion will be dark as black lacquer and firewood, and the blood has already stagnated."

(2) The Heart stores the spirit

The Heart stores the spirit, which can be also described by saying the Heart governs mental activity, or the Heart dominates the spirit and mind. The Heart dominates the life activity of the whole body and the functions of spirit, consciousness and thinking of humans.

The spirit of the human body has both broad and narrow meanings. In the broad sense, spirit refers to the external manifestation of the life activities of the whole body; in the narrow sense, spirit refers to the spirit, consciousness, and thinking of humans. Spirit being stored by Heart includes in the broad sense the spirit that dominates life activities of the human body, and in the narrow sense the spirit that dominates spirit, consciousness, and thinking.

The physiological action of the Heart storing the spirit, first means that it governs mental activity, and normalizes the consciousness, thinking and emotion. Secondly, it means to dominate and harmonize the life activity of the whole body, keep the functions of the zang-fu organs normalized, as well as those of the body constituents, sense organs and orifices, promote the mutual coordination and balance of various organs, and keep a healthy state for the whole body. Thus the Heart is named "the great master of the five zang organs and six fu organs".

The mental activity of humans is a physiological function of the brain, namely the reflection in the brain of external objects and information. In Chinese medicine, mental activities are distributed to the five zang organs and mainly belong to the function of the Heart storing the spirit. Thus the function of the Heart storing the spirit, mean, to some extent, that the Heart is taken as the brain.

The normal function of the Heart storing the spirit, on one hand, find its expression in normal spirit, consciousness and thinking of humans, in terms of inspired spirit, clear consciousness, prompt thinking and rapid response etc. On the other hand it dominates the physiological activities of zang-fu organs, body constituents, and sense organs and orifices and balances the physiological activity of the whole body in every aspect. Therefore, abnormal functions of the Heart storing spirit not only manifest as disorders of the spirit, emotions, consciousness, and thinking in terms of insomnia, too many dreams, delirium, insanity, lags in response time, and even a state of coma or unconsciousness etc., but also affect the function and activities of the zang-fu organs, body constituents, sense organs and orifices. (Table 2-1)

Plain Questions: Chapter Discussion on the Elucidation of Five-Qi (Sù Wèn: Xuān Míng Wǔ Qì Piān, 素问·宣明五气篇) says: "The Heart stores the spirit."

Plain Questions: Chapter Discussion on the Secret Classics Stored in Royal Library (Sù Wèn: Líng Lán Mì Diǎn Lùn, 素问·灵兰秘典论) says: "The Heart is like a monarch who controls the mental activity. Thus, if the monarch is bright, the officials will be calm. If the monarch is not bright, the twelve officers will be endangered."

Miraculous Pivot: Chapter Retention of the Evil Qi (Líng Shū: Xié Kè, 灵枢·邪客) says: "The Heart is the great master of the five zang organs and six fu organs; it is the place where the spirit resides; as it is firm, the exogenous pathogens can hardly intrude into it; if the exogenous pathogens penetrate, the Heart will be impaired, and then the spirit will be gone and the patient will die eventually."

Miraculous Pivot: Chapter The Diseases Caused by Spiritual Activities (Líng Shū: Běn Shén, 灵枢·本神) says: "The place to conceive things is named the Heart."

Correction of Errors in Medical Classics: Chapter Brain Marrow (Yī Líng Gǎi Cuò: Nǎo Suí Shuō, 医林改错·脑髓说) says: *"The intelligence and memory are not the function of the Heart but the brain."*

Elementary Medicine: Chapter Zang-fu Organs (Yī Xué Rù Mén: Zàng Fǔ, 医学入门·脏腑) says: *"The Heart is the dominator of the whole body and the monarch organ. The Heart of flesh and blood is lotus bud in its shape, and located below the Lung and above the Liver. There is spirit of Heart that is transformed by qi and blood and is the root of life. All things in the world grow by the function of spirit vigorously. It is not visible. If it exists, where is it? If it does not exist, there it is. It dominates everything in the world, that's because the empty spirit can't be clouded…However, the body constituents and the spirit are constantly interacting."*

Grand Materia Medica: Section Flos Magnoliae (Běn Cǎo Gāng Mù: Xīn Yí, 本草纲目·辛夷) says: *"The brain is the house of genuine spirit."*

Classified Classic: Chapter Class of Visceral Manifestations (Lèi Jīng: Zàng Xiàng Lèi, 类经·藏象类) says: *"The Heart is the monarch of the whole body, it functions with invisible spirit and possesses one truth in response to a myriad of things. The zang-fu organs and all the body constituents obey its commands. May cleverness and wisdom not be produced by it, so it is said that the Heart is where the mental activity out."*

② Relation of Heart to Body Constituents, Sense Organs and Orifices

Body constituents, sense organs and orifices primarily refer to the five body constituents, five sense organs and nine orifices. The five body constituents refer to vessels, sinew, meat, skin, and bone: five kinds of tissues. The five sense organs refer to the eyes, tongue, mouth, nose and ears: five kinds of organs. The five sense organs in the head have seven orifices, plus two lower orifices before and after, together making nine orifices. The structure and functions of different body constituents, sense organs and orifices vary. Yet, they have an indivisible relationship with the five *zang* organs. They are "what the five viscera control ", since the "five *zang* organs open at the orifices respectively."

(1) Heart dominates vessels

Vessels refers to blood vessels, are the house of blood and the passage where blood circulates, and they control the blood flow inside them.

The Heart dominates vessels. Structurally, the Heart connects with blood vessels; functionally, the Heart causes the blood to circulate inside the blood vessels, which indicates that the Heart and the vessels behave coherently. Namely, the impulse of Heart qi and the control of blood vessels guarantee the free circulation of the blood. Thereby, the illnesses of the Heart can be examined by pulse manifestations.

Plain Questions: Chapter Discussion on the Elucidation of Five-Qi (Sù Wèn: Xuān Míng Wǔ Qì Piān, 素问·宣明五气篇) says: *"Regarding the tissues that the five zang organs dominate, the Heart dominates the vessels."*

Plain Questions: Chapter Discussion on the Essentials of Pulse (Sù Wèn: Mài Yào Jīng Wēi Lùn, 素问·脉要精微论) says: *"Vessels are the house of blood."*

Miraculous Pivot: Chapter The Dredge of Qi (Líng Shū: Jué Qì, 灵枢·决气) says: *"The tissue converging and controlling the nutritive qi that can't escape is called the vessels."*

(2) The quintessence of the Heart appears on the face (Table 2-2)

This quintessence manifests in this case as a lustrous complexion. The five *zang* organs reside deep in the body, and their normal color (luster) manifests in different regions of the body surface. The color change of these regions reflects the wax and wane of the qi and blood of the five *zang* organs.

The quintessence of the Heart appears on the face, which indicates whether the action of the Heart governing blood and vessels is normal or not, and can be reflected by the color of the complexion. The face is rich in blood vessel networks, so the wax and wane of Heart qi and blood can be reflected by the color of the complexion. If Heart qi is abundant and blood vessels filled, facial complexion is be ruddy and lustrous. If the Heart qi and Heart blood are insufficient, one would have a pale and lusterless complexion; if the Heart vessels are obstructed

Table 2-2   The relation between the Heart and face

Foundation of the relationship	The Heart governs blood and vessels. The face is rich in blood vessel networks.
Physiological significance	If Heart qi is abundant and blood vessels filled, the facial complexion will be ruddy and lustrous.
Pathological significance	Insufficiency of Heart qi and blood: pale and lusterless complexion. Stagnation and blockage of Heart blood: greenish purple complexion

due to blood stasis, one would have a greenish purple complexion; if Heart fire is exuberant, one would have a red complexion; and if Heart yang suddenly collapsed, one would have a pale and dark complexion.

Plain Questions: Discussion on Six-Plus-Six System and the Manifestations of the Viscera (Sù Wèn: Liù Jié Zàng Xiàng Lùn, 素问·六节藏象论) says : *"Heart...its quintessence appears on the face."*

(3) *The Heart opens at the tongue (Table 2-3)*

The tongue is a gustatory organ, dominating taste; the movement of the tongue body can assist

Table 2-3   Relationship between Heart and tongue

Foundation of the relationship	The Heart governs the blood. The Heart stores the spirit.
Physiological significance	Therefore a ruddy tongue body, sensitive taste, prompt movement of the tongue body and fluent speech can indicate sufficient Heart blood and normal Heart spirit.
Pathological significance	Heart blood insufficiency: light pale tongue body, lack of taste; Stagnation of Heart blood: dark purple tongue body or petechia; Flaring-up of Heart-fire: a deep red tongue with ulceration; Abnormal Heart spirit: curled-up tongue, stiff tongue, retarded speech, or aphasia.

speech and is related to pronunciation.

For the relationship between the tongue and the Heart: structurally divergent collaterals of the Heart channel connect with the tongue. The physiological functions of the Heart governing blood circulation and housing the spirit are closely associated with the glossal color and luster, taste, the movement of the tongue body and speech. Therefore, ruddy tongue bodies, sensitive taste, prompt movement of the tongue body and fluent speech could indicate sufficient Heart blood and normal Heart spirit.

The pathological changes of the Heart can be reflected by the tongue manifestations. For instance: Heart blood insufficiency manifests as light pale tongue body and lack of taste in the mouth; stagnation of Heart blood manifests as a dark purple tongue body or petechia; flaring-up of Heart-fire manifests as a deep red tongue with ulcerations; abnormal Heart spirit manifests as a curled-up tongue, stiff tongue, retarded speech, or aphasia.

Plain Questions: Chapter Major Discussion on

the Theory of Yin and Yang and the Corresponding Relationships Among All the Things in Nature (Sù Wèn: Yīn Yáng Yìng Xiàng Dà Lùn, 素问·阴阳应象大论) says: *"The Heart opens at the tongue."*

Miraculous Pivot: Chapter Determining the Conditions of the Five Viscera by Examining the Five Sense Organs (Líng Shū: Wǔ Yuè Wǔ Shǐ, 灵枢·五阅五使) says: *"The tongue belongs to the Heart."*

Miraculous Pivot: Chapter On Channels (Líng Shū: Jīng Mài, 灵枢·经脉) says: *"The divergent collateral of the hand shaoyin channel...enters the Heart along with the channel and connects with the root of the tongue."*

Miraculous Pivot: Chapter The Length of Channels (Líng Shū: Mài Dù, 灵枢·脉度) says : *"The Heart qi connects with the tongue, so if the Heart is harmonious, the tongue can taste the five flavors."*

Miraculous Pivot: Chapter Dysphonia due to Melancholy and Resentment (Líng Shū: Yōu Guī Wú Yán, 灵枢·忧恚无言) says: *"The tongue is the pivot of tone and pronunciation."*

Treatment of Different Kinds of Diseases: Chapter Summarization of Internal Images (Lèi Zhèng Zhì

Cái: Nèi Jīng Zōng Yào, 类证治裁·内景综要) says: *"The tongue is the seedling of the Heart."*

③ Relationship of the Heart to the Five Minds and Five Fluids

"Five minds" refers to the five kinds of moods and states of mind in terms of happiness, anger, thought, sorrow and fear. The five minds belong to the five *zang* organs respectively. The mind of the Heart is happiness, the mind of the Liver is anger, the mind of the Spleen is thought, the mind of the Lung is sorrow, and the mind of the Kidney is fear.

The five fluids refer to five kinds of secretions: sweating, nasal discharge, tears, saliva and spit. The five kinds of secretions belong to the five internal organs, namely the fluid of the Heart is sweating, the fluid of the Lung is nasal discharge, the fluid of the Liver is tears, the fluid of the Spleen is saliva, and the fluid of the Kidney is spit. It is called "five secretions derived from the five *zang* organs" in *Internal Classic* (*Nèi Jīng*)

(1) The mind of the Heart is happiness

Happiness means joy and gladness. It is a happy mood and a benign response to external stimulation.

The mind of the Heart is happiness, which indicates the physiological function of the Heart

is related to happiness. Moderate happiness, a joyful spirit, and harmonious qi and blood are beneficial to the physiological functions of the Heart. Too much joy or happiness can impair the Heart and result in the pathological changes of mental and emotional disorders (See the section of seven emotions).

Plain Questions: *Chapter Major Discussion on the Theory of Yin and Yang and the Corresponding Relationships Among All the Things in Nature* (*Sù Wèn: Yīn Yáng Yìng Xiàng Dà Lùn*, 素问·阴阳应象大论) says: *"The mind of the Heart is happiness."*

(2) The body fluid of the Heart is sweat

Sweat is the liquid excreted from the pores after the transpiration and vaporization of the body fluid by yang qi.

"Sweat is the fluid of the Heart" means that the function of the Heart governing the blood is associated with the generation and excretion of sweat. Sweat is transformed from the body fluid that is the constituent of blood, and body fluid and blood are transformed by the same source, so as the sayings go "Fluid and blood share the same source", and "Blood and sweat share the same source." Actually, it is the Heart governing the blood that connects the complex relationship among blood, body fluid and sweat. (Fig. 2-4)

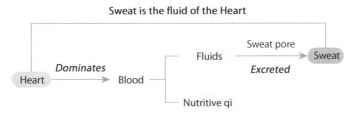

Fig. 2-4   Relationship between Heart and sweat

Therefore, the pathological changes of the Heart, blood and fluid would affect the generation and excretion of sweat. Insufficiency of the Heart blood and body fluid results in insufficiency of the sweat source, so it is not suitable to treat it with the method of diaphoresis. Superabundant sweating impairs body fluids and blood and injures the yang qi of the Heart, which manifests as palpitations; profuse sweating may result in

sudden collapse of Heart yang and the syndrome of yang exhaustion.

Plain Questions: *Chapter Discussion on the Elucidation of Five-Qi* (*Sù Wèn: Xuān Míng Wǔ Qì Piān*, 素问·宣明五气篇) says: *"Among the five secretions derived from the five zang organs, the one of the Heart is sweat."*

Plain Questions: *Chapter Separate Discussion On Yin and Yang* (*Sù Wèn: Yīn Yáng Bié Lùn*, 素

问·阴阳别论) says: "*If the yang pulse dominates over the yin pulse, sweating will be induced.*"

Required Readings for Medical Professionals: Section Sweat in (*Yī Zōng Bì Dú: Hàn*, 医宗必读·汗) says: "*What the Heart store inside is blood and what is dispersed outside is sweat, and sweat is the fluid of the Heart.*"

④ The Physiological Properties of the Heart

(1) The Heart is a yang organ and dominates yang qi

The Heart is located in the chest, belongs to fire, is the greater yang within yang, so it is a yang organ and dominates yang qi. Warmed and controllwed by the yang qi of the Heart, blood vessels are dredged by warmth, the spirit is inspired, the vital force cycles endlessly.

(2) The Heart communicates with and responds to the summer qi

According to the concept that the heavens and humankind are mutually responsive, the visceral functions and the activities of the human body communicate with and respond to the wax and wane of the yin and yang of the four seasons in the natural world. Heart qi communicates with summer qi, which means that the yang qi of the Heart is the most vigorous in summer with the strongest vital force. Summerheat qi is in season in summer. Thereby, it is important to prevent the summerheat pathogen from impairing the Heart in summer.

Plain Questions: Discussion on Six-Plus-Six System and the Manifestations of the Viscera (Sù Wèn: Liù Jié Zàng Xiàng Lùn, 素问·六节藏象论) says: "*The Heart is the greater yang within yang and communicates with the summer qi.*"

Appendix: Pericardium

The Pericardium (心包), also known as "*Dan Zhong, 膻中*", is the membrane which stores and protects the Heart.

The theory of visceral manifestations thinks that the Heart is the monarch organ and can't be affected by pathogens. Thus, when exogenous pathogens invade the Heart, they invade the Pericardium first; therefore the Pericardium has the action of "suffering pathogens instead of the Heart". Clinical manifestations of pathogesn invading the Pericardium primarily manifest as the dysfunction of the Heart in storing the spirit. For instances, syndromes of exogenous febrile diseases with high fever and abnormal mental activities like delirium and coma are called syndromes of "attack of the Pericardium by heat". The syndromes with pathological changes of unbalanced Heart spirit like vague consciousness and mental disorders are distinguished as syndrome of "phlegm turbidity covering the Pericardium". Actually, the pathological changes of the Pericardium being affected by pathogens manifest consistently as that of the dysfunction of the Heart storing the spirit. Thus, they are nearly the same in syndrome differentiation and treatment.

Miraculous Pivot: Chapter Retention of the Evil Qi (Líng Shū: Xié Kè, 灵枢·邪客) says: "*The Heart is the great master of the five zang organs and six fu organs and where the siprit resides, the organ is substantial. The exogenous pathogens can hardly intrude into it; if the exogenous pathogens penetrate, the Heart will be impaired, and then the spirit will be gone and the patient will die. Therefore, all the pathogens which attack the Heart would confront the resistance of Pericardium first.*"

The Lung

The lungs (肺) are located in the thoracic cavity, one lobe on the left and one on the right. They connect upward with the tracheae, larynx and nose, so the larynx is known as the door of the Lung and the nose as the exterior orifice of the lungs. The position of the Lung is the highest among the five *zang* organs and six *fu* organs and overlay the other organs, so it is called the "canopy".

The physiological functions of the lungs are dominating qi and respiration, promoting water metabolism, assembling hundreds of vessels, and dominating management and regulation.

The basic movements of the Lung qi (also known as the movement features of the Lung qi) manifest as diffusing, purifying and descending. The Lung functions of diffusing, purifying and descending run through every aspect of the physiological functions of the Lung. Thus, the movement of diffusion, purification or descending of the Lung qi accomplishes all the physiological functions of the Lung.

The Lung connects with the Large Intestine among *fu* organs, dominates the skin among the body constituents, its quintessence appears on the fine hair, it opens at the nose, its emotion is sorrow and its fluid is nasal discharge.

① The Physiological Functions of the Lung (Table 2-4)

(1) The Lung dominates respiration and qi

The Lung dominates qi means that the Lung governs the qi of the whole body, which include two aspects: dominating the qi of respiration and dominating the qi of the whole body.

a. **Dominating the qi of respiration:** the function of the Lung governing the qi of respiration is completed by the function of the Lung dominating breathing. The Lung is the place where the air exchanges between inside and outside the body: the clear qi of the natural environment is breathed in by the action of respiration of the Lung, and the turbid qi inside the body is expired, and then the exchange of the air inside and outside the body is completed. Therefore, it is said that the Lung governs the qi of respiration.

The Lung dominates the qi of respiration. It depends on the actions of diffusing, purification and descending of the Lung qi. The diffusion of the Lung qi is normal, and then the turbid qi can be exhaled. The purification and descent of the Lung qi are normal, and then the clear qi can be inhaled. Therefore, the respiratory movements can be normal. Failure of the Lung qi to diffuse and descend will affect the function of respiration, which results in respiratory movement disorders and pathological changes such as cough, dyspnea, an oppressed feeling in the chest and unsmooth breathing. (Table 2-4)

b. **Dominating the qi of the whole body:** the Lung dominating the qi of the whole body means that the qi of the whole body belongs to and is dominated by the Lung. It is mainly embodied in two aspects: the first aspect is the generation of pectorial qi. The clear qi in the natural environment inhaled by the Lung combines with the essence qi of water and food absorbed by the Spleen in the chest, which generates the gathering qi. The gathering qi is an important constituent of the qi of the whole body, and the generation of the gathering qi associates with the wax and wane of the qi of the whole body. The second aspect is the regulation of the qi dynamic of the whole body. The Lung governs breathing, diffusing, purifying and descending, and dominates the qi of the *zang-fu* organs, channels and collaterals of the whole body. It moves rhythmically in conjunction with the exhalation and inhalation of the Lung and keeps the qi dynamic free.

Therefore, dysfunction of the Lung in governing respiration, diffusing, purifying and descending, on the one hand, results in insufficient generation of qi manifesting as fatigue, lack of breath, lack of willingness to speak, low voice, fright due to deficiency of qi, feeble breathing, and dyspnea; on the other hand it influences the qi motion of the whole body, results in the abnormal qi circulation of the *zang-fu* organs, channels and collaterals, and brings about pathological changes of imbalanced qi dynamic. (Table 2-4)

Thus it can be known that the function of the Lung governing qi is determined by the function of the Lung dominating respiration. Through its respiratory function, the Lung acts to inhale clear qi, exhale turbid qi and govern the qi of respiration. Also through its respiratory function, the Lung inhales clear qi and generates gathering qi. The actions of expiration, inspiration, diffusion and descendence of the Lung regulate the qi dynamic and dominate the qi of the whole body. Thus, the function of the Lung governing qi is based on the function of respiration of the Lung. (Fig. 2-5)

Plain Questions: Chapter Major Discussion on the Theory of Yin and Yang and the Corresponding Relationships Among All the Things in Nature (Sù Wèn: Yīn Yáng Yìng Xiàng Dà Lùn, 素问·阴阳应象大论) says: *"The heaven qi communicates with the Lung."*

Plain Questions: Chapter Discussion on Various

Table 2-4 Table of the physiological functions of the Lung

Function	Meaning	Physiological action	Main pathological changes
The Lung governs qi and dominates breathing.	The Lung governs the qi of the body. By governing respiration, the Lung dominates the qi of respiration and the qi of the whole body.	The Lung dominates the qi of respiration: the Lung governs respiration, inhales clear qi, exhales turbid qi, and completes the air exchange inside and outside of the body. The Lung dominates the qi of the whole body: first, the Lung generates gathering qi by inhaling clear qi, which combines with the essence qi of water and food; second, the Lung regulates the qi dynamic of the whole body by the actions of expiration, inspiration, diffusing and descending.	The Lung fails to diffuse or descend and causes breathing disorders: cough, asthma, an oppressed feeling in the chest, or difficulty in breathing. Generation of gathering qi is insufficient: fatigue, dyspnea, lack of desire to talk, feeble breathing and voice, fright.
The Lung governs the regulating of water passage.	The diffusing, purifying and descending actions of the Lung qi distribute and excrete the water and fluids in the body.	Diffusing action of the Lung qi: to distribute water fluid upward and outward to moisten the body surface, skin and fine hair; the metabolic turbid fluid is excreted through the respiratory tract and sweat pores. The purifying and descending action of the Lung qi: to distribute the water fluid downward and inward, to moisten the *zang-fu* organs and tissues; through the action of the Kidney, the metabolic turbid fluid transforms into urine and is excreted out of the body.	Failure of the Lung in diffusing and descending, water passage obstruction and disharmony, disorders of distribution and excretion of water and fluids: anidrosis, oliguria, edema or retention of phlegm and fluid.
The Lung assembles all the vessels.	Convergence of all the vessels in the Lung refers to the function of the Lung in which all the blood of the body moves through the channels and vessels and gets oxygen in the lungs by its action of respiration, and then the blood istransported to the whole body through the channels and vessels.	The Heart governs blood circulation, the Lung governs qi, blood circulates with qi circulation. The Lung assembles all the vessels to assist the Heart in promoting blood circulation.	Insufficiency of Lung qi, obstruction of blood circulation: cough, asthma, oppressed feeling in chest, palpitations and cyanotic lips and tongue.
The Lung dominates administration and regulation	The administrative and regulatory actions of the Lung assist the Heart.	The action of the Lung governing administration and regulation is embodied as follows: first it is to manage and regulate respiratory qi; second is to manage and regulate the qi dynamic of the *zang-fu* organs of the body; third is to manage and regulate blood circulation; last is to manage and regulate water passage.	

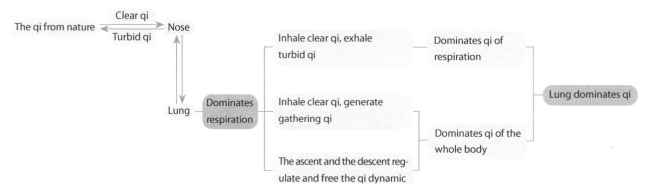

Fig. 2-5 Relationships between the Lung governing respiration and the Lung dominating qi

Relationships Concerning the Five Zang-Organs (Sù Wèn: Wǔ Zàng Shēng Chéng Piān, 素问·五脏生成篇) says: "All the qi belong to the Lung."

Plain Questions: Discussion on Six-Plus-Six System and the Manifestations of the Viscera (Sù Wèn: Liù Jié Zàng Xiàng Lùn, 素问·六节藏象论) says: "The Lung is the root of qi."

Book Compilation (Tú Shū Biān, 图书编) says: "The Lung is located above the other viscera and the qi of the other viscera are exhaled and inhaled by it."

Required Readings for Medical Professionals: Chapter Illustration and Explanation of Medical Discussions (Yī Zōng Bì Dú: Yī Lùn Tú Shuō, 医宗必读·医论图说) says: "The Lung lobes are white and jade-like and are called a canopy, which is used to cover other viscera. It is delicate like honeycomb, there are no opening orifices below, and so it is filled by inspiration and emptied by expiration. It breathes naturally when expiring and inspiring, dominates the transportation and transformation of the clear and the turbid, and is the bag and the flute of the body."

Easy Access to Medicine (Yī Xué Shí Zài Yì, 医学实在易) says: "Qi communicates with the Lung, all the qi of the zang-fu organs, channels and collaterals are diffused by the Lung qi."

Principle and Prohibition for the Medical Profession: Section The Lung Abscess and The Lung Wilt (Yī Mén Fǎ Lù: Fèi Yōng Fèi Wěi Mén, 医门法律·肺痈肺痿门) says: "The qi of the whole body obeys the commands of the Lung. If the Lung qi is clear and purified, the qi of the whole body will be obedient and circulate freely. If the Lung qi is obstructed and turbid, the qi of the whole body will easily and transversely invade the upper Jiao."

(2) The Lung governs regulating the water passage

The Lung governing the regulating of water passage as well as transportation means that the diffusing, purifying and descending functions of the Lung qi act on the distribution and drainage of body fluid inside the body. It is said that the Lung governs "clearing and regulating water passages" in the *Internal Classic (Nèi Jīng)*.

The function of the Lung governing the regulating of water passage is completed by the actions of the Lung qi to diffuse, purify and descend. On one hand, water moistens the tissues and organs through the diffusing function of the Lung which transports the water upward and outward to reach the orifices in the head and out through the skin and pores of the whole body. The metabolic turbid fluids are excreted via the respiratory tract or the pores on the skin in the form of sweat, which acts to regulate water metabolism. On the other hand, water moistens the tissues and *zang-fu* organs by the function of the purifying and descending function of the Lung which transports water inward and downward. Through the function of the Kidney governing water, the metabolic turbid fluid is transformed into urine, transported downward into the Bladder, and urinated outside the body, which keeps the metabolic balance of water and fluids. (Fig. 2-6)

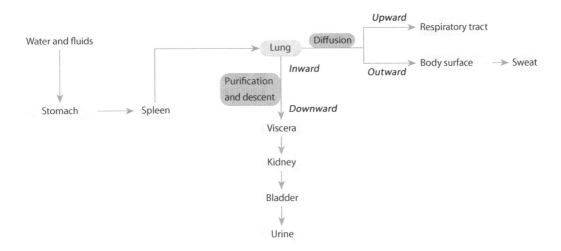

Fig. 2-6 Function of the Lung governing water circulation

If the Lung fails to diffuse and descend, water passage will not be free and harmonious, which will result in a disorder of the distribution and excretion of water and fluids, manifesting as pathological changes such as anhidrosis, oliguria, edema or retention of phlegm and fluid. (Table 2-4)

The Lung resides in the chest and possesses the highest position among the five *zang* organs and six *fu* organs. It has the function of purifying and descending water and fluids, so it is named as "the upper source of water".

Plain Questions: *Chapter Special Discussion on Channels and Vessels* (*Sù Wèn: Jīng Mài Bié Lùn Piān*, 素问·经脉别论篇) says: "*When water enters the Stomach, the Stomach evaporates the refined energy and spreads it upward to the Spleen; the Spleen spreads the essence upward into the Lung; the Lung qi communicates with water passage, and transports the essence to the Bladder. Therefore, water and essence are distributed to all the parts of the body and circulates in the five channels of the five zang organs.*"

(3) All the vessels converge in the Lung

Convergence of all the vessels in the Lung refers to the function of the Lung by which all the blood of the body moves through the channels and vessels and passes through the lungs, where it gathers oxygen through respiration and the air exchange in the Lung. After this, the blood is transported to the whole body through the channels and vessels.

The function of the Lung converging all the vessels indicates that blood circulation is a concurrent action of the Lung and the Heart. The Heart governs the blood, and the Heart qi is the fundamental impetus of the blood to circulate inside the vessels: the Lung dominates qi, and blood circulation also needs the assistance of the Lung qi, which means that blood circulates along with qi circulation. Thus, the convergence of all the vessels in the Lung refers to the action of the Lung in assisting the Heart to promote blood circulation.

Thereby, if insufficiency of the Lung qi results in a lack of ability to assist the Heart in promoting blood circulation, it results in disorders of blood circulation, which manifest as cough, asthma, an oppressed feeling in the chest, palpitations, and cyanotic lips and tongue. (Table 2-4)

Plain Questions: *Chapter Special Discussion on Channels and Vessels* (*Sù Wèn: Jīng Mài Bié Lùn Piān*, 素问·经脉别论篇) says: "*When food enters the Stomach, after being digested, the turbid qi enters the Spleen; the essence qi is soaked into the channels and blood. The vessel qi circulates and flows in the channels, and the channel qi pertains to the Lung. The Lung is the convergence of all the vessels, and the essence qi is transported to skin and hair.*"

(4) The Lung governs administration and regulation

The Lung governs administration and regulation refers to the administrative and regulatory effects of the Lung in assisting the Heart.

The action of the Lung governing administration and regulation is embodied as follows: first it manages and regulates respiratory qi; second it manages and regulates the qi dynamic of the *zang-fu* organs of the body; third it manages and regulates blood circulation; finally, it manages and regulates fluid metabolism. (Table 2-4)

Thus it can be seen that the Lung dominating administration and regulation is a generalization of the main physiological functions of the Lung, and emphasizes the importance of the functions of the Lung governing qi and respiration. The function of dominating qi and respiration of the Lung are closely related to the respiratory movement, generation of qi, regulation of qi dynamic, circulation of Heart blood, and the metabolism of body fluid. The theory of visceral manifestations emphasizes the dominance of the Heart for the whole body, while also stating that the Lung assists the Heart to manage and regulate.

Plain Questions: *Chapter Discussion on the Secret Classics Stored in Royal Library* (*Sù Wèn: Líng Lán Mì Diǎn Lùn*, 素问·灵兰秘典论) says: "*The Lung is the organ similar to the prime minister who is responsible for administration and regulation.*"

② The Relation of the Lung to the Body Constituents, Sense Organs and Orifices

(1) The Lung dominates the skin; its quintessence appears on the fine hair (Table 2-5)

Skin and hair include the tissues in terms of skin,

Table 2-5 Table of the relation of the Lung to the skin and body hairs

Foundation for relationship	The Lung qi diffuses and transports essence qi to the skin and body hairs.	The opening and closing of the sweat pores and the excretion of sweat influence the Lung.
Physiological significance	If the function of the Lung is normal, the skin and sweat pores will be tight and the fine hairs will be lustrous, the opening and closing of the sweat pores will be normal, and they will be powerful in resisting exogenous pathogens.	When the sweat pores open, close and excrete sweat normally, it will be helpful to the respiration of the Lung.
Pathological significance	Insufficiency of Lung qi: withered and yellow skin and fine hairs, failure of the sweat pores to open and close, debility of the defensive exterior which fails in repelling exogenous pathogens, being easy to suffer spontaneous sweating and susceptible to cold.	Exogenous pathogens visit the exterior of the body and are easy to be transmitted internally to the Lung: aversion to cold, fever, anhidrosis, cough, asthma.

sweat gland and body hair. Skin and hair form the exterior of the whole body and defend against exogenous pathogens, excrete sweat, regulate temperature and assist in respiration.

The Lung dominates the skin, which indicates the close relation of the Lung with skin and hair. There are two chief aspects.

One is the action of the Lung on skin and hair. The diffusing function of the Lung qi transports the essence, qi (defensive qi), blood and fluids to the skin and fine hairs, and the skin and fine hairs are warmed, nourished and moistened. If the Lung qi is sufficient, the exterior of the body (skin and pores) are tight, fine hairs are lustrous, sweat pores open and close normally, and therefore, the exterior of the body can exert its action of defending the body and repelling exogenous pathogens. Contrarily, deficiency of Lung qi results in the dysfunction of the Lung in distributing the essence qi to the skin and body hair, and then the body hair wilts and becomes lusterless. It results in the infirmness of the defensive exterior that fails to resist exogenous pathogens and manifests as spontaneous sweating and susceptibility to cold.

The luster and wilt of the body hair is intimately related to the Lung, so it is known that the Lung's "quintessence appears on the body hair".

Second is the action of the Lung on the skin and fine hairs. The opening and closing of skin pores and body hairs not only control and excrete sweat, but also process the air exchange inside and outside the body along with the diffusing and descending function of the Lung qi and assist the respiratory function of the Lung. Sweat pores are named "the door of qi" in *Internal Classic* (*Nèi Jīng*). Therefore, if the body surface is invaded by exogenous pathogens, the pathogens will attack the Lung internally via the skin and sweat pores, manifesting as aversion to cold, fever, anhidrosis, a stuffy nose, cough, and asthma. (Table 2-5)

Plain Questions: *Chapter Discussion on the Elucidation of Five-Qi* (*Sù Wèn: Xuān Míng Wǔ Qì Piān*, 素问·宣明五气篇) says: "*Among the five dominances... The Lung dominates skin.*"

Plain Questions: *Chapter Discussion on Various Relationships Concerning the Five Zang-Organs* (*Sù Wèn: Wǔ Zàng Shēng Chéng Piān*, 素问·五脏生成篇) says: " *The Lung coordinates with the skin and its splendor is reflected on the fine hairs.*"

Plain Questions: *Discussion on Six-Plus-Six System and the Manifestations of the Viscera* (*Sù Wèn: Liù Jié Zàng Xiàng Lùn*, 素问·六节藏象论) says: "*Lung... its quintessence appears on the fine hairs.*"

Plain Questions: *Chapter Special Discussion on Channels and Vessels* (*Sù Wèn: Jīng Mài Bié Lùn Piān*, 素问·经脉别论) says: "*The Lung assembles all the vessels and distributes the essence qi to the skin and fine hairs.*"

Classic of Questioning: *The Twenty-fourth Question* (*Nàn Jīng: Èr Shí Sì Nàn*, 难经·二十四难) says: "*Taiyin refers to the Lung which circulates qi and warms the skin and fine hairs.*"

Miraculous Pivot: Chapter On Channels (Líng Shū: Jīng Mài, 灵枢·经脉) says: "*If the qi of the hand taiyin channel is exhausted, the skin and the fine hairs will wilt.*"

(2) The Lung opens at the nose

The nose is the passageway where the qi of respiration goes in and out, is the door of breathing and is also a sense organ. Therefore, the nose has the actions of aeration and olfaction.

Relationship between the Lung and the nose: Structurally, the Lung connects with the nose via the tracheae and throat, and the nose is the upper orifice of the respiratory tract. Physiologically, the function of the Lung dominating qi and governing breathing closely relates to the aeration and olfaction capabilities of the nose. Therefore, if the Lung qi is sufficient and respiratory function is normal then the nose will be free and have sensitive olfaction. If the Lung is sick, the nose will be symptomatic of the Lung problem. For example, failure of the Lung in diffusing manifests as a stuffy and running nose and poor sense of smell; Lung heat manifests as yellow nasal discharge, poor sense of smell, or flaring of the nares; Lung dryness manifests as dry nasal cavities, etc. (Table 2-6)

Table 2-6   Table of relationship between the Lung and the nose

Foundation of relationship	The Lung dominates qi and governs breathing.
Physiological significance	If the Lung qi is sufficient and the respiratory function is normal then the nasal cavity will be free from obstruction and have sensitive olfaction.
Pathological significance	Failure of the Lung in diffusing: stuffy and running nose, inefficacious smelling. Lung-heat: yellow nasal discharge, lack of sense of smell or flaring of the nares; Lung dryness: dry nasal cavities etc.

Plain Questions: Chapter Discussion on Important Ideas in the Golden Chamber (Sù Wèn: Jīn Guì Zhēn Yán Lùn, 素问·金匮真言论) says: "*The Lung opens at the nose.*"

Miraculous Pivot: Chapter Determining the Conditions of the Five Viscera by Examining the Five Sense Organs (Líng Shū: Wǔ Yuè Wǔ Shǐ, 灵枢·五阅五使) says: "*The nose is the officer of the Lung.*"

Miraculous Pivot: Chapter The Treating Therapy from Oral Inquiry (Líng Shū: Kǒu Wèn, 灵枢·口问) says: "*The mouth and nose are the doors of qi.*"

Miraculous Pivot: Chapter The Length of Channels (Líng Shū: Mài Dù, 灵枢·脉度) says: "*If the Lung qi communicates with the nose, the Lung and the nose can distinguish different odors.*"

③ Relation of the Lung to the Five Minds and Five Fluids

(1) The mind of the Lung is sorrow

Sorrow refers to grief and anxiety. Saying that the mind of the Lung is sorrow means that emotional activities like sorrow and grief are closely related to the Lung. The Lung dominates qi, so excessive grief can impair the Lung and result in the pathological changes of Lung qi stagnation and depression. (See the section on the seven emotions)

Plain Questions: Chapter Major Discussion on the Theory of Yin and Yang and the Corresponding Relationships Among All the Things in Nature (Sù Wèn: Yīn Yáng Yìng Xiàng Dà Lùn, 素问·阴阳应象大论) says: "*The Lung… its mind is sorrow.*"

(2) The fluid of the Lung is nasal discharge

Nasal discharge is the mucus secreted by the nasal cavity and has the action of moistening the nasal cavity.

Saying that the fluid of the Lung is nasal discharge means that the generation and pathological changes of nasal discharge have a close relationship with the Lung. The nose is the orifice of the Lung, and nasal discharge is secreted by the nasal cavity, therefore, it is said that "nasal discharge is the fluid of the Lung" (Fig. 2-7). For normal Lung function with qi and yin sufficiency, the secretion of nasal discharge moistens the nasal cavity rather than flowing out of it. Invasion of the Lung by wind cold pathogens manifests as clear nasal discharge;

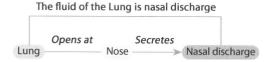

Fig. 2-7   Chart of relationship between the Lung and nasal discharge

invasion of the Lung by heat pathogens manifests as turbid nasal discharge; dryness of the Lung manifests as a dry nose with very little nasal discharge.

Plain Questions: *Chapter Discussion on the Elucidation of Five-Qi* (*Sù Wèn: Xuān Míng Wǔ Qì Piān*, 素问·宣明五气篇) says: *"The five fluids are transformed by the five zang organs…that of the Lung is nasal discharge."*

④ Physiological Properties of the Lung

(1) The Lung dominates diffusion, purification and descending (Table 2-7)

Table 2-7   The Table of the Lung qi actions of diffusing, purifying and descending

Characteristic	Meaning	Physiological action	Main pathological changes
Diffusing, purifying and descending	Outward and upward diffusion, inward and downward purification and descending	Embodied by the actions of diffusion, purification and descending: 1) Diffusing and descending the qi of respiration and keeping the respiratory tract free from obstruction 2) Diffusing and descending water and regulating water metabolism 3) Diffusing and descending the essence from water and food and transporting and distributing it to the whole body; diffusing and descending the defensive qi	Diffusing and descending disorders: 1) Abnormal respiration 2) Failure of the water passage to be ventilated and regulated 3) Influencing qi and blood circulation

Diffusion means dispersing, inhaling and exhaling. Purification and descending mean clearing, purifying and descending. Saying that the Lung dominates diffusion, purification and descending refers to the actions of the Lung qi to diffuse and disperse both upwards and outward, and to purify and descend both inward and downward. The actions of diffusion, purification and descending of the Lung are the movement features of the Lung qi and are accomplished by the ascending and descending movement of the Lung qi, so it is said, "the Lung qi diffuses and disperses" and "the Lung qi purifies and descends".

The actions of the Lung qi to diffuse, purify and descend are mainly embodied in the following aspects. First, the qi of respiration is diffused, purified and lowered to exhale turbid qi and inhale clear qi to keep a free and clear respiratory tract and normal respiratory movement. Second, the fluids are diffused, purified and lowered, and water is transported and distributed to the whole body, regulating the metabolic balance of water. Third, the essence qi from water and food are diffused, purified and descended and are transported and distributed to the whole body, which disperse the defensive qi to the skin, body hairs and striae.

If the function of diffusion, purification and descending of the Lung is abnormal, it will affect the physiological function of the Lung and result in pathological changes of abnormal Lung functions. (See the Table of physiological functions of the Lung)

The diffusion, purification, and descending are aspects that mutually restrict one another. To balance diffusion, descent, and purification, the respiratory movement, water metabolism and transportation and distribution will be normal. If the Lung fails to diffuse, purify and descend, then the respiratory movement would be abnormal, the waterway would be obstructed, and the circulation of qi and blood would be blocked. (Table 2-7)

(2) The Lung is a delicate organ

The Lung has a clear and empty form, coordinates externally with the skin and fine hairs, opens at the nose and communicates with the heaven qi of the external environment. The six exogenous pathogens easily attack the Lung via the skin and sweat pores or via the nose and mouth and result in the diseases of the Lung. The Lung is the convergence of all the vessels, so pathological changes to the other viscera are easily spread to the Lung and result in Lung disease. Owing to the delicate Lung lobes that are easily affected by pathogens, resulting in sickness, the Lung is called a delicate organ.

(3) The Lung communicates with and responds to the autumn qi

Both the Lung and autumn belong to metal among the five phases. The Lung, autumn and metal dominates descending, and since types of qi with same properties help each other, the Lung qi responds to the autumn qi. Therefore, the Lung qi is vigorous in autumn when its actions of descending and converging are stronger.

Autumn is dominated by dry qi and the climate is usually dry in autumn, resulting in autumn-dryness. The Lung is a clear and empty organ and prefers moistening. Lung qi communicates with and responds to the autumn qi, therefore, the autumn dryness pathogen is easily communicated to the Lung. Therefore, it is easy to see the syndrome of Lung dryness in autumn.

Plain Questions: Discussion on Six-Plus-Six System and the Manifestations of the Viscera (Sù Wèn: Liù Jié Zàng Xiàng Lùn, 素问·六节藏象论) says: "The Lung belongs to taiyin within yang and communicates with the autumn qi."

The Spleen

The Spleen (脾) is located in the abdomen and connects with the Stomach via a membrane. The Spleen and Stomach dominate digestion together, and are the chief organs to digest and to absorb water and food, as well as transport and distribute their essence. After birth the essence substances needed for life activity and the generation and transformation of qi, blood and fluids depend on the digestion of the Spleen and Stomach, so it is said that the Spleen and the Stomach are "the root of acquired constitution" and "the source of growth and development of qi and blood".

The chief physiological functions of the Spleen are to dominate transportation and transformation, and controlling blood.

The Spleen connects with the Small Intestine among the *fu* organs, dominates muscles among the body constituents, opens to the mouth, its quintessence appears on the lips, its emotion is thinking, and its fluid is saliva.

① The Physiological Function of the Spleen(Table 2-8)

(1) The Spleen dominates transportation and transformation

To say that the Spleen dominates transportation and transformation means that the Spleen has the function of digesting water and food, absorbing essential substances and water from them, and transporting this to the Lung and the Heart to further transport and distribute the essential substances and water to the whole body.

The function of the Spleen dominating transportation and transformation is the action of the Spleen to warm and promote movement. Therefore, the normal function of the Spleen to transport and transform is called the healthy transportation of the Spleen qi. The transportation and transformation of the Spleen include two aspects: transporting and transforming food; and transporting and transforming water and fluids. (Fig. 2-8)

a. Transportation and transformation of water and food: water and food, in this case, refers mainly to food. Saying that the Spleen dominates transporting and transforming water and food refers to the function of the Spleen to digest and absorb food and transport the resulting essence. After the elementary digestion by the Stomach, the food needs further digestion by the Spleen and is transformed into the essential substances

Table 2-8   The physiological function of the Spleen

Function	Meaning	Physiological action	Main pathological changes
The Spleen dominates transportation and transformation	The Spleen has the function of digesting water and food, abosorbing the essential substances and water and transporting them to the Lung and the Heart.	Transporting and transforming water and food: the Spleen digests and absorbs water and food and transports the essence to the Lung and the Heart where the qi and blood are transformed and generated to nourish the whole body. Transporting and transforming water: based on the Spleen's function of transporting and transforming the essence of water and food, the Spleen absorbs the water in the essence of water and food and generates fluid that nourishes the tissues and *zang-fu* organs of the whole body. The function of the Spleen dominating transportation and transformation is the action of the Spleen to warm and promote movement & digestion.	Dysfunction of the Spleen in transporting, dysfunction of digestion and absorption: poor appetite, flatulence, loose stools or diarrhea, fatigue and emaciation. Dysfunction of the Spleen in transporting water causing fluid retention: retention of phlegm and fluid, edema.
The Spleen dominates controlling blood	The Spleen has the function of keeping the blood circulating inside the vessels instead of overflow out of the vessels.	The Spleen controlling the blood primarily refers to the consolidating action of the Spleen qi. Vigorous Spleen qi can control the blood, keeping it in the vessels, so there is no bleeding.	Deficient Spleen qi can't control blood: subcutaneous hemorrhage, bloody stools, bloody urine, metrorrhagia and metrostaxis (failure of the Spleen in controlling blood).

of water and food. The Spleens absorbs the food essence and transport it to the Lung and the Heart where the food essence is transformed into qi and blood that is transported and distributed to the whole body and nourishes the tissues and *zang-fu* organs of the body. Water and food are the primary source of the nutrient substance required for supporting all life activities after birth, and are the material basis for generating qi and blood. However, the transportation and transformation of water and food are dominated by the Spleen, so, it is known that the Spleen is the acquired root, and is the source of the transformation and generation of qi and blood.

A weakened function of the Spleen in transporting and transforming results in dysfunction of digestion and absorption: this is called dysfunction of the Spleen in transportation. It manifests as poor appetite, flatulence, loose stool or diarrhea, even fatigue, or emaciation, all pathological changes of insufficient transformation and generation of qi and blood. (Table 2-8)

b. **Transportation and transformation of water and fluids:** saying that the Spleen dominates the transportation and transformation of water and fluids refers to the action of the Spleen absorbing the water which is in the essence of water and food and generating fluids to be transported and distributed to the whole body based on the Spleen's function of transporting and transforming the essence of water and food. In the metabolic processes involving body fluid, the Spleen plays a central role in the generation and transportation of the body fluid. When the Spleen is functioning normally in transporting and transforming water and fluids, the fluids moisten the tissues and *zang-fu* organs of the whole body and there is no abnormal fluid retention.

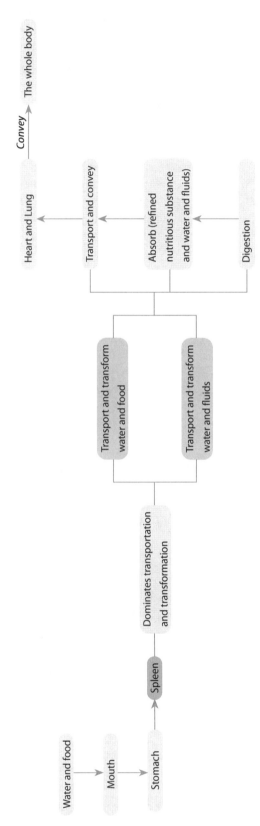

Fig. 2-8　Chart of the actions of the Spleen dominating transportation and transformation

Dysfunction of the Spleen in transportation will result in a dysfunction of the Spleen in transporting and transforming water and bring about pathological changes like retention of phlegm and fluid, and edema. (Table 2-8) Therefore, there are sayings that Spleen deficiency generates dampness, Spleen deficiency results in edema, and that the Spleen is the source of generating phlegm.

Plain Questions: *Chapter Discussion on the Secret Classics Stored in Royal Library* (*Sù Wèn: Líng Lán Mì Diǎn Lùn*, 素问·灵兰秘典论) says: "*The Spleen and the Stomach are the officials of the granary and are responsible for the digestion, absorption and transportation of the five flavors.*"

Plain Questions: *Chapter Discussion on Special Diseases* (*Sù Wèn: Qí Bìng Lùn*, 素问·奇病论) says: "*The five flavors are taken into the mouth and stored in the Stomach, and their essence qi is transformed and transported by the Spleen.*"

Plain Questions: *Chapter Discussion on Jue Syndrome* (*Sù Wèn: Jué Lùn*, 素问·厥论) says: "*The Spleen governs transporting water and fluids for the Stomach.*"

Plain Questions: *Chapter Special Discussion on Channels and Vessels* (*Sù Wèn: Jīng Mài Bié Lùn Piān*, 素问·经脉别论) says: "*When food qi is taken into the Stomach, the turbid qi is transported to the Heart… when the fluid is taken into the Stomach, the essence qi is transported to the Spleen, and the Spleen distributes the essence qi upwards to the Lung…The essence of water is distributed all through the body and to the five channels.*"

Annotatations and Explanations of the Discussion of Cold Damage (*Zhù Jiě Shāng Hán Lùn*, 注解伤寒论) says: "*The Spleen belongs to Kun earth. The Spleen helps the Stomach qi to digest food, and if the Spleen fails to transport, the food stored in the Stomach won't be digested.*"

Required Readings for Medical Professionals: *Chapter Treatise on the Kidney Being the Innate Root and the Spleen the Acquired Root* (*Yī Zōng Bì Dú*, 医宗必读) says: "*When one is born, one must depend on the support of water and food. When water and food are taken into the Stomach, they are transported to the six fu organs and qi is generated. The essence qi of water and food coordinates with the five zang organs,*

and then the blood is generated. The human being depends on the support of the qi and the blood. So it is said that the acquired root is Spleen."

(2) The Spleen dominates controlling blood

The Spleen governs controlling blood means that the Spleen has the function of controlling the blood and keeping it circulating inside the vessels instead of overflowing out of the vessels.

The dominant mechanism of the Spleen controlling the blood is the consolidating action of the Spleen qi, also called the action of controlling blood by the Spleen qi. Therefore, vigorous Spleen qi can forcefully control the blood, keeping it circulating inside the vessels and preventing bleeding.

If the deficient Spleen qi can't control the blood, the blood will not remain in the channel and bleeding occurs. Clinically, it manifested as subcutaneous hemorrhage (ecchymosis or petechia), bloody stools, hematuria, metrorrhagia and metrostaxis, caused by the failure of the Spleen in controlling blood (Table 2-8). Failure of the Spleen to control blood is usually caused by Spleen-qi deficiency and usually belongs to bleeding due to deficiency, and is always accompanied by qi deficiency symptoms and signs.

Classic of Questioning: *The Forty-second Question* (*Nàn Jīng: Sì Shí Èr Nàn*, 难经·四十二难) says: "*The Spleen governs swathing blood.*"

Treatment of Different Kinds of Diseases: *Chapter General Remarks on Blood Diseases* (*Lèi Zhèng Zhì Cái: Xuě Zhèng Zǒng Lùn*, 类证治裁·血症总论) says: "*The Heart dominates blood, the Liver stores blood and the Spleen controls blood.*"

Notes of Vol. 16 in *Synopsis of Golden Chamber* (*Jīn Guì Yào Lüè*, 金匮要略) by Shen Mu-nan (沈目南): "*All the blood of the five zang organs and six fu organs are controlled by the Spleen qi.*"

2 The Relationship of the Spleen to the Body Constituents, Sense Organs and Orifices

(1) The Spleen dominates muscles and the four extremities (Table 2-9)

Muscle generally refers to the muscles of the body, as well as fat and subcutaneous tissue. Muscular contraction produces force and relates

Table 2-9   Relationship of the Spleen to the muscles and four limbs

Foundation of relationship	Physiological significance	Pathological significance
The Spleen dominates transportation and transformation.	If the Spleen qi is healthy in transportation, the nutrition is abundant, the muscles will be plump, strong and firm, and the four limbs will be forceful and prompt to respond.	Failure of the Spleen in transportation, and insufficient nutrition: emaciation, loose muscles, fatigue of the four limbs, or debility and flaccidity of the four limbs.

to motor functions.

The Spleen dominating muscle primarily refers to the actions of transportation and transformation of the Spleen that intimately relate to the strength of the muscles. The Spleen dominates transformation and transportation of water and food, and then absorbs the essence of water and food to nourish the muscles. Therefore, if Spleen qi is healthy in transporting and sufficiently absorbs the essence of water and food, the muscles will be plump and strong, and the movements of the muscles will be forceful. Malnutrition and dysfunction of the Spleen in transporting will manifest as muscular wasting and weakness, or even pathological changes of flaccidity and atrophy.

The four extremities are the terminal ends of the body compared to the trunk, so the four extremities are also called the "Four Terminals". The Spleen dominating the four extremities refers to the function of the Spleen dominating transformation and transportation of water and food, and absorbing the essence of water and food to nourish the muscles. Therefore, if the Spleen qi is healthy in transporting and nutrition is sufficient, the four limbs will be forceful and quick to respond. Malnutrition and dysfunction of the Spleen in transporting will manifest as fatigue and weakness in the four limbs, or even the pathological changes of muscle flaccidity and atrophy.

Plain Questions: Chapter Discussion on the Elucidation of Five-Qi (Sù Wèn: Xuān Míng Wǔ Qì Piān, 素问·宣明五气篇) says: *"Among the five dominances of the five zang organs, the Spleen dominates muscles."*

Plain Questions: Chapter Discussion on Flaccidity (Sù Wèn: Wěi Lùn, 素问·痿论) says: *"The Spleen dominates the muscles of the whole body."*

Variorum of Plain Questions: Chapter Discussion on Various Relationships Concerning the Five Zang-Organs (Sù Wèn Jí Zhù: Wǔ Zàng Shēng Chéng Piān, 素问集注·五脏生成篇) says: *"The Spleen governs transporting and transforming the essence of the water and food to generate and nourish the muscles, and therefore, it dominates muscles."*

Treatise on Spleen and Stomach: Chapter Discussion on the Excess and Decline of the Spleen and Stomach (Pí Wèi Lùn: Pí Wèi Shèng Shuāi Lùn, 脾胃论·脾胃胜衰论) says: *"When both Spleen and Stomach are vigorous, one will have a good appetite and be plump; when both Spleen and Stomach are deficient, one will have a poor appetite and be emaciated."*

Plain Questions: Chapter Discussion on Taiyin and Yangming (Sù Wèn: Tài Yīn Yáng Míng Lùn, 素问·太阴阳明论) says: *"The four limbs are nourished by the Stomach, but Stomach qi cannot reach them directly. Thus the four limbs have to depend on the Spleen to provide nourishment. When the Spleen qi is in disorder, it is unable to transport fluid for the Stomach. The four limbs cannot get nutrients and become weaker and weaker. The channels become obstructed, thus the sinews and muscles become atrophic. That is why the four limbs cannot move normally."*

(2) The Spleen opens to the mouth and its quintessence appears on the lips (Table 2-10)

The Spleen opening at the mouth refers to the intimate connection between the transformation and transportation fucntions of the Spleen with appetite and taste. If the Spleen qi is healthy in transportation, one will have a good Stomach and normal taste. Dysfunction of the Spleen in transportation manifests as poor appetite, and a lack of taste when eating; obstruction of the Spleen by turbid dampness manifests as poor appetite and a greasy or sweet taste in the mouth.

The Spleen's quintessence appearing on the

Table 2-10   Table of relationship between the Spleen, mouth and lips

Foundation of the relationship	Physiological significance	Pathological significance
The Spleen dominates transportation and transformation.	When Spleen qi is healthy in transportation, transformation and generating sufficient qi and blood, it will manifest as a vigorous appetite, normal taste sensations and ruddy and lustrous mouth and the lips.	Dysfunction of the Spleen in transportation: poor appetite, tastelessness. Obstruction of the Spleen by turbid dampness: poor appetite, greasy and sweet taste in mouth. Dysfunction of the Spleen in transportation, and insufficient transformation and generation of qi and blood: pale lusterless lips, even becoming pale and yellowish.

lips refers to the intimate connection of the actions of the Spleen that dominates transformation and transportation with the color and shape of the mouth and lips. If the Spleen qi is healthy in transporting, it absorbs the essence of the water and food and transforms and generates qi and blood, causing nutrition to be sufficient, so the mouth and the lips will be ruddy in color. Dysfunction of the Spleen in transportation, or insufficient qi and blood, or malnutrition manifests as pale and lusterless lips, even being pale or yellowish.

Plain Questions: Chapter Discussion on Important Ideas in the Golden Chamber (Sù Wèn: Jīn Guì Zhēn Yán Lùn, 素问·金匮真言论) says: *"The Spleen opens at the mouth."*

Miraculous Pivot: Chapter Determining the Conditions of the Five Viscera by Examining the Five Sense Organs (Líng Shū: Wǔ Yuè Wǔ Shǐ, 灵枢·五阅五使) says: *"The mouth and lips are the officials of the Spleen."*

Miraculous Pivot: Chapter The Length of Channels (Líng Shū: Mài Dù, 灵枢·脉度) says: *"The Spleen qi communicates with the mouth, so if the Spleen qi is harmonious, the mouth can distinguish the flavor of the five cereals."*

Plain Questions: Chapter Discussion on Various Relationships Concerning the Five Zang-Organs (Sù Wèn: Wǔ Zàng Shēng Chéng Piān, 素问·五脏生成篇) says: *"The Spleen coordinates with muscles externally and its quintessence appears on the lips."*

③ Relation of the Spleen to the Five Minds and Five Fluids

(1) The mind of the Spleen is thinking

Thinking means meditation and thoughtfulness.

It is an emotional activity focusing on cogitation.

Saying that the mind of the Spleen is thinking refers to the physiological function of the Spleen that correlates to emotion and thinking. Overall, the Heart governs the spirit and emotions; therefore, it said that thought originates from the Heart and the Spleen. Normal thinking is an emotional activity every one has. Over thinking can impair the Heart and the Spleen and result in the pathological changes of Spleen qi depression and uneasy Heart spirit. (See the section on seven emotions)

Plain Questions: Chapter Major Discussion on the Theory of Yin and Yang and the Corresponding Relationships Among All the Things in Nature (Sù Wèn: Yīn Yáng Yìng Xiàng Dà Lùn, 素问·阴阳应象大论) says: *"The Spleen… its mind is thinking."*

(2) The fluid of the Spleen is saliva

Saliva is the fluid in the mouth, and the clear and thin part of sputum. Saliva has the function of moistening the oral cavity and protecting oral mucosa, is secreted more when eating and is helpful in swallowing and digesting food.

The fluid of the Spleen is saliva refers to the function of the Spleen that dominates transformation and transportation, and opens at the mouth. The saliva is secreted by the oral cavity, so it is said that "the saliva is the fluid of the Spleen" (Fig. 2-9). When the actions of the

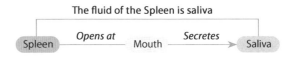

The fluid of the Spleen is saliva

Spleen — *Opens at* — Mouth — *Secretes* → Saliva

Fig. 2-9   Chart of relationship between the Spleen and saliva

Spleen and Stomach are normal, and qi and yin are sufficient, then the saliva can be secreted to moisten the oral cavity instead of overflowing outside the mouth. Lack of co-ordination between the Spleen and the Stomach or insufficiency of Spleen-qi resulting in a failure to control can result in increased secretion of saliva, and manifest as the overflow of the saliva out from the mouth: as well, yin deficiency of the Spleen and Stomach may result in less secretion of the saliva and manifest as a dry mouth and tongue.

Plain Questions: *Chapter Discussion on the Elucidation of Five-Qi* (*Sù Wèn*: *Xuān Míng Wǔ Qì Piān*, 素问·宣明五气篇) says: "*Among the five fluids transformed by the five zang organs…the one of the Spleen is saliva.*"

④ Physiological Properies of the Spleen

(1) The Spleen qi dominates ascending (Table 2-11)

The Spleen qi dominating ascending refers to

Table 2-11　Table of actions of the Spleen qi dominating ascending

Chief manifestations	Meaning	Physiological action	Main pathological changes
The Spleen dominates lifting the clear yang	The Spleen absorbs the essence of water and food and transports them upward to the Heart and the Lung where the qi and blood are transformed and generated to nourish the whole body.	It is one aspect of the function of the Spleen dominating transformation and transportation. Whe the Spleen qi is healthy in transportation and the action of lifting the clear is normal, the Spleen qi will absorb the essence of water and food, as well as transform and generate qi and blood to nourish the whole body.	Dysfunction of the Spleen in transportation results in failure of the clear qi in being lifted: resulting in flatulence, diarrhea, fatigue, dizziness and vertigo occurring (failure of the Spleen to lift the clear).
The Spleen dominates lifting the viscera	The Spleen dominating the lifting of the viscera refers to the actions of the Spleen qi to consolidates organs and keeps them in a relatively stable position instead of prolapsing.	The Spleen qi is vigorous and it can lift and consolidate organs.	Insufficiency of the Spleen-qi fails to lift: enteroptosis, chronic diarrhea, prolapse of anus (collapse of the Spleen-qi)

the movement features of the Spleen qi, which chiefly moves upward. The Spleen qi dominates ascending, by primarily finding its expression in lifting the clear yang and viscera.

a. Dominating the lifting of clear yang

The clear yang refers to the essential substances from water and food. The Spleen dominating the lifting of the clear refers to the Spleen functions of absorbing the essence of water and food and transporting it upward to the Heart and the Lung to transform and generate qi and blood and nourish the whole body.

The Spleen dominating the lifting of the clear is one aspect of the function of the Spleen dominating transformation and transportation. When the Spleen qi is healthy in transporting and its action of lifting the clear yang is normal, then it can absorb the essential substances of water and food. The essential substances are transported to the Heart and the Lung where qi and blood are transformed and generated, and the life activity is vigorous as a result. Dysfunction of the Spleen in transportation results in failure of the water and food to be transported and transformed, and then the clear qi will fail to lift, and symptoms of flatulence, diarrhea, fatigue, dizziness and vertigo occur. This is called the failure of the Spleen to lift the clear.

b. Dominating lifting the viscera

The Spleen dominating lifting the viscera refers to the actions of the Spleen qi to consolidating the organs, keeping them in a relatively stable position instead of prolapsing. Deficiency of Spleen-qi that fails to consolidate and lift would result in the pathological changes of prolapse of the organs (i.e. gastroptosis, nephroptosis and hysteroptosis), or chronic diarrhea and prolapse of anus. It is distinguished as "the collapse of Spleen-qi" (also known as "the sinking of the qi of the middle-*Jiao*").

(2) The Spleen likes dryness and dislikes dampness

The characteristics of the Spleen liking dryness and disliking dampness are related to the function of the Spleen dominating the transformation and the transportation of water and fluid. When the Spleen qi is healthy in transporting it has the normal actions of transporting and transforming water and fluid. This means that the water and food essence will be distributed to all the parts of the body, and there will be no retention of damp phlegm. Insufficiency of Spleen-qi results in dysfunction of the Spleen in transporting and transforming water and fluid, and then the endogenous retention of water dampness and phlegm fluid occur. This is insufficiency of the Spleen generating dampness. The endogenous water dampness due to insufficiency of the Spleen obstructs and inhibits the transporting and transforming actions of the Spleen, therefore it is the obstruction of the transportation of the Spleen by dampness. In addition, after invasion of the body by exogenous dampness, the Spleen is easily obstructed and the Spleen qi will stagnate, which influences the Spleen's actions of transportation and transformation. For both the generation of dampness due to Spleen deficiency, and inhibition of the transportation of the Spleen by dampness, the syndromes can manifest as poor appetite, flatulence, loose stools or retention of phlegm and fluid, and edema. Methods of strengthening the Spleen and eliminating dampness can be used to treat the diseases, and then the symptoms of the disease can be relieved. Therefore, it is said that the Spleen likes dryness and hates dampness.

(3) The Spleen communicates with long summer qi

Long summer is the third month of summer (June in the lunar calendar): it is the time of the joining of summer and autumn. The climate at the time is rainy and wet.

The Spleen communicates with and responds to long summer. On the one hand, it responds seasonally, since Spleen qi is vigorous in long summer and the physiological functions of the Spleen are at their most vigorous in this season. On the other hand, from the aspect of climate, the Spleen dominates transformation and transportation of water and fluid, and its nature likes dryness and dislikes dampness. Damp qi is in charge in long summer and the damp pathogen is easy to impair humans and attack the Stomach. It is manifested as flatulence, poor appetite, fatigue, and loose stools, all symptoms of the syndrome of dampness obstructing the Spleen.

The Spleen communicates with and responses to long summer qi (damp qi), and its nature like dryness and dislike dampness. From the aspect of pathogenesis, the Spleen has special susceptibility to the damp pathogen.

The Liver

The Liver (肝) is located in the abdomen, below the diaphragm, and in the right flank.

The main physiological functions of Liver are dominating free movement of qi and storing blood.

The Liver connects with the Gallbladder among *fu* organs, dominates sinews among the body constituents, its quintessence appears on the nails, it opens at the eyes, its mind is anger and its fluid is tears.

① The Physiological Functions of the Liver(Table 2-12)

(1) The Liver dominates free coursing, or movement of qi

"Free coursing" means dredging and smoothing. To say that the Liver dominates free coursing refers to the actions of the Liver that dredge and free the qi dynamic of the whole body.

When free coursing actions of the Liver are normal, then the qi dynamic is harmonious and free, and therefore the activities of the tissues, organs and *zang-fu* organs are normal. When the

Table 2-12 The physiological functions of the Liver

Actions	Meaning	Physiological action	Main pathological changes
The Liver dominates free coursing.	It refers to the actions of the Liver to dredge and smoothe the qi dynamic of the whole body.	**Regulating the mental and emotional activities:** if the qi dynamic is harmonious and free, one will be happy, outgoing, and will not be depressive or irritable.	**Failure of the Liver in free coursing, and Liver qi depression:** lack of sociability, unhappiness, sentimentality, sorrow and sighing. **Excessive free coursing by the Liver, and hyperactivity of the Liver qi:** irritability, testiness, headache and insomnia, etc.
		Promoting digestion and absorption: when the ascent and descent of the qi dynamic of the Spleen and Stomach is harmonious and free, then the bile secretion and excretion is normal, which is helpful to digestion and absorption.	**Disharmony of the Liver and Stomach:** distending pain, poor appetite, hiccups, belching and acid regurgitation. **Disharmony of the Liver and Spleen:** distending pain in the abdomen, diarrhea, and indigestion. Failure of the Liver and Gallbladder in free coursing: hypochondriac pain, bitter taste, anorexia and jaundice.
		Maintaining blood circulation: when the qi dynamic is harmonious and free, the blood is not congestive or stagnant and doesn't overflow (the qi circulates, and then the blood circulates accordingly)	**Qi stagnation and blood stasis:** pain in chest and hypochondrium, or tumors. **Blood overflow due to qi reversal:** hemorrhagic changes of hematemesis, emptysis, profuse menstruation, metrorrhagia and metrostaxis.
		Regulating metabolism of water and fluids: when the qi dynamic is harmonious and free, the transportation, distribution and excretion of water and fluids is normal (Qi circulates, and then the water circulates accordingly).	**Unsmooth qi dynamic, and difficulty of transportation, distribution and excretion of water and fluids:** retention of phlegm and fluid, edema.
		Regulating menstruation and ejaculation: when the qi dynamic of the Liver is harmonious and free, then the blood can fill the uterus, thus menstruation will be free and harmonious; when the free coursing of the Liver is normal, ejaculation will be free.	**Failure of the Liver in free coursing:** irregular menstruation, obstructive or overactive ejaculation.
The Liver governs storing blood.	This refers to the actions of the Liver to store blood and regulate the volume of blood.	**Storing blood:** The abundant storage of blood by the Liver can moisten and nourish the Liver, constrain the Liver yang and prevent bleeding. **Regulating the blood volume:** in company with the static or active movement of the body, the Liver regulates the peripheral blood volume and nourishes correlative tissues and organs.	**Failure of the Liver in storing blood:** hematemesis, nosebleed, emptysis, profuse menstruation, metrorrhagia and metrostaxis. **Liver-blood deficiency:** dizziness, vertigo, muscle spasms, numbness in the limbs, scanty menses, or amenorrhea.

free coursing action of the Liver is not functioning smoothly, it will result in the pathological changes of disharmonious qi dynamics of the *zang-fu* organs.

The Liver dominating free coursing mostly finds its expression in regulating mental activities, promoting digestion and absorption, maintaining blood circulation, regulating water metabolism, and regulating menstruation and seminal excretiosn. (Fig. 2-10)

a. Regulating emotional and mental activities

Chinese medicine thinks that the mental and emotional activities of the human body are based on the qi and blood of the *zang-fu* organs and are the external manifestations of the actions of the *zang-fu* organs. When the free coursing action of the Liver is normal, the qi dynamic is harmonious and free, and the qi and blood of the *zang-fu* organs is balanced, then mental and emotional activities will be normal and manifested by happiness, good moods and lack of irritability.

If the Liver's action of free coursing is not functioning, the qi dynamic will not be smooth, thus it easily causes disorders of both mental and emotional activities. If the Liver doesn't move fully and freely, it manifests as Liver qi depression, unsociability, unhappiness, sentimentality, sorrow, and sighing. If the function of the Liver is excessive in free coursing, the Liver qi will be excited and manifest as irritability and short-temperedness accompanied by headaches, insomnia etc. (Table 2-12)

b. Promoting digestion and absorption

The digestion and absorption of water and food are affected by *zang-fu* organs like the Spleen, Stomach, Gallbladder etc. The actions of the Liver in free coursing and smoothing the qi dynamic, on the one hand, regulate the qi dynamic of the Spleen and Stomach, keeping a balance in the ascending and descending of the qi dynamic of the Spleen and Stomach, therefore allowing the Spleen and the Stomach to digest and absorb water and food normally. On the other hand, the free coursing action of the Liver can promote the secretion and excretion of bile which is good for the digestion and absorption of water and food. Therefore, when the free coursing action of the Liver is normal, the qi dynamic of the Spleen and Stomach is harmonious and free, bile secretion and excretion are normal, and digestion and absorption will function normally.

If the free coursing action of the Liver is abnormal, it can affect digestion and absorption. Hyperactive Liver qi attacking the Stomach results in the failure of descending of the Stomach-qi, manifesting as distending pain, eructation, hiccups and acid regurgitation (the syndrome of disharmony of the Liver and the Stomach). If the Liver qi attacks the Stomach, it will result in dysfunction of the Spleen in transportation, with symptoms of distending pain in the abdomen and diarrhea, belonging to the syndrome of disharmony of the Liver and Spleen. If the Liver qi attacks the Gallbladder, it will influence the secretion and excretion of bile and manifest as distending pain in the hypochondrium, a bitter taste, poor appetite, and jaundice, belonging to the syndrome of disharmony of the Liver and Gallbladder. (Table 2-12)

c. Keeping the blood circulating

Blood circulation depends not only on the promoting action of qi, but also a harmonious and free qi dynamic, or what is meant by saying, "The qi circulates, and then the blood circulates accordingly". The action of free coursing as well as harmonizing and smoothing the qi dynamic of the Liver maintains a free qi circulation of the *zang-fu* organs, as well as the channels and collaterals of the whole body. As a result, the blood circulation is free from stagnation and stasis, and will not overflow out of the vessels; therefore, normal blood circulation is kept.

Failure of the Liver in free coursing results in a problem with the qi dynamic and definitley affects blood circulation. Stagnation of Liver qi manifests as pain in the chest and hypochondrium, or masses and tumors belonging to the syndrome of qi stagnation and blood stasis. Ascending invasion of Liver qi would result in blood overflow due to qi reversal, which manifests as the hemorrhagic changes of hematemesis, emptysis, profuse menstruation, metrorrhagia and metrostaxis. (Table 2-12)

d. Regulating water metabolism

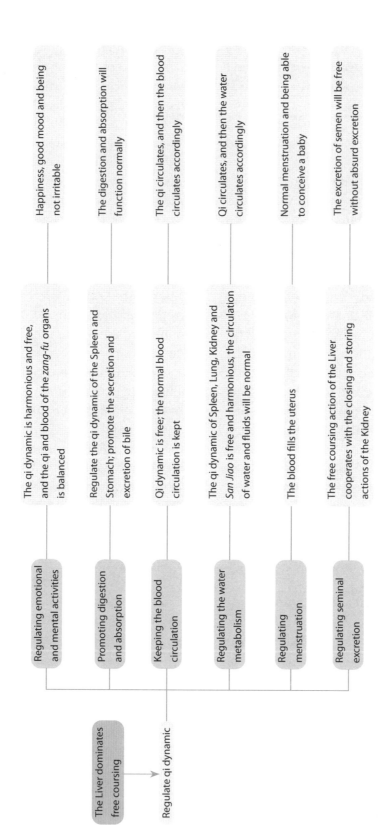

Fig. 2-10　Chart of the actions of the Liver that dominate free coursing

The absorption, distribution and excretion as part of the metabolic processing of water and fluids in the body is completed by the combined actions of the *zang-fu* organs in terms of the Spleen, Lung, Kidney, *San Jiao* etc. The free coursing action of the Liver smoothes the qi dynamic of the body, and then smooths the qi dynamic of the *zang-fu* organs of the Spleen, Lung, Kidney and *San Jiao*, thereby keeping normal metabolism of water and fluids. Essentially, qi circulates, and then water circulates accordingly.

If the free coursing action of the Liver malfunctions and the qi dynamic is disharmonious, it will affect the distribution and drainage of water and fluids and result in the pathological changes of water metabolism in terms of retention of phlegm and fluid, and edema. (Table 2-12)

e. Regulating menstruation and seminal excretion
Menstruation is a physiological phenomenon of the cyclic congestion and bleeding of the uterus. Menstruation is the combined action of many *zang-fu* organs. When the free coursing action of the Liver is normal, the qi dynamic is harmonious and free, and the blood vessels are not obstructed, then blood can fill the uterus, and menstruation can be free and harmonious with a normal cycle. If the free coursing action of the Liver malfunctions, the pathological change of irregular menstruation occurs, manifesting as irregular menstrual cycles, dysmenorrhea, profuse menses, or even metrorrhagia and metrostaxis, etc. (Table 2-12)

Semen is stored in the testes and the opening and closing of the testes controls the excretion of semen. Chinese medicine thinks that this is the combined action of both the Kidney and Liver. The storage of the semen is controlled by the Kidney, specifically by the action of storing Kidney essence; the excretion of semen is controlled by the Liver, namely by the free coursing action of the Liver. If the inter-coordination of the free coursing action of the Liver and the closing and storing actions of the Kidney are normal and the testes open and close properly, the excretion of semen will be free and not of too large a volume. If the action of free coursing of the Liver is not functioning, the opening and closing of the testes will be in disorder, and it will result in semen drainage difficulty or over excretion of semen. (Table 2-12)

Women's menstruation and men's ejaculation influence their reproductive functions. Therefore, the free coursing action of the Liver is also related to reproductive functions.

Further Discourses on the Properties of Things: *Chapter Discussion on Superabundance of Yang and Insufficiency of Yin* (*Gé Zhì Yú Lùn: Yáng Yǒu Yú Yīn Bù Zú Lùn*, 格致余论·阳有余阴不足论) says: "*The organ that governs closing and storage is the Kidney; the organ that governs free coursing is the Liver.*"

Zhang's Treatise on Medicine (*Zhāng Shì Yī Tōng*, 张氏医通) says: "*The Liver stores the qi of generation and sprout, the vital qi is vigorous, the qi of five zang organs circulate freely, the vital qi is obstructed, and the qi of the five zang organs stagnate.*"

Vol. 4 of *Essays of Reading Medical Works* (*Dú Yī Suí Bǐ*, 读医随笔) says: "*For qi transformation of the twelve channels of the zang-fu organs, they all need encouragement by the qi transformation of the Liver qi and Gallbladder qi, and then they can be harmonious and free and not easily get sick.*"

Discussion of Blood Syndromes: *Section Discussion on Pathogenesis of Zang-Fu Organs* (*Xuè Zhèng Lùn: Zàng Fǔ Bìng Jī Lùn*, 血证论·脏腑病机论) says: "*The property of wood dominates free coursing, the food that enters the Stomach depends on the qi of the Liver wood to course freely, and then water and food can be digested. If the clear yang of the Liver fails to lift, it will fail to cause water and food to course freely, and patients will suffer symptoms of diarrhea and fullness in the middle Jiao.*"

Requisite Readings for Wise Doctors: *Section Discussion on Liver Qi* (*Zhì Yī Bì Dú: Lùn Gān Qì*, 知医必读·论肝气) says: "*Hyperactive Liver qi will over-restrain the Spleen earth and result in distending pain and diarrhea in a severe case; or attack the Stomach earth and send it upwards, resulting in vomiting due to qi reversal and hypochondriac pain.*"

(2) The Liver governs storing blood
The Liver storing blood refers to the actions of the Liver storing blood and regulating the volume of blood.

The physiological action of the Liver that stores blood is embodied in two aspects: storing the blood and regulating the blood volume. (Fig. 2-11)

a. Storing blood: the abundant storage of blood by the Liver can moisten and nourish the Liver and prevent bleeding. Blood belongs to yin, and the yin blood of the Liver can restrain the Liver yang and nourish the Liver qi. Thus, the Liver yang and the Liver qi will not be hyperactive or move in a reversed way. This means that it can prevent bleeding.

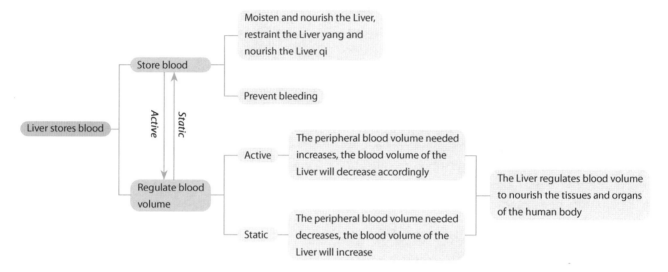

Fig. 2-11   Chart of the actions of the Liver that store blood

b. Regulating blood volume: based on the storage of blood, and according to physiological needs, the Liver regulates the blood volume of every part of the body. In company with the static or active movements of the boy, the blood volume needed by each part changes accordingly. When the body moves violently or if a person is in an excited or agitated mood, the blood volume correspondingly increases, and the blood stored in the Liver is transported out of the Liver, so the blood volume of the Liver will decrease accordingly. When the body is static or one is in a stable mood, the peripheral blood volume correspondingly decreases, and some blood returns to the Liver, therefore the blood volume of the Liver will increase. The Liver regulates blood volume to nourish the tissues and organs of the human body. In particularly nourishes the tissues and organs of the uterus, eyes, sinews and nails, which need nourishment by Liver blood to maintain normal physiological activities.

Failure of the Liver in storing blood may result in pathological changes in two aspects.

First, if the Liver fails in storing blood and is incapable of preventing bleeding, hemorrhage occurs. Reversal and hyperactivity of the Liver qi and yang would result in hyperactivity of Liver fire that manifests as hemorrhagic diseases of hematemesis, nosebleeds, emptysis, profuse menstruation, metrorrhagia and metrostaxis. Second, if the storage of blood in the Liver is insufficient (Liver-blood deficiency); the Liver is incapable of regulating the blood volume as well as the demands of the body. Thus the correlative tissues and organs can't be nourished by blood, and then the pathological changes of Liver-blood deficiency occur. Failure of the blood in nourishing the eyes manifests as dizziness, vertigo, blurred eyes, night blindness etc.; failure of the blood in nourishing sinews manifests as muscle spasms, numbness in the limbs, difficulty in extension and flexion etc.; failure of the blood in filling the uterus manifests as scanty menses that is light in color, amenorrhea etc. (Table 2-12)

Plain Questions: *Chapter Discussion on the Regulation of Channels* (*Sù Wèn: Tiáo Jīng Lùn*, 素

问·调经论) says: "The Liver stores blood."

Plain Questions: Chapter Discussion on Various Relationships Concerning the Five Zang-Organs (Sù Wèn: Wǔ Zàng Shēng Chéng Piān, 素问·五脏生成篇) says: "When one lies down, the blood returns to the Liver. Nourished by the blood, the eyes can see; nourished by the blood, the feet can walk; nourished by the blood, the palms can grasp; nourished by the blood, the fingers can take things."

Wang Bing (王冰) from the Tang Dynasty explained in his notes that "When one lies down, the blood returns to the Liver" and that the "Liver stores the blood that is circulated by the Heart. When one exercises, blood is transported and distributed to all the channels; when one rests, blood returns to the Liver. Why? That's because the Liver dominates the sea of blood."

② The Relation of the Liver to the Body Constituents, Sense Organs and Orifices

(1) The Liver dominates the sinews and its quintessence appears on the nails (Table 2-13)

Table 2-13   Relationship of the Liver, sinews and nails

Foundation of the relationship	Physiological significance	Pathological significance
The Liver governs storing blood.	When sufficient Liver blood nourishes the sinews and nails normally, the joint movements will be prompt and forceful, and the nails will be firm, ruddy and lustrous.	Insufficiency of Liver blood, with malnourishment of the sinews and nails: numbness in the four limbs, difficulties in extension and flexion, muscle spasms, tremors or cramps in the hands and feet, or, nails which are soft, thin, withered distorted or fragile.

Sinew, also called fasciae, include tendons and ligaments, and connect muscle, bone and joints. The contraction and relaxation of the sinews determines the smooth movement of the joints. Therefore, sinews have an intimate connection with the motor functions of the limbs.

Saying that the Liver dominates sinew primarily refers to the action of the Liver-blood nourishing the sinews. When sufficient Liver-blood nourishes the sinews, then joint movement will be prompt and forceful. Insufficient Liver-blood can result in malnourishment of the sinews and difficulties of joint movements, manifesting as numbness in the four limbs, difficulties in extension and flexion, muscle spasms, tremors in the hands and feet, all part of the syndrome of "endogenous wind due to blood deficiency". Blazing pathogenic heat can burn the yin blood of the Liver and result in malnourishment of the sinews, manifested by the pathological changes of convulsions of the four limbs, lockjaw, or opisthotonus, part of the syndrome of "endogenous wind due to extreme heat".

"Claws", referring to nails, include the nails of the hands and feet. Nails are the continuation of sinew, thus there is the saying that "Claws are the surplus of sinew." The relationship between the Liver and the nails is based on the action of the Liver storing blood, since the Liver blood nourishes the nails. Therefore, if the Liver-blood is sufficient, the nails will be ruddy, lustrous and firm. If the Liver-blood is insufficient, the nails will be soft, thin and withered, even distorted and fragile. Therefore, it is known that the quintessence of the Liver appears on the nails.

Plain Questions: Chapter Discussion on the Elucidation of Five-Qi (Sù Wèn: Xuān Míng Wǔ Qì Piān, 素问·宣明五气篇) says: "Among the five dominances of the five zang organs...the Liver dominates sinews."

Plain Questions: Chapter Discussion on Various Relationships Concerning the Five Zang-Organs (Sù Wèn: Wǔ Zàng Shēng Chéng Piān, 素问·五脏生成篇) says: "The Liver coordinates with the sinews externally, its quintessence appears on the nails...all the sinews belong to the joints."

Plain Questions: Chapter Major Discussion on the Theory of Yin and Yang and the Corresponding Relationships Among All the Things in Nature (Sù Wèn: Yīn Yáng Yìng Xiàng Dà Lùn, 素问·阴阳应象大论) says: "Liver generates sinews".

Plain Questions: Discussion on Six-Plus-Six

System and the Manifestations of the Viscera (Sù Wèn: Liù Jié Zàng Xiàng Lùn, 素问·六节藏象论) says: "Liver is the root of the four limbs…its quintessence appears on the nails, and its function is to nourish sinews."

Plain Questions: Chapter Ancient Ideas on Flow to Preserve Natural Healthy Energy (Sù Wèn: Shàng Gǔ Tiān Zhēn Lùn, 素问·上古天真论) says: "Man… his Liver qi will decline after he is at the age of fifty-six, and his musculature will become inflexible."

(2) The Liver opens at the eyes (Table 2-14)

Table 2-14   Relationship between the Liver and the eyes

Foundation for relationship	Physiological significance	Pathological significance
The Liver governs storing yin blood.	When the yin blood of the Liver is sufficient, the eyes can see things clearly and discriminate colors normally.	**Liver blood insufficiency:** blurred eyes or night blindness **Liver yin insufficiency:** dry eyes, diminution of vision **Flaming-up of the** Liver **fire:** conjunctival congestion **Endogenous** Liver **wind stirring:** squinting of the eyes, or even the eyes rolling back in the head

The eye is the organ of vision, and has the action of seeing things.

The relationship between the Liver and the eyes: Structurally, the Liver channel connects with the eyes. Physiologically, the function of the Liver storing blood primarily and closely relates to the visual actions of the eyes. Namely, normal vision depends on the nourishment of the Liver yin blood, so that the eyes can exert their functions of seeing things and discriminating colors. If the Liver is sick, the eyes will be symptomatic of Liver disease. Thus, liver blood insufficiency manifests as blurred eyes or night blindness; Liver yin insufficiency manifests as dry eyes and diminution of vision; flaming-up of the Liver fire manifests as conjunctive congestion; damp-heat in the Liver and the Gallbladder manifests as yellow sclera; and endogenous stirring of Liver wind manifests as squinting of the eyes or even the eyes rolling back in the head. (Table 2-14)

Plain Questions: Chapter Discussion on Important Ideas in the Golden Chamber (Sù Wèn: Jīn Guì Zhēn Yán Lùn, 素问·金匮真言论) says: "Liver…it opens at the eyes."

Miraculous Pivot: Chapter Determining the Conditions of the Five Viscera by Examining the Five Sense Organs (Líng Shū: Wǔ Yuè Wǔ Shǐ, 灵枢·五阅五使) says: "Eyes are the officials of the Liver."

Miraculous Pivot: Chapter On Channels (Líng Shū: Jīng Mài, 灵枢·经脉) says: "The Liver channel of foot jueyin connects with the eyes."

Plain Questions: Chapter Discussion on Various Relationships Concerning the Five Zang-Organs (Sù Wèn: Wǔ Zàng Shēng Chéng Piān, 素问·五脏生成篇) says: "The blood returns to the Liver, and nourished by the blood, the eyes can see."

Miraculous Pivot: Chapter The Length of Channels (Líng Shū: Mài Dù, 灵枢·脉度) says: "The Liver qi communicates with the eyes, the Liver is coordinative, and then the eyes can distinguish the five colors."

③ Relation of the Liver to the Five Minds and Five Fluids

(1) The mind of the Liver is anger

Anger is a kind of emotional activity when one is angry or enraged.

Saying that the mind of the Liver is anger means that for emotional activity, anger is closely related to the physiological functions of the Liver. When the free coursing action of the Liver is normal, it can adjust depression and anger. If excessive anger impairs the Liver, it will result in the failure of the Liver in free coursing, with pathological changes of depression and anger. (See the section on seven emotions)

Plain Questions: Chapter Major Discussion on the Theory of Yin and Yang and the Corresponding Relationships Among All the Things in Nature (Sù Wèn: Yīn Yáng Yìng Xiàng Dà Lùn, 素问·阴阳应

象大论) says: "*Liver... its mind is anger.*"

(2) The fluid of the Liver is tears

Tears are the secretion of the eyes, moistening and protecting the eyes.

The Liver opens at the eyes and tears are secreted by the eyes, therefore it is said that "Tears are the fluid of the Liver." (Fig. 2-12) Under normal conditions, the secretion of tears moistens the eyes but does not overflow. If the Liver is sick, the secretion of tears can be abnormal. Insufficiency of Liver yin blood results in decreased secretion of tears and manifests as dry eyes: Liver channel wind-heat manifests as excess tears induced by wind, with increased eye secretion.

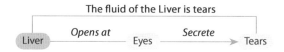

Fig. 2-12 Chart of relationship between Liver and tears

Plain Questions: Chapter Discussion on the Elucidation of Five-Qi (Sù Wèn: Xuān Míng Wǔ Qì Piān, 素问·宣明五气篇*)* says: "*Among the five fluids transformed by the five zang organs...that of the Liver is tear.*"

④ Physiological Properties of the Liver

(1) The Liver governs ascent and dispersion, likes order and extension, and dislikes depression

The Liver belongs to wood among the five phases, and the property of the wood governs ascent and dispersion. The Liver dominates free coursing and its qi is apt to be harmonious and smooth. The Liver governs ascent and dispersion, likes order and extension, and dislikes depression. This refers to the property of the Liver qi that send up gently and disperse smoothly, which in turn keep its physiological functions normal. Over-ascent and dispersion of the Liver qi manifests as impatience, testiness, a feeling of fullness of the head, headaches, dizziness and vertigo: insufficient ascent and dispersion of the Liver qi manifests as unhappiness, depression, and distending pain in the chest and hypochondrium. Thus, the ascent and dispersion of the Liver qi must keep the features of moving qi smoothly,

and gently but firmly. On the other hand, over-depression of Liver qi can impair the Liver and result in the disorder of the free coursing of the Liver qi. Therefore, it is said that the Liver likes order and extension and dislikes depression.

(2) The Liver is a firm zang organ, its form belongs to yin, and its functions belong to yang

The Liver is a firm *zang* organ, which refers to the properties of the Liver as strong, firm and irritable. Liver qi governs ascent and dispersion and the Liver qi, and Liver yang is easy to move and ascend, which reflects the features of the Liver to be firm, strong and irritable. Liver diseases also always manifests with symptoms of the over-ascent and dispersion of Liver qi and Liver yang in terms of vertigo, blushing, impatience, testiness, spasms, tics, opisthotonos etc., which are the counterevidence of the unyielding and irritable properties of the Liver.

The form of the Liver belonging to yin refers to the condition that the Liver stores yin blood. Yin and blood belong to yin, so it is known that form belongs to yin. The function of the Liver belonging to yang refers to the fact that the physiological function of the Liver governs free coursing, and the Liver qi and Liver yang govern motion and ascent, and since all these functions belong to yang, thus it is knows that the Liver's functions belongs to yang. The Liver is an unyielding *zang* organ, Liver qi and Liver yang are easy to move and ascend and must be nourished by Liver yin and Liver-blood to keep softness and harmony and exert its normal physiological actions. Among the pathological changes of the Liver, the yin blood is easy to be consumed and manifests as insufficiency of yin blood. Yang qi easily becomes hyperactive and reverses, manifesting as excess. Therefore, it is known that "the Liver yin and Liver-blood are always insufficient, the Liver qi and Liver yang always excessive."

(3) The Liver communicates with and responses to spring qi

The Liver dominates free coursing, and its qi dominates motion and ascent. Springtime is the beginning of each year and it is when the yang qi ascends and everything in the natural world is vigorously growing and flourishing. The Liver communicates with and responds to the spring qi, which means that the ascent and dispersion of the Liver qi is in tune with the spring qi, and the Liver qi is most vigorous in the springtime. The Liver relates to spring, wind, wood, the color blue, and sour tastes, all of which have certain significance in guiding the prevention and treatment of Liver diseases.

Plain Questions: Discussion on Six-Plus-Six System and the Manifestations of the Viscera (Sù Wèn: Liù Jié Zàng Xiàng Lùn, 素问·六节藏象论) says: "*Liver…is shaoyang within yang and communicates with the spring qi.*"

The Kidney [Appendix: The Life Gate (*Ming Men*)]

The two Kidneys (肾) are located at either sides of the spine at the waist, one on the left and one on the right.

The main physiological functions of the Kidney are governing the storage of essence, dominating water, and governing receiving qi. The Kidney stores innate essence and dominates reproduction. It is the root of the life of the human body, so it is known that the Kidney is the root of congenital constitution.

The Kidney connects with Bladder among the *fu* organs, dominates bone among body constituents, opens at the ears and two lower orifices, its quintessence appears on the hair, its mind is fear, and its fluid is spit.

① The physiological function of the Kidney (Table 2-15)

(1) The Kidney stores essence

The concept of the Kidney storing essence: the Kidney storing essence means that the Kidney

Table 2-15 The physiological functions of the Kidney

Function	Meaning	Physiological action	Main pathological changes
The Kidney governs the storage of essence.	Essence, also called essence qi, is the refined nutritious substance that constitutes the form and maintains the life activity of the human body. The Kidney storing essence means that the Kidney has the function of storing and sealing essence qi.	Governing growth and development: The essence qi in the Kidney is the material basis and driving force of the Kidney governing growth and development. When the essence qi in the Kidney is sufficient, the growth and development of the body will be normal.	Insufficiency of the essence qi in the Kidney: retarded or delayed growth in infants or premature senility in adults.
		Dominating reproduction: The essence qi in the Kidney dominates reproduction by its action of generating *Tian gui*. When essence qi in the Kidney is sufficient, the reproductive function will be normal.	Deficiency of the essence qi in the Kidney: maldevelopment of the reproductive organs, sexual hypofunction and sterility.
		Governing generating marrow, supplementing brain and transforming blood: when the Kidney essence is sufficient, the brain marrow will be suffused, which is represented by being full of energy, prompt thinking, good hearing and eyesight. The essence generates the marrow and marrow transforms into blood. Thus if the essence is sufficient, the blood will be sufficient too.	Insufficiency of Kidney essence, empty brain marrow: amnesia, dull thinking, dizziness and tinnitus. Insufficiency of essence: deficiency of blood.
		Transforming and generating the Kidney yin and the Kidney yang: the Kidney yin moistens and nourishes the yin of each *zang-fu* organs and the Kidney yang warms the yang of each *zang-fu* organ. The Kidney yin and the Kidney yang are the root of the yin and yang of the human body and regulate the balance between yin and yang for the whole body.	Deficiency of the yin and yang of the Kidney: the physiological function of the Kidney declines and results in pathological changes of endogenous heat due to yin deficiency or endogenous cold due to yang deficiency. Therefore, it will result in the yin deficiency or yang deficiency of the rest of the *zang-fu* organs.

Continued

Function	Meaning	Physiological action	Main pathological changes
The Kidney dominates water.	It refers to the action of the Kidney that presides over and regulates the metabolic balance of water and fluids of the whole body.	The action of qi transformation of the Kidney on water and fluids includes two aspects: separating the clear and turbid and governing the opening and closing. The action of the Kidney governing the water and fluids is completed via the actions of the Kidney yang and the Kidney qi. The yang qi of the Kidney is sufficient and then the qi transformation will be normal. Thus the clear part of water and fluids ascends and is consolidated inside the body; the turbid part descends and is discharged outside the body, which keeps the metabolic balance of water and fluids.	Deficiency of yang qi of the Kidney: Dysfunction of qi transformation and metabolic disturbance of water and fluids. Unconsolidation of the Kidney due to qi deficiency- the Kidney opens more and closes less, so diuresis, enuresis, and urinary incontinence occur; disturbance in qi transformation- the Kidney closes more and opens less, so oliguria and edema occur.
The Kidney governs reception of air.	It refers to the action of the Kidney that receives the qi inhaled by the Lung and assists respiration.	The Kidney governing receiving qi is the embodiment of its actions of sealing and storing for the respiratory movements. When the essence qi in the Kidney is sufficient and its action of reception is normal, it can assist the Lung to receive qi, which manifests as normal, regular and harmonious respiration.	Insufficient of the essence qi in the Kidney and failure of the Kidney in receiving qi: shallow respiration with more expiration and less inspiration, and dyspnea when doing activities.

has the function of storing and holding essence qi. Essence, also named essence qi, is the primary substance that constitutes the form and maintains the life activity of the human body. (Regarding the concept of essence, see the Chapter of essence qi, blood and fluids) Because essence (essence qi) is stored in the Kidney, it is called the Kidney essence or the essence qi in the Kidney.

The source of Kidney essence includes two aspects; innate and acquired. The innate essence roots in the essential substance for reproduction of the parents, it is innate and stored in the Kidney. The acquired essence is the refined nutrition absorbed from water and food by the body after birth, and transported and distributed to the Kidney. Innate essence continuously supports acquired essence; acquired essence also continuously nourishes innate essence, so they depend on and promote each other to keep sufficient essence qi in the Kidney.

The primary functions of Kidney essence are: governing growth and development, dominating reproduction, generating marrow, supplementing the brain, transforming blood, transforming and generating the Kidney yin and Kidney yang etc. (Fig. 2-13)

a. Governing growth and development (Table 2-16)

Kidney essence (also called essence qi in the Kidney), is the material basis and energy of the Kidney governing growth and development. The law of life (birth, growth, strength, growing old and death) is closely related to the wax and wane of the essence qi in the Kidney. Along with an increase in age, all the physical changes and different physiological status changes emerging in the course of growth and development of the body are determined by the wax and wane of the essence qi in the Kidney. From birth to juvenile stage, the essence qi in the Kidney become vigorous gradually, hair grows faster and thicker, permenant teeth starts to replace baby teeth, bones grow, and the height of the body increases. In the adolescent stage, the essence qi in the Kidney become more vigorous, the upgrowth of the body nears maturity, the wisdom teeth grow, bones are fully grown, and the body is able to reproduce. In the adult stage, the essence qi in the Kidney is sufficient and prosperous, bones and muscles are strong, the body is robust and energized. In the senile stage, the essence qi in the Kidney decreases gradually, hair and teeth starts to fall out, the physique is weakened and the body loses reproductive capacity. Thereby, the

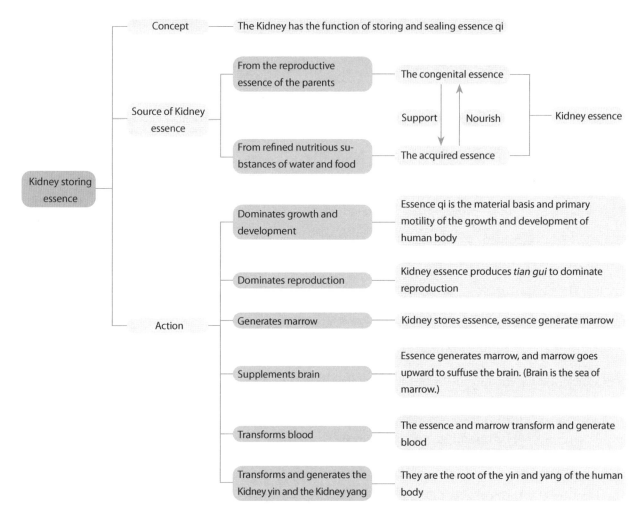

Fig. 2-13   Chart of the concept and action of the Kidney storing essence

Table 2-16   Relation of the essence qi in the Kidney to growth, development and reproduction

Essence qi in the Kidney	Age	Growth and development	*Tian gui*	Reproductive function
Comparatively vigorous and sufficient	Juvenile stage	Hair growth, dental transition, bone growth, increase in body height.	Not arrived yet	Naught
Gradually sufficient and vigorous	Adolescent stage	Being near maturation, growth of wisdom teeth, and full growth of bone.	Arrived	Begin to have the capability
Extremely sufficient and vigorous	Adult Stage	Bones and muscles are strong, the body is robust and energized.	Strong	Normal
Gradually decline and decrease	Senile stage	Falling out of hair and teeth, physical decline	Exhausted	Gradually lost

essence qi in the Kidney plays a very important role in the course of the growth and development of the human body.

If the essence qi in the Kidney is insufficient, it manifests as retarded or delayed growth of infants or premature senility of adults. (Table 2-15)

b. Dominating reproduction (Table 2-16)

The development of the reproductive organ of the human body and its reproductive capacity take the essence qi in the Kidney as their material basis. After birth, in company with the essence qi in the Kidney becoming more and more vigorous, *tian gui* (天癸) is generated in the adolescent stage. *Tian gui* is a sort of refined nutritious substances that is generated when the essence qi in the Kidney is sufficient to a certain degree. It has the action of promoting the development and maturation of the reproductive organs of the human body and maintaining reproductive functions. From the time the *tian gui* is generated, the menstruation of females and seminal fluid discharge of males starts, and the reproductive organs mature and are of reproductive capacity. Along with increase of age, from midage to senility, the essence qi in the Kidney gradually decreases. At the same time, gradually, *tian gui* attenuates, reproductive organs wilt, and reproductive function declines. Finally, *tian gui* is exhausted and reproductive capacity is lost. This fully indicates that the essence qi in the Kidney has a decisive effect on the reproductive function, and is the root of human reproduction.

If the essence qi in the Kidney is deficient, it can result in maldevelopment of the reproductive organs, sexual hypofunction and sterility. (Table 2-15)

The theory that the Kidney stores essence and governs growth, development and reproduction, plays a role in guiding the prevention and treatment of retarded growth, sterility, and impaired fetal development, as well as health preservation, health protection and prevention of decline of health, etc.

c. Generating marrow, supplementing brain and transforming blood (Table 2-15)

Marrow includes brain marrow, spinal cord marrow and bone marrow: all three marrows are transformed and generated by Kidney essence. The spinal cord connects upward with the brain. As soon as the essence is formed, the brain marrow is generated. Thus, if the Kidney essence is sufficient, the brain marrow will be suffused, which is demonstrated by being full of energy, with prompt thinking, and good hearing and eyesight. As well, if the Kidney essence is insufficient, the brain marrow will be empty and insufficient, amnesia; dull thinking, dizziness and tinnitus etc demonstrate that.

Kidney essence transforms blood, namely it is the action of the Kidney that generates essence and transforms blood. (See the section on Generation of the Blood)

Kidney essence can generate marrow, supplement the brain, and transform blood, but also has a close relation with the generation of teeth and hair, etc., since all the tissues and organs take the Kidney essence as their material basis. (Fig. 2-14)

d. Transformation and generation of the Kidney yin and the Kidney yang (Table. 2-15)

Internal Classic (*Nèi Jīng*) thinks that: "*At the beginning of human life, the essence is formed first.*" The essence is the origin of life activities. Among the physiological activities of the Kidney, the Kidney yin and the Kidney yang play central roles in the activities of life of the human body and they rooted in the essence qi of the Kidney. The essence qi of the Kidney is known as genuine essence and genuine qi. The Kidney yin and Kidney yang generated by the Kidney essence are known as genuine yin and genuine yang. Among the physiological activities of the Kidney, the Kidney yin has the actions of moistening, nourishing and inhibiting, and the Kidney yang has the actions of warming and promoting. The Kidney yin and Kidney yang depend on each other, interact, and mutually restrict, which keeps a harmonious balance to maintain the normal physiological function of the Kidney.

Comparison of the Kidney yin and Kidney yang to the yin and yang of the *zang-fu* organs: the Kidney yin (primordial yin, genuine yin, and genuine water) is the root of the yin fluid of

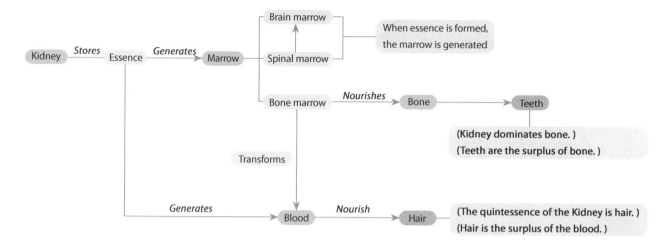

Fig. 2-14 Chart of relationship of Kidney to brain, marrow, bone, teeth, blood and hair

the human body and continually supplies and moistens the yin of each *zang-fu* organs. The Kidney yang (primordial yang, genuine yang, and genuine water) is the root of the yang fluid of the human body and continually supplies and warms the yang of each *zang-fu* organs. Therefore, if the Kidney yin and the Kidney yang are sufficient, the yin and yang of *zang-fu* organs is sufficient too. Thus it is said that the Kidney yin and Kidney yang are the root of the yin and yang of the *zang-fu* organs of the human body. In comparison, the essence qi, yin and yang in the Kidney, besides the innate part, also depend on the nourishment, transformation and generation of the essence qi, yin and yang of the *zang-fu* organs, so that they can keep their sufficiency. Therefore, the Kidney yin and Kidney yang interact with the yin and yang of the *zang-fu* organs of the human body.

Thus the insufficiency of the Kidney yin or yang not only appears as yin deficiency or yang deficiency of the Kidney itself, but also results in yin deficiency or yang deficiency of other *zang-fu* organs. Long-term yin or yang insufficiency of other *zang-fu* organs can also involve the Kidney and waste the essence qi, yin and yang of the Kidney. Therefore, there is the saying "The thorough impairment of the five *zang* organs would surely involve the Kidney."

Plain Questions: *Discussion on Six-Plus-Six System and the Manifestations of the Viscera* (*Sù Wèn: Liù Jié Zàng Xiàng Lùn*, 素问·六节藏象论) says: "The Kidney governs hibernation, is the root of

sealing and store, and is the site of essence."

Miraculous Pivot: *Chapter The Diseases Caused by Spiritual Activities* (*Líng Shū: Běn Shén*, 灵枢·本神) says: "The substance enabling the development of the human body is called the essence of life," and "The Kidney stores essence."

Miraculous Pivot: *Chapter The Dredge of Qi* (*Líng Shū: Jué Qì*, 灵枢·决气) says: "When the yin and yang essences approach each other, they combine and form a new body, the substance generated before the body is called the essence."

Plain Questions: *Chapter Discussion on Important Ideas in the Golden Chamber* (*Sù Wèn: Jīn Guì Zhēn Yán Lùn*, 素问·金匮真言论): "Essence is the root of life."

Miraculous Pivot: *Chapter On Channels* (*Líng Shū: Jīng Mài*, 灵枢·经脉) says: "At the beginning of human life, the essence is formed first, and then the brain marrow is generated."

Plain Questions: *Chapter Ancient Ideas on Flow to Preserve Natural Healthy Energy* (*Sù Wèn: Shàng Gǔ Tiān Zhēn Lùn*, 素问·上古天真论) says: "For a woman, her Kidney qi becomes prosperous and her teeth begin to change at the age of seven. At the age of fourteen, Tian gui begins to appear, and the Ren Channel and Penetrating vessel are vigorous in function. Then she begins to have menstruation and is able go conceive a baby. At the age of twenty-one, as Kidney qi is in vigor, the wisdom teeth begin to grow and the body has fully developed. At the age of twenty-eight, her musculature and bones become strong, and her hair grows long. Her body has reached the summit of development. At the age of thirty-five, the Yangming Channel starts to decline, her face begins to wither and her hair starts to be lost. At the age of forty-two, as the three Yang Channels are deficient in both blood and qi, her countenance becomes faded and her hair begins to turn grey. At the age of forty-nine, as both the Ren Channel and Penetrating vessel become deficient and menstruation stops, she becomes physically feeble and is no longer able to conceive a baby.

For a man, at the age of eight, his Kidney qi becomes prosperous and his teeth begin to change. At the age of sixteen, as Kidney qi is abundant and Tian gui occurs, he begins to experience spermatic emission. If he has copulated with a woman at this period, he can have a baby. At the age of twenty-four, his Kidney qi is full, his musculature and bones become strong, the wisdom teeth appear and his whole body is fully developed. At the age of thirty-two, his musculature and bones are well developed and are very strong. At the age of forty, as Kidney qi declines, his hair begins to fall out and his teeth start to wither. At the age of forty-eight, Yang qi in the upper part of the body collapses, his face starts to wither and his hair begins to turn grey. At the age of fifty-six, as his Liver qi declines, his musculature becomes inflexible. With the exhaustion of Tian gui and the reduction of Kidney qi, his Kidneys are weakened and his body becomes very weak, his teeth and hair begin to fall out. The Kidney controls water. It receives and stores essence from the five zang organs and the six fu organs. Thus only when the five zang organs and the six fu organs

are vigorous can the Kidney have enough essence to discharge. When the five zang organs have declined, the bones become weak and the Tian gui is exhausted, his hair turns grey and his body becomes clumsy, then he walks with difficulty and is unable to have a baby."

Plain Questions: Chapter Discussion on Flaccidity (Sù Wèn: Wěi Lùn, 素问·痿论) says: "The Kidney dominates the bone marrow of the whole body."

Origin of Medicine: Chapter Treatise on Inter-generation and Inter-restraint among Five Phases (Yī Yuán: Wǔ Xíng Shēng Kè Lùn, 医原·五行生克论) says: "The genuine yang qi in the Kidney warms, nourishes and communicates upwards with the yang of all the zang-fu organs. By the steaming and transporting action of the genuine yang-qi of the Kidney, the genuine yin-qi of the Kidney communicates with the yin of all the zang-fu organs."

Attached Supplementary to the Classified Classic: Chapter Great Treasures (Lèi Jīng Fù Yì: Dà Bǎo Lùn, 类经附翼·大宝论) says: "The generation of all things depends on yang essence; the growth of all the things depends on yin essence, they are called the original yang and original yin, and also named genuine yang and genuine yin."

Classified Differentiation of Luxiantang (Lǚ Shān Táng Lèi Biàn, 侣山堂类辨) says: "The Kidney is a water zang organ, dominates essence and transforms blood."

(2) The Kidney dominates water (Table 2-15)

The Kidney dominating water refers to the action

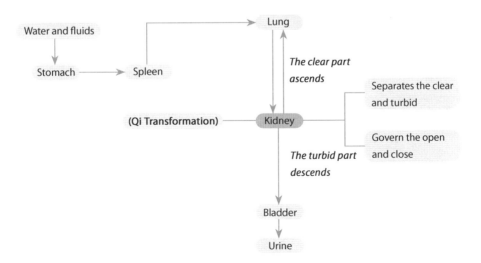

Fig. 2-15 **The Chart of the function of the Kidney that governs water**

of the Kidney that presides over and regulates the metabolic balance of water and fluids of the whole body. Therefore, it is known that the Kidney is a "water *zang* organ".

The action of the Kidney that dominates water is also known as the vaporizing action or the qi transforming action of the Kidney on the water and fluids. This include two primary aspects:

a. The qi transformation of the Kidney penetrates the entire metabolic course of water and fluids. The entire metabolic process of water and fluids includes the absorption and distribution of water and fluids, and the excretion of turbid fluids of the body, completed by the combined actions of the *zang-fu* organs of the Spleen, Lung, Kidney and *San Jiao*. Yet, all these actions depend on the qi transformation of the Kidney, therefore, the metabolism of water and fluids can be kept in a harmonious balance.

b. It refers to the action of the Kidney itself that distributes and excretes water and fluids. The water and fluids utilized by the *zang-fu* organs of the human body come to the Kidney eventually. Through the qi transformation of the Kidney, the Kidney separates the clear part and excretes the turbid part of water and fluids, and governs opening and closing. The water and fluids flowing into the Kidney are a mixture of the clear and turbid parts, and the Kidney separates the clear part (useful part) from the turbid part (useless part) of the water and fluids. It is the action of the Kidney that separates the clear and turbid. Opening (*Kai*) means to afford unobstructed water passage and Closing (*He*) means to bar access to the water passage. After the clear and turbid part of the water and fluids are separated from each other in the Kidney, the action of closing can lift the clear part and keep it inside the body; the action of opening can drop the turbid part and excrete it outside the body. It is the action of the Kidney that governs the opening and closing (Fig. 2-15). The action of the Kidney itself to distribute and excrete water and fluids mostly refers to the action of the Kidney that secretes and excretes urine.

The action of qi transformation of the Kidney on water and fluids is also completed via the actions of the Kidney yang and the Kidney qi. The clear part of the water and fluids is warmed by Kidney yang and consolidated by Kidney qi, which keeps it inside the body, so it is called "*He* (closing)"; the turbid part of water and fluids is warmed by Kidney yang and promoted by the Kidney qi, which drops it and forms urine which is discharged outside the body, so it is named "*Kai* (opening)". Therefore, the metabolic balance of water and fluids in the human body is maintained. (Fig. 2-16)

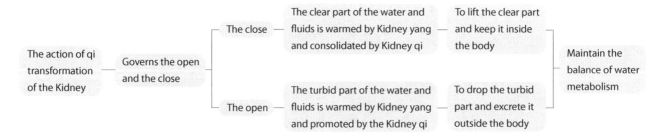

Fig. 2-16   The conclusive chart of the action of Kidney yin and Kidney yang in the course of vaporization of water and fluids

Therefore, if the yang qi of the Kidney is deficient and qi transformation is abnormal, it can result in pathological changes of metabolic disturbances of water and fluids. Unconsolidation of the Kidney due to qi deficiency (disability to consolidate) results in the Kidney opening more and closing less, which manifests as diuresis, enuresis, and urinary incontinence. Disturbance in qi transformation (disability to impulse) results in the Kidney closing more and opening less, which manifests as oliguria and edema. (Table 2-15)

Plain Questions: Chapter Discussion on Disharmony (Sù Wèn: Nì Tiáo Lùn, 素问·逆调论*)* says: "*The Kidney is a water zang organ, and dominates water and fluids.*"

Plain Questions: Chapter Discussion on Water and Heat Diseases (Sù Wèn: Shuǐ Rè Xuè Lùn, 素问·水热穴论*)* says: "*The Kidney is the pass of the Stomach. Dysfunction of the pass will result in accumulation of water, and manifests as a disorder of water that will overflows upwards and downwards to the skin. Therefore, edema occurs: edema is sickness caused by the accumulation of water.*"

(3) The Kidney governs receiving qi (Table 2-15)

The Kidney governing receiving qi refers to the action of the Kidney to receive the qi inhaled by the Lung and assist respiration.

The Lung governs the respiration of the body. Turbid qi is exhaled by the diffusing action of the Lung qi, and clear qi is inhaled by the purifying and descending action of the Lung qi. However, it also needs the reception of the Kidney to keep the depth of inspiration and to prevent shallow respiration. Therefore, it is known that "the Lung is the dominator of qi; and the Kidney is the root of qi."

The Kidney governing reception of air is the embodiment of its action of sealing and storing in the respiratory movement. When the essence qi in the Kidney is sufficient and its action of reception is powerful, it can help the Lung receive qi, which manifests as normal, regular and harmonious respiration. When the essence qi in the Kidney is deficient and its action of reception is forceless, it can't help the Lung to receive qi, which manifests as pathological changes of the Kidney failing to grasp qi in terms of shallow respiration with more expiration and less inspiration, and dyspnea when doing activities. (Table 2-15)

Treatment of Different Kinds of Diseases: Chapter Panting Syndrome (Lèi Zhèng Zhì Cái: Chuǎn Zhèng, 类证治裁·喘证*)* says: "*The Lung is the dominator of qi and the Kidney is the root of qi. The Lung governs exhalation, and the Kidney governs inhalation or receiving qi. Yin and yang communicate, and then breathing will be harmonious and normal.*"

Danger Zone of Medicine: Section Qi in Miscellaneous Diseases (Yī Biān: Zá Zhèng, 医碥·杂症*)* says: "*Qi roots in Kidney and pertains to Kidney, so the Kidney governs receiving qi, its breathing is very deep.*"

② The relation of the Kidney to the body constituents, sense organs and orifices

(1) The Kidney dominates bone (Table 2-17)

Bone generally refers to the skeleton of the human body. The bones constitute the bracket of the human body that supports the body, shields viscera and connects with sinews and muscles to perform kinetic actions.

Table 2-17   Relationship of the Kidney to brain, marrow, bone, teeth, blood and hair

Foundation of the relationship	Physiological significance	Pathological significance
The Kidney stores essence, generates marrow and nourishes the bone	When the essence and marrow are sufficient, then the skeleton is stout and firm and not easily fractured (The Kidney dominates bone)	Insufficiency of Kidney essence and empty bone marrow: retarded growth of the bone, fragility of the bones which are easily broken in elders
Kidney essence nourishes teeth	If the Kidney essence is sufficient and the growth and development of teeth is normal, the teeth will be stout and firm (Teeth are the branch of the Kidney)	Insufficiency of Kidney essence: retarded growth of teeth in infants, teeth looseness and loss in adults
The Kidney essence transforms to blood; and the essence and blood nourish the hair	When the essence and blood are sufficient, then the hair is jet black and lustrous (the hair is the surplus of the blood)	Insufficiency of essence and blood: limp and sparse hair with early loss and premature grey (The hair is the external sign of the Kidney)

The Kidney dominating bone refers to the normal growth and development, and the exertion of the actions of the bone demand the supplementation and nourishment by Kidney essence. The Kidney stores essence, essence generates marrow, and bone marrow or medulla nourishes the bone. Therefore, if the Kidney essence is sufficient, the medullae is suffused, the bone will be nourished by the medulla, and the skeleton will be stout and firm and not easily fractured, and the movement of the limbs will be forceful. If the kidney essence is insufficient and bone marrow is empty, it will result in malnourishment of the bones and the pathological changes of retarded growth of bone, delayed fontanel closure, forceless and soft bones in infant, as well as fragile bones that are easily broken in elders.

Teeth are the surplus of bone, share the same source with bone and are supplemented and nourished by Kidney essence. (Fig. 2-14) Therefore, it is known that the teeth are "the branch of the Kidney and the root of bone". Therefore, the retarded growth of teeth in child, and teeth looseness and loss in adults, are both related to the insufficiency of Kidney essence. (Table 2-17)

(2) The quintessence of the Kidney appears on the hair (Table 2-17)

The growth of hair depends on the nourishment of the blood, so it is known that "the hair is the surplus of the blood." However, the vital force of the hair is rooted in the Kidney. The Kidney stores essence and essence transforms to blood. Thus if the essence and blood are vigorous, the hair will be thick and lustrous, so, it is said that the Kidney's "quintessence appears on the hair". The growth and slough, luster and wilt of the hair always reflect the wax and wane of the Kidney essence, so, it is said that "the hair is the external sign of the Kidney." In the stage of adolescence and postadolescence, when essence and blood are vigorous, the hair is jet black and lustrous. In the senile stage, the essence and blood are insufficient and begin to decline, and hair is grey and begins to fall out. These are normal physiological phenomena. In a long-standing case where hair is sparse, withered and falling out; or if a person is prematurely senile and his or her hair is withered, prematurely falling out and becoming grey, then this is related to the insufficiency of the Kidney essence.

Plain Questions: Chapter Discussion on the Elucidation of Five-Qi (Sù Wèn: Xuān Míng Wǔ Qì Piān, 素问·宣明五气篇*) says: "Among the five dominances of five zang organs…that of the Kidney is bone."*

Plain Questions: Chapter Major Discussion on the Theory of Yin and Yang and the Corresponding Relationships Among All the Things in Nature (Sù Wèn: Yīn Yáng Yìng Xiàng Dà Lùn, 素问·阴阳应象大论*) says: "Kidney generates bone and marrow."*

Plain Questions: Chapter Discussion on the Abstruse Theory (Sù Wèn: Jiě Jīng Wēi Lùn, 素问·解精微论*) says: "Marrow is that which fills the cavity of the bone."*

Plain Questions: Discussion on Six-Plus-Six System and the Manifestations of the Viscera (Sù Wèn: Liù Jié Zàng Xiàng Lùn, 素问·六节藏象论*) says: "Kidney…its quintessence appears on the hair and is in charge of nourishing bone."*

Plain Questions: Chapter Discussion on Various Relationships Concerning the Five Zang-Organs (Sù Wèn: Wǔ Zàng Shēng Chéng Piān, 素问·五脏生成篇*) says: "The Kidney is related to the bone, and its quintessence is reflected by the hair."*

(3) The Kidney opens at the ears and the two lower orifices (Table 2-18)

a. The Kidney opens at the ears

Ears are hearing organs and dominate hearing. The Kidney opening at the ears primarily means that whether the hearing is normal or not is closely related to the wax and wane of the Kidney essence. This means that the ears dominating hearing depends on the supplement and nourishment of the Kidney essence. The two ears connect with the brain, and the sounds being heard are transmitted to the brain. Therefore, if the Kidney essence is sufficient and the sea of the medulla is nourished, hearing will be sensitive. If the Kidney essence is insufficient, it will result in malnourishment of the sea of the medulla and manifest as hearing loss, deafness, or tinnitus. Hearing loss in elders is caused by the

Table 2-18 Relationship of the Kidney to the ears and the two lower orifices

Relationship	Foundation of link	Physiological significance	Pathological significance
Kidney and the ears	The Kidney governs the storage of essence.	When the Kidney essence is sufficient and the sea of themedulla is filled, the hearing will be sensitive.	When Kidney essence is insufficient and the sea of the medulla is empty: hearing loss, deafness, and tinnitus.
Kidney and the external genitals	The Kidney dominates reproduction	The Kidney essence is sufficient and generates *Tian gui*, and then the reproductive function will be normal.	Kidney essence deficiency: reproductive hypofunction, for instance, impotence, premature ejaculation, spermatorrhea, irregular menstruation, cold uterus and sterility.
	The Kidney dominates water.	When the qi transformation of water and fluids by the Kidney is normal, then the secretion and excretion of the urine will be normal.	Abnormal qi transformation of the Kidney: abnormal discharge of the urine, for instance, frequent urination, urinary incontinence, enuresis and blocked urination.
Kidney and the anus (posterior lower orifice)	The essence qi, yin and yang in the Kidney	When the Kidney yin and Kidney yang are sufficient, they can moisten and warm the bowel *fu* organ, and then defecation will be normal.	Deficiency of Kidney yin, exhaustion of fluid in the intestine: constipation. Deficiency of Kidney yang qi: difficult defecation or fecal incontinence, chronic diarrhea.

insufficiency and decline of the Kidney essence. (Table 2-18)

Plain Questions: *Chapter Major Discussion on the Theory of Yin and Yang and the Corresponding Relationships Among All the Things in Nature* (*Sù Wèn: Yīn Yáng Yìng Xiàng Dà Lùn*, 素问·阴阳应象大论) says: "*The Kidney...opens at the ears.*"

Miraculous Pivot: *Chapter The Length of Channels* (*Líng Shū: Mài Dù*, 灵枢·脉度) says: "*The Kidney qi communicates with the two ears, so if the Kidney qi is cooperative, the ears can hear the five sounds.*"

Miraculous Pivot: *Chapter On the Four Seas* (*Líng Shū: Hǎi Lùn*, 灵枢·海论) says: "*If the sea of the marrow is insufficient, it will result in vertigo and tinnitus.*"

b. The Kidney opens at the two lower orifices

Two lower orifices refer to the external genitalia and anus. "External genitalia" is the generic term for the exterior genitals and urethra, related to the actions of reproduction and urination. The anus (the posterior lower orifice), is also called the door of draff, and is the passway for discharging feces and related to the action of defecation.

The relationship between the Kidney and the genital orhifices: we can explain the theory through the function of the Kidney dominating reproduction and water. The Kidney dominates reproduction, so when the essence qi in the Kidney is filled to a certain degree, *tian gui* will be generated. *Tian gui* promotes the maturation of the reproductive organs and maintains reproductive functions. If the essence qi in the Kidney is deficient, it can result in maldevelopment of the reproductive organs, or reproductive incompetence or hypofunction.

The Kidney dominates water. The qi transformation of the Kidney completes the work of the secretion and discharge of urine. If the yang qi of the Kidney is insufficient and the qi transformation is abnormal, pathological changes of frequent urination, urinary incontinence, enuresis and blocked urination will occur.

Relationship between the Kidney and anus: this is related to defecation and mainly refers to the action of transportation of the Large Intestine. However, it is also closely related to the Kidney yin and Kidney yang. The Kidney yin and Kidney yang are the yin and yang of the *zang-fu* organs of the human body. The moistening action of the Kidney yin and the warming action of the Kidney yang is beneficial to the transportation of the Large Intestine, and defecation. When the Kidney yin is insufficient and the fluid in the intestine is exhausted, the constipation will occur. When the yang qi of the Kidney is deficient and declined and fails to warm and move, difficulties will occur in defecation. If the Kidney qi is weak and fails to consolidate, it manifests as fecal incontinence and chronic diarrhea that is difficult to be controlled. (Table 2-18)

Plain Questions: Chapter Discussion on Important Ideas in the Golden Chamber (Sù Wèn: Jīn Guì Zhēn Yán Lùn, 素问·金匮真言论) says: *"The Kidney opens at the two lower orifices (genital orifice and anus)."*

③ Relationship of the Kidney to the five minds and five fluids

(1) The mind of the Kidney is fear
Fear, or dread, is a kind of mental and emotional activity of being afraid or scared. The essence qi in the Kidney transforms and generates fear, therefore, it is known that fear is the mind of the Kidney. Excessive fear may impair the Kidney and result in unconsolidation of the Kidney

qi and pathological changes of the qi being discharged downward. (See the section on seven emotions)

Plain Questions: Chapter Major Discussion on the Theory of Yin and Yang and the Corresponding Relationships Among All the Things in Nature (Sù Wèn: Yīn Yáng Yìng Xiàng Dà Lùn, 素问·阴阳应象大论) says: *"Kidney... its mind is fear."*

(2) The fluid of the Kidney is spit
Spit is the thick part in the sputa and is also called spittle. Spit has the actions of moistening the oral cavity, dissolving and mixing food, and nourishing the Kidney essence. Spit is transformed and generated by the Kidney essence, goes upward along the Kidney channel of foot *shaoyin* via the throat, through the root of the tongue, and comes out under the tongue. Thus, it is said that spit is the fluid of the Kidney (Fig. 2-17). Spit is transformed by the Kidney essence, so if one spits for a long time or suffers from profuse spit; it is easy to waste the Kidney essence. Thus, there comes the saying that to swallow the spit can nourish the Kidney essence.

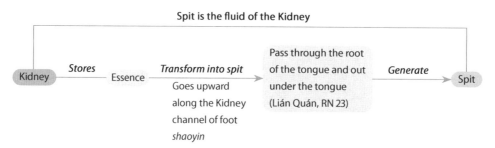

Fig. 2-17 Chart of relationship between Kidney and spit

Spit and saliva are the fluids secreted in the mouth and known as sputa; they are closely related to the actions of digestion and absorption of the Spleen and Stomach. There are differences between them: saliva refers to slobber, is relatively dilute and clear, overflows and dribbles from the angles of the mouth, and is generated by the Spleen. Spit refers to spittle, is relatively thick, is generated under the tongue and is spit out from the mouth, and is transformed by the Kidney essence.

Plain Questions: Chapter Discussion on the Elucidation of Five-Qi (Sù Wèn: Xuān Míng Wǔ Qì

Piān, 素问·宣明五气篇) says: *"Among the five fluids transformed by the five zang organs... that of the Kidney is spit."*

Miraculous Pivot: Chapter On Channels (Líng Shū: Jīng Mài, 灵枢·经脉) says: *"The Kidney channel of foot shaoyin... goes upward via the throat, through the root of the tongue."*

④ Physiological Properties of the Kidney

(1) The Kidney governs sealing and storing
Sealing and storing means hold in and keep. The Kidney is the root of congenital constitution and the root of life. It is a *zang* organ of water and

fire, stores genuine yin and contains genuine yang. The Kidney governs storing essence, sicne the essence is suitable to be stored but not discharged. The Kidney dominates the fire from the life gate, and the fire is suitable to be hidden but not exposed. Therefore, *Internal Classic (Nèi Jīng)* calls the Kidney *"the root of sealing and storing"*. The physiological property of the Kidney governs sealing and storing embodied by its actions of storing essence, dominating water and grasping qi. Pathological changes of the Kidney like spermatorrhea, premature ejaculation, morbid leukorrhea, threatened abortion, enuresis, urinary incontinence, and asthma of deficient type are mainly caused by deficiency of Kidney qi and dysfunction of the Kidney in sealing and storing. According to the physiological property of the Kidney governing sealing and storing, predecessors put forward the academic viewpoints that the Kidney essence can't be reduced and the fire from the life gate can't be cut, so the Kidney has no excess to be reduced for the treatment of Kidney diseases.

Plain Questions: Discussion on Six-Plus-Six System and the Manifestations of the Viscera (Sù Wèn: Liù Jié Zàng Xiàng Lùn, 素问·六节藏象论) says: *"The Kidney dominates hibernation, is the root of sealing and storing, and is the site of essence."*

(2) The Kidney communicates with and responds to the winter qi

The Kidney qi communicating with and responding to the winter qi means that the Kidney relates to winter, coldness, closure and storage. In winter, all creatures in nature respond to the frigid climate and are in the stage of being static, closed and hidden to living through the wintertime. The Kidney is the *zang* organ of water, stores essence, and is the root of sealing and storing, so the Kidney responds to the winter. Winter is a season of frigid climate, so the rule of life should conform to the season and preserve the Kidney qi.

Plain Questions: Discussion on Six-Plus-Six System and the Manifestations of the Viscera (Sù Wèn: Liù Jié Zàng Xiàng Lùn, 素问·六节藏象论) says: *"Kidney is shaoyin within yin and communicates with winter qi."*

Appendix: The Life Gate (*Ming Men*, 命门)

The earliest records of the term *Ming Men* can be seen in *Internal Classic (Nèi Jīng)* and means the eyes. *Classic of Questioning (Nàn Jīng)* first took *Ming Men* as internal *zang* organs. The physicians in the *Ming* and *Qing* Dynasties did in-depth research on *Ming Men* and put forward different kinds of views, and created the Theory of *Ming Men*. Since then, the significance of *Ming Men* has attracted extensive attention.

The location of *Ming Men*: there were theories that the right Kidney was *Ming Men*, that *Ming Men* was the general name for both Kidneys, and that *Ming Men* was located in the region between the two Kidneys. [For detailed information, please refer to ancient books like *Classic of Questioning (Nàn Jīng)*.]

The function of *Ming Men*: there were theories of *Ming Men* dominating fire, *Ming Men* dominating water and fire, and *Ming Men* bing the qi stored between the Kidneys. [For detailed information, please refer to the ancient books like *Classic of Questioning (Nàn Jīng)*.]

Different physicians have different views of *Ming Men*, but all of them believe that *Ming Men* is intimately related to the Kidney; *Ming Men* is the gate of life, the root of life. The Kidney is the root of congenital constitution, dominates reproduction and is the source of life. The Kidney is the *zang* organ of water and fire. *Ming Men* has both water and the fire. Therefore, it can be concluded: fire from the gate of life is equivalent to Kidney yang; the water from the gate of life is equivalent to Kidney yin. The ancient physicians put forward *"Ming Men"* theories for emphasizing the importance of the Kidney yin and the Kidney yang in life activities.

Miraculous Pivot: Chapter The Beginning and End of the Channel (Líng Shū: Gēn Jié, 灵枢·根结) says: *"The Bladder channel of foot taiyang begins from the zhì yīn point (BL 67) and ends at Ming Men (actually it refers to the jīng míng point, BL 1), Ming Men means the eyes."*

Classic of Questioning: The Thirty-ninth Question (Nàn Jīng: Sān Shí Jiǔ Nàn, 难经·三十九难) says: *"It is said that the Kidney has two organs:*

the left one is the Kidney and the right one is Ming Men. Ming Men is the house where the spirit and essence resides. It is the place where the male stores essence and an organ that connects with uterus in female. The qi of Ming Men communicates with the Kidney."

Elementary Medicine: Chapter Mnemonic Rhyme of Ming Men (Yī Xué Rù Mén: Mìng Mén Fù, 医学入门·命门赋) [written by Li Ting (李梴) in *Ming* Dynasty] says: "Ming Men is located in the right Kidney, its collateral passes roundabout through the Bladder and connects upward with the Pericardium where the diaphragm connects with it transversely and fat distributes. It is accompanied by the left Kidney to store genuine essence and is different according to man, woman, yin and yang. It assists the monarch fire to maintain the original qi. Whether a disease will recover or get worse depends on the Ming Men."

Medical Subject under Discussion: Chapter Some Medical Questions (Yī Xué Zhèng Zhuàn: Yī Xué Huò Wèn, 医学正传·医学或问) [written by Yu Tuan (虞抟) in the *Ming* Dynasty] says: "The two Kidneys are the root of the genuine original qi and the pass of life. Although they are the water zang organs, ministerial fire is contained in them, like the dragon fire in the water that is activated because of the motion of the fire. I think that Ming Men is the generic name for the two Kidneys, the Ming Men point just like the pivot in the door that governs opening and closing."

Attached Supplementary to the Classified Classic: Section Differentiation of San Jiao, Pericardium Collateral and Ming Men, Chapter Records of Proofs (Lèi Jīng Fù Yì: Sān Jiāo Bāo Luò Mìng Mén Biàn, Qiú Zhèng Lù, 类经附翼·求正录·三焦包络命门辨) [written by Zhang Jie-bin(张介宾) in the *Ming* Dynasty] says: "Ming Men is the generic name of the two Kidneys and the two Kidneys belong to Ming Men. Thus, Ming Men is the residence of water and fire, the mansion of yin and yang, the sea of essence qi and the whole of life and death."

Key Link of Medicine: Chapter Discussion on Twelve Officials in the Internal Classic (Yī Guàn: Nèi Jīng Shí Èr Guān Lùn, 医贯·内经十二官论) [written by Zhao Xian-ke (赵献可) in the *Ming* Dynasty] says: "Ming Men is located in the middle of two Kidneys that are 1.5 cun lateral to the midline of the body. *Internal Classic (Nèi Jīng)* says: 'There is

a xiaoxin in the place next to the seventh vertebrae', it is named after Ming Men and is the genuine monarch and owner. It is the taiji of the whole body and can't be seen. The place between the two Kidneys is where it resides." It also says: "Gallop light…there is only one tongue of flame in it. If the fire is vigorous, it moves faster; if the fire is weak, it moves slower; if the fire is extinguished, it stops moving… So Ming Men is called the gate of life, and the fire from Ming Men is the most precious treasure of the body."

Secret Records in a Stone Room (Shí Shì Mì Lù, 石室秘录) [written by Chen Shi-duo (陈士铎) in the *Qing* Dynasty] says: "Ming Men is the congenital fire."

Jing-yue's Complete Works: Section Supplementary Discussion on the Life Gate, Chapter Chuan Zhong Lu (Jīng Yuè Quán Shū: Mìng Mén Yú Yì, Chuán Zhōng Lù, 景岳全书·传忠录·命门余义) [written by Zhang Jie-bin(张介宾) in the *Ming* Dynasty] says: "Ming Men is the root of the original qi, the house of water and fire. The yin qi of the five zang organs is nourished by it; the yang qi of the five zang organs is pushed by it."

Remainder of Medical Lemma: Chapter Illustration of Ming Men (Yī Zhǐ Xù Yú: Mìng Mén Tú Shuō, 医旨绪余·命门图说) [written by Sun Yi-kui (孙一奎) in the *Ming* Dynasty] says: "Qin Yue-ren (秦越人) also said that 'the active qi between the two Kidneys is the life of the human body, is the root of the five zang organs and six fu organs. It is the root of the twelve regular channels and the gate of respiration, it is the origin of the San Jiao.' The meaning of Ming Men should originate from this…Ming Men is the active qi between the two Kidneys, it is neither water nor fire, it is the pivot of transformation and generation, is the root of yin and yang, it is the congenital taiji."

Section 2 The Six-*fu* Organs

The six-*fu* organs are the generic name for the Gallbladder, Stomach, Small Intestine, Large Intestine, Bladder and *San Jiao*. Their common physiological function is to "transport, digest, and absorb water and food", their physiological features are "*discharge without storage*", and "*being filled instead of being substantial".*

In the course of receiving, transporting and digesting water and food, the actions of the six-*fu* organs seem like six doors of the alimentary tract where water, food and residue must pass, and they are named the *"seven important portals, 七冲门"* in *Classic of Questioning (Nàn Jīng).*

The six-*fu* organs transport and digest water and food, and have the features of being in favor of being unobstructed and descending, therefore, there is the saying that *"The six-fu organs take being unobstructed and descent as their action."*

Plain Questions: Chapter Different Discussion on the Five-zang Organs (Sù Wèn: Wǔ Zàng Bié Lùn, 素问·五脏别论) says: *"The six-fu organs transport and transform water and food but do not store them, so the six-fu organs can be filled but not substantialized. Why it is so? That's because after the water and food are taken into the mouth, the Stomach is filled but the intestine is empty. When food enters the intestine, the intestine is filled but the Stomach is empty."*

Classic of Questioning: The Forty-fourth Question (Nàn Jīng: Sì Shí Sì Nàn, 难经·四十四难) says: *"Where are the seven important portals? Lips are the feimen (flying portal, 飞门), teeth are the humen (door portal, 户门), the epiglottis is the ximen (portal of breath, 吸门), the Stomach is the penmen (portal of diaphragm, cardia, 贲门), the lower port of Stomach is youmen (deep portal, pylorus, 幽门), the conjunction of the large and Small Intestine is the lanmen (terminal portal, appendix, 阑门), the lowest port is pomen (portal of draff, anus, 魄门)."*

The Gallbladder

The Gallbladder (胆) is located at the right hypochondrium, connects with the Liver and attaches to the left lobe of the Liver. The Gallbladder and the Liver connect with each other via channels and have and exterior and interior relationship.

The Gallbladder is a cyst-like and hollow organ and also is named cholecyst. The bile is stored in the Gallbladder, and is also called the extract succus or clear fluid, and therefore, the Gallbladder also is named after "the palace of storing essence in the middle", "the palace of the middle clear", and "the palace of cleaning".

Like other *fu*-organs, the Gallbladder is hollow in shape, and it also stores bile that can assist digestion, which indicates that it shares the common physiological function of the six-*fu* organs. Thus, the Gallbladder is one of the six-*fu* organs. However, the Gallbladder stores the bile, which is similar to the functional characteristic of "storing essence qi" of the five-*zang* organs. There is no food or residue to pass through the Gallbladder, which is different from other *fu*-organs, so the Gallbladder also belongs to the extraordinary *fu*-organs.

The main physiological functions of the Gallbladder are to store and excrete bile and dominate making decisions (Table 2-19).

Table 2-19   **The physiological functions of the Gallbladder**

Gallbladder		
Actions	Storing and excreting bile	Dominating making a decision
Physiological action	Bile originates from the Liver and is stored in the Gallbladder. The free coursing of the Gallbladder-qi promotes the excretion of the bile into the intestine to assist with the digestion of water and food.	To judge things and make decisions. It is related to the courage, bravery, and timidity of people.
Main pathological changes	Imbalance in the storage and excretion of bile: anorexia, fullness in the abdomen, diarrhea.	Deficiency of Gallbladder-qi: abnormal mental activities like timidity, being easily frightened.

① Storing and Excreting Bile

Bile originates from the Liver and is transformed

and generated by the surplus qi of the Liver. The bile converges into and is stored in the

Gallbladder after its generation. Through the free coursing action of the Liver, bile is excreted into the intestine to assist with the digestion of food.

If the actions of the Gallbladder of storing and excreting bile malfunction, it will affect the transportation and transformation of the Spleen and Stomach, and symptoms of dyspepsia will occur in terms of the anorexia, fullness in the abdomen, diarrhea or constipation. If damp-heat accumulates in the Liver and Gallbladder and results in the failure of the two organs in free coursing, the bile will overflow and infiltrate the skin, and then jaundice will occur, and manifests as yellow sclera, yellow skin of the whole body and yellow urine. If the qi of the Gallbladder is not free and the qi dynamic reverses, symptoms of bitter taste, nausea, and vomiting of yellowish green bitter fluid will occur.

② Dominating Decision-making

The Gallbladder controlling the power of decision-making refers to the action of the Gallbladder that judges things and makes decisions, among mental and conceptual activities.

The action of the Gallbladder in controlling the power of decision-making plays a role in preventing and relieving the effects of negative stimulation on the mind, maintaining the normal circulation of qi and blood, and ensuring harmonious relationships among the *zang-fu* organs. The person with brave and stout Gallbladder qi easily recovers from the effects of terrifying stimulations on the mind, and so the vicious effects become relatively small. The person with deficient Gallbladder qi is easy to suffer pathological changes of timidity, being easily frightened, insomnia and dreamfulness etc. Thus, the action of the Gallbladder controlling the power of decision-making is related to the courage, braveness and timidity of people.

Miraculous Pivot: Chapter On Acupoints (Líng Shū: Běn Shū, 灵枢・本输): "*The Gallbladder is a clean hollow organ that rejects all the turbids.*"

Classic of Questioning: The Forty-second Question (Nàn Jīng: Sì Shí Èr Nàn, 难经・四十二难) says: "*The Gallbladder is attached to the left lobe of the Liver, its weight is 3 liang (两) 2 zhu (铢), and it contain bile three he.*"

Precious Mirror of Oriental Medicine (Dōng Yī Bǎo Jiàn, 东医宝鉴) says: "*The surplus qi of the Liver overflows into the Gallbladder in where the surplus qi converges and forms the extract (bile).*"

Plain Questions: Chapter Discussion on the Secret Classics Stored in Royal Library (Sù Wèn: Líng Lán Mì Diǎn Lùn, 素问・灵兰秘典论) says: "*The Gallbladder is the official of righteousness, and it is where decisions are made.*"

The Stomach

The Stomach (胃) is located in the upper part of the abdominal cavity. It connects upwards with the esophagus and downwards with the Small Intestine. The Stomach is also called the gastric cavity (*Wei Wan*, 胃脘), and is classified into the upper, middle and lower gastric cavity (*shang wan, zhong wan* and *xia wan*, 上脘, 中脘, 下脘): the upper gastric cavity (*shang wan*) refers to the upper part of the Stomach including the cardia; the lower gastric cavity (*xia wan*) refers to the lower part of the Stomach including pylorus; the part between the upper and the lower gastric cavity is where the middle gastric cavity (*zhong wan*) is located at, and the region is where the Stomach body is. The cardia connects upwards with esophagus, and the pylorus connects downwards with the Small Intestine, and they are the two portals for the water and food that enter and exit the Stomach. Both the Stomach and the Spleen are located in the middle *Jiao*, connect with each other via channels, and have the exterior and interior relationship.

The main physiological function of the Stomach is to receive and digest water and food. The physiological property of the Stomach is to be unobstructed and descend. It likes moistness and hates dryness.

① The Physiological Function of the Stomach (Table 2-20)

(1) Dominating receiving and containing water and food

The function of the Stomach to receive food refers

Table 2-20 Physiological functions and properties of the Stomach

	Actions	Physiological action	Main pathological changes
Stomach	Receiving and containing water and food	Receiving and containing water and food, and assisting digestion	**Failure of the tomach to receive and contain:** loss of appetite, anorexia, epigastric fullness
	Rotting and ripening water and food	Elementarily digesting water and food	**Dysfunction of rotting and ripening of the Stomach:** distending pain in the Stomach, eructation with foul smell
	Characteristics: The Stomach dominates being unobstructed and descending.	If the Stomach keeps its unobstructed and descending movement, the actions of the Stomach to receive, contain, rot and ripen water and food will be normal.	**When the Stomach fails to be unobstructed and descend:** retention of food in the Stomach that manifests as distending pain in Stomach; Adverse rising of the Stomach qi that manifests as nausea, hiccups and eructation; failure of intestines in transporting manifests as constipation.

to the action of the Stomach that receives and contains water and food. After being taken into the mouth, water and food pass the esophagus, enter the Stomach and are received and contained by the Stomach. Therefore, the Stomach is named "the great storehouse", and "the sea of water and food". The transformation and generation of qi and blood, and the functional activities of the *zang-fu* organs depend on the nutritional substances in the water and food, so the Stomach is also known as "the sea of water, food, qi and blood", and "the root of the five-*zang* organs".

If the Stomach is sick, it will affect the receiving and containing action of the Stomach and result in the symptoms of loss of appetite, anorexia and Stomach fullness.

(2) Dominating digesting (fu shu, 腐熟) of water and food

Digesting (*fu shu*) means to rot and ripe. The action of the stomach dominating rotting and ripening water and food refers to the action of the Stomach that initially digests the water and food and forms chyme. The water and food contained in the Stomach, after being rotted and ripened, is initially digested and changed into chyme. Then the chyme is transported downward into the Small Intestine to be further digested.

If the Stomach's action of rotting and ripening water and food malfunctions, the symptoms of food retention in the Stomach will occur in terms of distending pain in epigastria, eructation with fetid odor etc.

The combination of the actions of the Stomach to receive, contain, rot and ripen water and food with the actions of the Spleen to transport and transform promotes the transformation of the water and food into refined nutritious substances. The refined nutritious substances further form and generate qi, blood and body fluids to support and nourish the whole body. Thus, it is said that the Spleen and Stomach are the acquired root of the constitution and are the source of the transformation and generation of qi and blood.

② The Physiological Properties of the Stomach

(1) The Stomach dominates being unobstructed and descnding

The Stomach dominating being unobstructed and descending refers to the motional features of the Stomach qi that are in favor of being kept unobstructed and descending. After entering the Stomach, and being driven by the Stomach qi, water and food are initially digested and changed into chyme. Then the chyme is transmitted downwards into the Small Intestine and is further digested and absorbed there. Only the qi dynamic of the Stomach keeps a free and descending motion, allowing the digestion of the food to be normal. Therefore, there are the sayings that the Stomach dominates being unobstructed and descending; that the Stomach takes being unobstructed as harmony, and takes descent as favorableness; and the Stomach dominates harmony and descent. The receiving, containing, rotting and ripening actions of the Stomach are based on the actions of the Stomach qi. Therefore, the Stomach dominating being unobstructed and descending is also known as that the Stomach qi governing being unobstructed and descending.

The Stomach's function of freeing and descending is embodied by the physiological function of the Stomach. If the Stomach qi is free and descends normally, the Stomach can receive, contain and elementarily digest water and food, and then the chyme formed by the rotting and ripening action of the Stomach can be transported into the Small Intestine. The Stomach's action of being unobstructed and descending also has effects on the transportation of food by the intestine, and the discharge of feces. If the Stomach fails to be unobstructed and descend, it will result in retention of food in the Stomach and manifest as loss of appetite, epigastric fullness, and Stomachache. If the Stomach qi fails to descend and reverses, it will result in nausea, vomiting, hiccups, eructation etc. Failure of the Stomach qi in descending may also affect the conduction of the intestines and result in constipation.

(2) The Stomach likes moistness and dislikes dryness

To say that the Stomach likes moistness and dislikes dryness means that the Stomach needs to keep adequate fluids in it to promote the reception, containment, rotting and ripeness of the water and food in it. The receiving, containing, rotting and ripening actions of the Stomach not only rely on the propelling and steaming action of the Stomach qi, but also demand to be moistened by the fluids in the Stomach. If the fluids in the Stomach are sufficient, the normal functions of receiving, containing, rotting and ripening of the Stomach can be kept. The Stomach belongs to yang earth, its property is apt to be unobstructed and to descend, it likes moistness and dislikes dryness. Vomiting caused by the reversal of Stomach qi can consume the fluids in the Stomach. Invasion of the Stomach by dry-heat can consume and impair the Stomach yin and result in the impairment of the Stomach yin. Thus, the Stomach yin should be protected when

treating Stomach diseases.

Miraculous Pivot: *Chapter On the Four Seas* (*Líng Shū: Hǎi Lùn*, 灵枢·海论) says: "*The Stomach is the sea of water and food.*"

Miraculous Pivot: *Chapter Plate of Jade* (*Líng Shū: Yù Bǎn*, 灵枢·玉版) says: "*Humans receive qi from food, and the Stomach is where the food pours into. Thus, the Stomach is the sea of water, food, qi and blood.*"

Plain Questions: *Chapter Discussion on Genuine-Zang Pulses* (*Sù Wèn: Yù Jī Zhēn Zàng Lùn*,素问·玉机真脏论) says: "*All the five-zang organs receive their qi from the Stomach. Thus, the Stomach is the root of the five-zang organs.*"

Miraculous Pivot: *Chapter The Fast of an Ordinary Man* (*Líng Shū: Píng Rén Jué Gǔ*, 灵枢·平人绝谷) says: "*The Stomach… it is where the water and food are received.*"

Classic of Questioning: *The Thirty-first Question* (*Nàn Jīng: Sān Shí Yī Nàn*, 难经·三十一难) says: "*The middle Jiao is located at the middle part of the Stomach (zhongwan), not upward or downward, and it dominates rotting and ripening water and food.*"

Plain Questions: *Chapter Different Discussion on the Five Zang-Organs* (*Sù Wèn: Wǔ Zàng Bié Lùn*, 素问·五脏别论) says: "*The Stomach is the sea of water and food and is the great source of the six-fu organs. Food with five flavors are taken into the mouth and stored in the Stomach to nourish the qi of the five-zang organs…So, the qi and flavor of the five-zang organs and six-fu organs originate from the Stomach.*"

Plain Questions: *Chapter Discussion on the Secret Classics Stored in Royal Library* (*Sù Wèn: Líng Lán Mì Diǎn Lùn*, 素问·灵兰秘典论) says: "*The Spleen and Stomach are the officials of the granary where the five flavors produce.*"

The Small Intestine

The Small Intestine (小肠) is located in the abdominal cavity, its upper port connects with Stomach by the pylorus, and its lower port connects with the Large Intestine with the ileocecal conjunction. It is a relatively long organ in which food is further digested. The Small

Intestine and the Heart connect with each other via channels and have an exterior and interior relationship.

The main physiological functions of the Small Intestine are receiving, containing and digesting water and food, and separating the clear and turbid (Table 2-21).

Receiving, containing and digesting water and food: receiving and containing (*shoucheng*) means to accept, store and fill. Digesting (*huawu*) means to digest water and food and to transform them into refined nutritious substances. The Small Intestine governs receiving, containing and transforming water and food in two ways. First,

Table 2-21 The physiological functions of the Small Intestine

	Actions	Physiological action	Main pathological changes
Small Intestine	Receiving, containing and digesting water and food. Separating and excreting the clear and turbid	It receives and contains the chyme being elementarily digested by the Stomach and further digests and absorbs it and transforms it into refined nutritious substances. It absorbs refined nutritious substances and fluids, and transports the food residue down to the Large Intestine. The redundant water is transformed into urine via the Kidney and Bladder.	Indigestion and malabsorption: abdominal fullness, borborygmus, diarrhea, loose stools etc.

it refers to the actions of the Small Intestine to receive and contain the water and food digested elementarily by the Stomach. Second, it refers to the action of the Small Intestine to further digests the chymes that is elementarily digested by the Stomach and transform it into refined nutritious substances.

Excreting and separating the clear and turbid: excreting means to excrete the fluid contained inside the body. Separating means to differentiate and separate different substances. The clear refers to the essence of water and food (including fluid). The turbid refers to the food residue (including fluid). The separation of the clear and turbid by the Small Intestine means that the Small Intestine separates refined nutritious substances, water and residue, contained in the water and food (chyme) that is elementarily digested by the Stomach, from each other. 'The separation of the clear' means the separation and absorption of the refined nutritious substances (including fluids) in the water and food. The separation of the turbid refers to two things. First, it means to transport the food residue down to the Large Intestine. Second, it means to transport the turbid fluid that is utilized by the tissues and *zang-fu* organs down to the Kidney and Bladder and form urine.

The Small Intestine absorbs water and attends to the metabolic processes of water and fluid in the human body, so it is said that "The Small Intestine dominates fluids."

The action of receiving, containing, and digesting water and food, and the action of separating the clear and turbid of the water and food in the Small Intestine are an indivisible whole. The action of receiving, containing and digesting water and food is the preparation for the separation of the clear and turbid; the action of separating the clear and turbid is based on the action of receiving, containing and digesting water and food and is the goal of digesting water and food. Digestion primarily refers to digesting water and food; the separation of the clear and turbid primarily refers to the absorption of refined nutritious substances. Therefore, the primary function of the Small Intestine is digestion and absorption. Pathological changes of Small Intestine are usually malabsorption and indigestion, and manifest as abdominal fullness, borborygmus, diarrhea and loose stool etc.

When the action of separating the clear and turbid of the Small Intestine is normal, the water and fluid will go their own way, and then the urination and defecation will be normal. When the separation of the clear and turbid of the Small Intestine is in malfunctions, the clear and turbid can't be separated, the water will go with draff, and it will result in the mixing of water and food, manifest as loose stools and scanty urine. The function of the Small Intestine is also related to the urinary volume. Thereby, in the early stage of diarrhea, the method of "*promoting urination to harden the stool*" is always adopted.

Regarding the theory of visceral manifestations, the digestion and absorption functions of the Small Intestine are always attributed to the scope of the transformation and transportation actions of the Spleen. The pathological changes of indigestion and malabsorption of the Small Intestine, such as abdominal fullness, diarrhea and loose stool etc., fall under the category of dysfunction of the Spleen in transportation, and are treated with the method of strengthening the Spleen.

Plain Questions: *Chapter Discussion on the Secret Classics Stored in Royal Library* (*Sù Wèn: Líng Lán Mì Diǎn Lùn*, 素问·灵兰秘典论) says: "*The Small Intestine is the official controlling containment where the water and food are digested and absorbed.*"

Classified Classic: *Chapter Class of Visceral Manifestations* (*Lèi Jīng: Zàng Xiàng Lèi*, 类经·藏象类) says: "*The Small Intestine is located below*

the Stomach. It receives the water and food from the Stomach, and separates the clear part from the turbid, and then the water and fluids infiltrate into the organ in front of it (the Bladder), and the organ behind it (the Large Intestine). The clear qi is lifted by the action of transformation of the Spleen qi, and the turbid is lowered by the transformation of the Small Intestine, so the Small Intestine is where water and food are further digested: it absorbs the essence and transmits the dregs into the Large Intestine.*"

The Large Intestine

The Large Intestine (大肠) is located in the abdominal cavity: the upper port connects with the Small Intestine with the ileocecal conjunction, and the lower port connects with the anus. The upper segment of the Large Intestine is called the ileum (*hui chang*, 回肠), and the lower segment is called the broad intestine (*guang chang*, 广肠). The broad intestine includes the colon and rectum in modern anatomy. The Large Intestine and the lungs connect with each other via channels and have an exterior and interior relationship.

The primary function of the Large Intestine is to transport and transform draff (Table 2-22).

Table 2-22   The physiological functions of the Large Intestine

	Actions	Physiological action	Main pathological changes
Large Intestine	Transforming and changing draff	In the conduction course, the Large Intestine absorbs water, transforms the food residue into solid feces, and discharges it outside the body.	Disorder of transportation and change of the Large Intestine: diarrhea or constipation

To transport and to transform (*chuan hua*, 传化) means conducting and changing. Transportation or conduction means transmission or guiding. It refers to the actions of the Large Intestine that receive, transport, guide and excrete the food residue from the Small Intestine. Change refers to the function of the Large Intestine to absorb the redundant water in the food residue and changes it into solid feces.

When the Large Intestine transport and transform, it absorbs water and participate in the water metabolism. Therefore, it is said that "the

Large Intestine dominates fluid."

The function of the Large Intestine in transporting and changing draff refers to the action of the Large Intestine of absorbing partial water in the food residue, and forming and storing feces for a short period of time, and then discharging it out of the body. Therefore, dysfunction of the transportation and change of the Large Intestine manifests as disorders of the stool. If the water and fluid can't be absorbed and are conducted downward together with thes draff, diarrhea will occur. If the fluid in the Large

Intestine is not sufficient, the intestinal tract is not moistened, and constipation will occur.

Plain Questions: Chapter Discussion on the Secret Classics Stored in Royal Library (Sù Wèn: Líng Lán Mì Diǎn Lùn, 素问·灵兰秘典论) says: "The Large Intestine is the official of transportation and is responsible for change and transformation."

Treatise on Spleen and Stomach (Pí Wèi Lùn, 脾胃论) says: "The Large Intestine dominates the clear diluted fluid, the Small Intestine dominates the thick fluids. The large and Small Intestines receive the nutrient qi from the Stomach, and then they can transmit the fluids to the upper Jiao, nourish and moisten the skin and fine hairs, and the interstitial striae."

The Bladder

The Bladder (膀胱) is located in the lower abdomen, below the Kidney and anterior to the Large Intestine, and is a cyst-like and hollow organ. It connects with the Kidney via the ureter and downward via the urethra, and opens at the anterior lower orifice (the genital orifice). The Bladder and the Kidney connect with each other via channels and have an exterior and interior relationship.

The main physiological function of the Bladder is to store and discharge urine (Table 2-23).

Table 2-23　The physiological functions of the Bladder

	Actions	Physiological actions	Main pathological changes
Bladder	Store and discharge urine	When the qi transformation of the Kidney and the Bladder is normal, its actions of storing and discharging will be normal.	**Disorder of qi transformation of the Bladder:** dysuria, anuresis. **Bladder qi deficiency fails to restrain:** frequent urination, urgency of urination, enuresis and urinary incontinence.

The water and fluids of the human body, through the actions of *zang-fu* organs like the Spleen, Lung, Kidney and *San Jiao*, are transported and distributed to the whole body and nourish the tissues and *zang-fu* organs. After the metabolism of water and fluids, the turbid fluid is transported downward to the Kidney. Through the qi transformation of the Kidney, the turbid part of water and fluid is transformed into urine, and urine is transported into the Bladder and is stored there. After storing a certain volume of urine, through the action of the qi transformation of the Kidney, the Bladder discharges the urine outside of the body.

The storage and discharge of the urine by the Bladder depends on the qi transformation of the Kidney. If the qi transformation of the Kidney is abnormal, it can result in the pathological changes of failure of the Bladder to store and discharge urine. If the Bladder has a disorder in qi transformation, it manifests as dysuria or anuresis. If qi deficiency of the Bladder fails to restrain, it manifests as frequent urine, urgency of urination, enuresis and urinary incontinence.

Plain Questions: Chapter Discussion on the Secret Classics Stored in Royal Library (Sù Wèn: Líng Lán Mì Diǎn Lùn, 素问·灵兰秘典论) says: "The Bladder is the Official in charge of the reservoir and is where the fluids are stored, and discharges the turbid part by qi transformation."

Classic of Questioning: The Forty-second Question (Nàn Jīng: Sì Shí Èr Nàn, 难经·四十二难) says: "The Bladder… can contain urine 9 sheng(升) 9 he(合)."

General Treatise on Causes and Manifestations of All Diseases: Chapter Diseases of the Bladder (Zhū Bìng Yuán Hóu Lùn: Páng Guāng Bìng Hòu, 诸病源候论·膀胱病候) says: "The surplus part of the fluids entering the Bladder is urine."

The *San Jiao*

① Basic Concept of the *San Jiao*

The *San Jiao* (三焦) is the combined name for the

upper *Jiao*, middle *Jiao* and lower *Jiao*, and it is one of the six-*fu* organs.

Regarding the concept of the *San Jiao*, there has been a great deal of dispute about this for generations. *Internal Classic* (*Nèi Jīng*) first puts forward the name of the *San Jiao* and states that the *San Jiao* belongs to the six-*fu* organs. *Classic of Questioning* (*Nàn Jīng*) puts forward that the *San Jiao* "has name without form". Therefore, the dispute that the *San Jiao* "has name without form" versus "has name with form" was engendered.

The application of the word "*San Jiao*" in Chinese medicine:

a. "The *San Jiao* of the *zang-fu* organs" belongs to the six-*fu* organs. It is a large official residence located in the chest and abdominal cavity, and includes all the viscera. There is no one organ that can match it, therefore, it is also known as the "large official residence" and the "solitary official residence".

b. "The *San Jiao* of location" refers to the regional division that the chest and abdominal cavity were divided into the three regions in terms of the upper *Jiao*, the middle *Jiao* and the lower *Jiao*.

The division of the *San Jiao* is generally considered as follows: the upper *Jiao* refers to the region above the diaphragm, including the Heart and the Lung. Some also attribute the upper extremity and head to the upper *Jiao*. The middle *Jiao* refers to the epigastric region below the diaphragm and above the umbilicus, including the Spleen, Stomach, Liver and Gallbladder. The lower *Jiao* refers to the lower abdomen, and the region below the umbilicus, including the Kidney, Bladder, Small Intestine and Large Intestine. Some attribute the lower extremities to the lower *Jiao*.

c. "The *San Jiao* of channel" refers to the *San Jiao* channel of hand *shaoyang*. (For detailed information see the section about the channels and collaterals.)

d. "The *San Jiao*s of syndrome differentiation" refers to the syndrome differentiation of the three *Jiao*s. It is one of the guiding principles for syndrome differentiation of warm-heat diseases. (For detailed information please see the section

on syndrome differentiation.)

Classic of Questioning: The Thirty-eighth Question (*Nàn Jīng: Sān Shí Bā Nàn*, 难经·三十八难) says: "*The sixth fu organ is the San Jiao, which is the divergence of the original qi. It manages all the qi and has name without form.*"

Miraculous Pivot: Chapter On Acupoints (*Líng Shū: Běn Shū*, 灵枢·本输): "*The San Jiao is the house of the center ditch where the water passage produces, and it connects with the Bladder and is called the solitary organ.*"

Classified Classic: Chapter Class of Visceral Manifestations (*Lèi Jīng: Zàng Xiàng Lèi*, 类经·藏象类) says: "*Among the twelve organs, the San Jiao is the largest one, there is no one can match it among them, that's why it is called the solitary organ... Generally it is outside all the zang-fu organs, inside the human body, and it embraces all the zang fu organs and is the largest fu organ in the cavity of the body.*"

② The Main Physiological Functions of the *San Jiao* (Table 2-24)

As one of the six-*fu* organs, the *San Jiao* has the function of transmitting the original qi, and transporting water, food, and fluids.

(1) Transmitting the original qi

Original qi (source qi) originates from the Kidney, is the root qi of the human body, and is the driving force of life activities. The original qi is transported to the five *zang*-organs and six *fu*-organs and distributed to the whole body to excite and motivate the functions and activities of all the tissues and *zang-fu* organs via the *San Jiao*. Therefore, it is said that the *San Jiao* is the passageway for the circulation of the original qi.

(2) Transporting water, food and fluids

Transporting water and food: as one of the six-*fu* organs, the *San Jiao* is the official house of transportation, and can transport water and food. It is described in detail in *Classic of Questioning* (*Nàn Jīng*): the upper *Jiao* "dominates receiving", the middle *Jiao* "dominates rotting and ripening", and the lower *Jiao* "dominates separating the clear and turbid". The actions of the *San Jiao* embody the course of digesting, absorbing and discharging water and food by the Spleen, Stomach and intestines. Therefore, it is said that the *San Jiao* is "the passageway of water and food."

Transporting water and fluids: the water and fluid metabolism is an intricate physiological process of the human body, and is completed by the combined actions of the Spleen, Lung and Kidney. However, the *San Jiao* must be taken as a passage for the water and fluids to ascend, descend, enter, exit and circulate all over the body. Therefore, it is said that the *San Jiao* is the passageway for the circulation of water and fluids. The action of the *San Jiao* circulating water and fluids is also known as the "qi transformation of the *San Jiao*". If the qi transformation of the *San Jiao* is normal, the water metabolism will be kept in harmony and balance. Dysfunction of qi transformation of the *San Jiao* can result in the disturbance of transporting, distributing and discharging water and fluids by the Lung in the upper *Jiao*, the Spleen in the middle *Jiao*, and the Kidney in the lower *Jiao*. Therefore, one might say that the action of the *San Jiao* in transporting water and fluids is the summarization of the actions of the Spleen, Lung and Kidney being in charge of the metabolism of water and fluids.

Plain Questions: *Chapter Discussion on the Secret Classics Stored in Royal Library* (*Sù Wèn*: *Líng Lán Mì Diǎn Lùn*, 素问·灵兰秘典论) says: "*The San Jiao is like the officer in charge of dredging river and is where the water passage produces.*"

Classic of Questioning: *The Thirty-first Question* (*Nàn Jīng*: *Sān Shí Yī Nàn*, 难经·三十一难) says: "*The San Jiao is the passage of water and food, and is where the qi starts and ends.*"

Classic of Questioning: *The Sixty-sixth Question* (*Nàn Jīng*: *Liù Shí Liù Nàn*, 难经·六十六难) says: "*The San Jiao is the divergence of the original qi, and dominates dredging and circulating the three qi to bypass all the five-zang and six-fu organs.*"

(3) The physiological features of the upper, the middle and the lower *Jiaos* (Table 2-24)

The three *Jiao*s have dissimilar functional characteristics in the course of circulating the original qi, and transporting food, water and fluids. *Internal Classic* (*Nèi Jīng*) summarizes it as: "The upper *Jiao* resembles a sprayer, the middle *Jiao* resembles a fermentation cask, the lower *Jiao* resembles water passages." *Classic of Questioning* (*Nàn Jīng*) describes it as: The upper *Jiao* "dominates receiving", the middle *Jiao* "dominates rotting and ripening water and food", and the lower *Jiao* "dominates separating the clear and turbid and dominates discharging but not receiving".

Table 2-24 The main physiological function of *San Jiao*

	Actions	Physiological action	Main pathological changes
San Jiao	Transmitting the original qi, circulating food, water and fluids.	The *San Jiao* is the passageway for the circulation of the original qi. The *San Jiao* is the passageway for the transportation of water and food. The *San Jiao* is the passageway for the transportation of water and fluids.	It influences the qi circulation of the whole body and the transportation of water, food and fluids. If the upper *Jiao* is not ruled, the water will attack the Heart and the Lung. If the middle *Jiao* is not ruled, the water will be retained in the Stomach and Spleen. If the lower *Jiao* is not ruled, the water will disturb the urine and feces.
	Features: The upper *Jiao* resembles a sprayer. The middle *Jiao* resembles a fermentation cask. The lower *Jiao* resembles water passages.	The Heart and Lung in the upper *Jiao* disperse and distribute the qi and blood to warm and nourish the whole body. The Stomach and the Spleen in the middle *Jiao* rot, ripen, transport and transform water and food to transform and generate qi and blood. The Kidney and Bladder in the lower *Jiao* exert the action of qi transformation on the water and fluids to generate and discharge urine.	

(1) The upper Jiao resembles a sprayer

The upper *Jiao* refers to the chest region where the Heart and the Lung sit. To resemble a sprayer means that the function of the upper *Jiao* seems to be similar to diffusive fog and dew. The upper *Jiao* resembles a sprayer means that the Heart and the Lung in the upper *Jiao* disperse and distribute the qi and blood, like the irrigation of fog and dew, to the whole body, to warm and nourish the tissues and *zang-fu* organs. Because the upper *Jiao* accepts the refined nutritious substances, so *Classic of Questioning* (*Nàn Jīng*) states that the upper *Jiao* "dominates receiving".

(2) The middle Jiao resembles a fermentation cask

The middle *Jiao* refers to the epigastric region, including the Spleen, Stomach, Liver and Gallbladder. To act as fermentation cask means to soak. The middle *Jiao* resembling a fermentation cask refers to the actions of the Stomach and the Spleen in the middle *Jiao* that rot, ripen, transport and transform water and food to transform and generate qi and blood. Therefore, *Classic of Questioning* (*Nàn Jīng*) states that the middle *Jiao* "dominates rotting and ripening water and food".

(3) The lower Jiao resembles water passages

The lower *Jiao* refers to the lower abdomen, including the Kidney, Bladder, Small Intestine and Large Intestine. Water passage means the furrow or ditch where water and fluid flow through. The lower *Jiao* resembling water passages refers to the qi transformation of the Kidney and Bladder that act on water and fluids to generate and discharge urine.

The lower *Jiao* "dominates the separation of the clear and the turbid and the discharge of urine". Comparatively speaking, the clear refers to urine and the turbid refers to stool. The lower *Jiao* dominates the separation of the clear and turbid, and the discharge of urine refers to the actions of the Kidney, Bladder, Small Intestine and Large Intestine that transform the turbid fluid into urine and transform food residue into feces and discharge them outside the body.

Miraculous Pivot: Chapter The Issue of Distribution and Operation of The Defensive Qi and Nutritive Qi (*Líng Shū: Yíng Wèi Shēng Huì*, 灵 枢·营卫生会*) says: "The upper Jiao resembles a sprayer. The middle Jiao resembles a fermentation cask. The lower Jiao resembles water passages."*

Classic of Questioning: The Thirty-first Question (*Nàn Jīng: Sān Shí Yī Nàn*, 难经·三十一难*) says: "The upper Jiao is located below the Heart and goes downward through the diaphragm, and bypasses the upper port of the Stomach, dominates receiving but not discharging… The middle Jiao is located at the middle part of the Stomach* (*zhongwan*), *not upward or downward, and dominates rotting and ripening water and food… The lower Jiao is located at the upper port of the Bladder, dominates separating the clear and the turbid, and dominates discharge but not containment."*

Classified Classic: Chapter Class of Visceral Manifestations (*Lèi Jīng: Zàng Xiàng Lèi*, 类经·藏 象类*) says: " If the upper Jiao is not ruled, the water will attack the Heart and the Lung. If the middle Jiao is not ruled, the water will be retained in the Stomach and Spleen. If the lower Jiao is not ruled, the water will disturb the urine and feces."*

Section 3　The Extraordinary *Fu* Organs

The Extraordinary *fu* organs are the generic name for the brain, marrow, bone, vessel, Gallbladder and uterus. Although the six organs are named after *fu*, functionally, they are different from the physiological features of the six-*fu* organs in terms of "receiving and containing", "transporting and digesting water and food" and "discharging without storage", and they are similar to the physiological features of the five-*zang* organs in terms of "storing essence without discharge". They are similar to *zang* organs but are not *zang* organs, and are similar to *fu* organs but are not *fu* organs, so *Internal Classic* (*Nèi Jīng*) calls them the extraordinary *fu* organs.

The marrow, bone, vessel and Gallbladder have been discussed in the related section of *zang-fu* organs. In this section, we deal only with brain and uterus.

Plain Questions: Chapter Different Discussion on the Five Zang-Organs (*Sù Wèn: Wǔ Zàng Bié Lùn*,

素问・五脏别论) says: *"Brain, marrow, bone, vessel (pulse), Gallbladder and uterus are generated by the influence of earth qi; all of them store yin substances just like the earth that contains everything. Thus, they store essence without discharge, and are called the extraordinary fu organs."*

The Brain

The brain (脑) is located in the head and resides in the cranial cavity; the outside tissues are the head and face, the inside is the brain marrow. The brain is the convergence of the marrow and connects with the spinal cord, so it is also known as the sea of marrow.

Plain Questions: Chapter Discussion on Various Relationships Concerning the Five Zang-Organs (Sù Wèn: Wǔ Zàng Shēng Chéng Piān, 素问・五脏生成篇) says: *"All the marrows belong to the brain."*

Miraculous Pivot: Chapter On the Four Seas (Líng Shū: Hǎi Lùn, 灵枢・海论) says: *"The brain is the sea of marrow, its upper important acupoint is bǎi huì (DU 20), and the lower one is fēng fǔ (DU 16)."*

① The Physiological Functions of the Brain (Table 2-25)

(1) Dominating life activities

The brain dominating life activity means that the brain is the vital center of the human body and

Table 2-25　The physiological functions of the brain

Actions	Physiological significance	Pathological significance
Dominating life activities	The brain is the vital center of life activity of the human body	If the brain is impaired, it will endanger life.
Dominating mental activities	If the action of the brain dominating mental activities is normal, one will be freshened and conscious, as well as have prompt thinking, good memory, fluent and clear speech and normal emotional activities.	Abnormal mental activities will result in disorders of vital spark, consciousness, thinking and emotion.
Dominating sense and motion	The vision, hearing, speech, and motion of the human body are dominated by the brain. When the brain marrow is sufficient, the different kinds of sensations and motor function will be normal.	If the sea of marrow is insufficient, it will result in disorders of vision, hearing, speech and motion.

dominates the life activities of the human body. The brain is transformed and generated by the innate essence. The spirit generated along with the formation of the brain is called the original spirit and hides in the brain, therefore the brain is also known as the house of the original spirit. The brain stores the original spirit and is the dominator of life. If the brain is impaired, it will endanger life. Therefore it is said that one will live with spirit, and one will die without spirit.

Miraculous Pivot: Chapter On Channels (Líng Shū: Jīng Mài, 灵枢・经脉) says: *"At the very beginning of the human life, essence qi is generated first. When the essence is formed, the brain marrow is generated."*

Miraculous Pivot: Chapter The Diseases Caused by Spiritual Activities (Líng Shū: Běn Shén, 灵枢・本神) says: *"The original substance which enables the evolution of the human body is called the essence of life; when the yin essence and the yang essence combine, it produces the activities of life which are collectively called the spirit."*

Plain Questions: Chapter Discussion on the Contraindication of Needling Therapy (Sù Wèn: Cì Jìn Lùn, 素问・刺禁论) says: *"When pricking the head, if the nǎo hù point (DU 17) is hurt erroneously, the patient will die immediately."*

Grand Materia Medica: Section Flos Magnoliae (Běn Cǎo Gāng Mù: Xīn Yí, 本草纲目・辛夷) says: *"The brain is the house of genuine spirit."*

(2) Dominating mental activities

The mental activities of the human body

including thinking, consciousness and emotion etc, are the outcome of the reflections in the brain of the impersonal things in the environment. The brain is the house of the original spirit, so the brain dominates the mental activities of thinking, consciousness, memory and emotion. When the action of the brain dominating mental activities is normal, one will be fresh and conscious, have prompt thinking, good memory, fluent and clear speech, and normal emotional activities. Otherwise, one will suffer disorders of spirit, consciousness, thinking and emotion.

Plain Questions: *Chapter Discussion on the Essentials of Pulse* (*Sù Wèn: Mài Yào Jīng Wēi Lùn*, 素问·脉要精微论) says: "*The head is where the spirit is located; if the head hangs down or tilts with eyes caving in, it shows the spirit will decline soon.*"

Correction on Errors in Medical Classics: *Chapter Brain Marrow* (*Yī Lín Gǎi Cuò: Nǎo Suí Shuō*, 医林改错·脑髓说) says: "*The intelligence and memory is not the function of the Heart but the brain.*"

Records of Medicine Root in Chinese Medicine and Referred to Western Medicine: *Chapter Explanation on the Spirits of the Human Body* (*Yī Xué Zhōng Zhōng Cān Xī Lù: Rén Shēn Shén Míng Quán*, 医学衷中参西录·人身神明诠) says: "*The spirit in the brain is the original spirit and the one in the Heart is cognitive spirit. The original spirit is stored in the brain: without thinking and consideration, it is natural and empty. The cognitive spirit sets out from the Heart with thinking and consideration; it is prompt but not empty.*"

(3) Dominating sense and motion

All the five sense organs including the eyes, tongue, mouth, nose and ears, are located in the head and face and connect with the brain. The sensations of vision, hearing, smelling and taste, as well as speech and motion are closely related to the brain. The brain is the house of the original spirit, and the brain spirit governs the motion of the limbs. When the sea of marrow is full, the functions of sensation and motion would be normal, then it manifests as normal vision and hearing, sensitive olfaction, normal feeling, fluent speech and smooth movement. If the sea of marrow is insufficient, it will result in failure of the brain in dominating sensation and motion

and manifest as blurred vision, impaired hearing and smelling, blunt sensations, speech disorder, akinesia, lassitude, sleepiness, and so on.

Miraculous Pivot: *Chapter On the Four Seas* (*Líng Shū: Hǎi Lùn*, 灵枢·海论) says: "*When the sea of marrow is surplus, it will cause one to feel light and vigorous in the body, and he can do harder work; when the sea of marrow is insufficient, one's brain will feel like turning and he will have the symptoms of tinnitus, sore legs, dizziness, seeing nothing, fatigue and sleepiness.*"

The Origin and Start of Medicine: *Chapter Discussion on Memory by Heart* (*Yī Xué Yuán Shǐ: Jì Xīn Biàn*, 医学原始·记心辩) says: "*The five sense organs are located in the upper part of the body, and are the organs in charge of sensations. The ears, eyes, mouth and nose gather in the head where the highest and outstanding position is, and is convenient for them to sense things. Because the ears, eyes, mouth and nose are close to brain in location, all that is sensed by the ears, eyes, mouth and nose are received by the brain first, and then the brain feels, deposits, analyzes and memorizes them. Thus, it is said that the memory of the Heart is memorized by the brain.*"

Correction on Errors in Medical Classics: *Chapter Brain Marrow* (*Yī Lín Gǎi Cuò: Nǎo Suí Shuō*, 医林改错·脑髓说) says: "*The two ears connect with the brain, so the sounds heard are transmitted to the brain…The two eyes connect with the brain with two threads, so the things seen are transmitted to the brain…The nose communicates with the brain, so the flavors smelled are transmitted to the brain…At birth, the brain of the infant is not completely grown, the fontanel is soft, the eyes are not prompt, the ears can hear nothing, nose can smell nothing, and tongue can speak nothing. When people are one year old, the brain is gradually grown, the fontanel gradually closes, the ears can hear a little, eyes moves more promptly, nose smell a little, and thetongue can speak one or two words…Why do the infants have no memory? That's because the brain marrow is not suffused. The memory of the elders gradually decline, that's because the brain marrow is gradually empty.*"

② Relationship of the Brain with the Five-*zang* Organs

The brain is an organ of vital importance in the

human body. However, the theory of visceral manifestations takes the five-*zang* organs as core, therefore, the physiological functions of the brain mainly refer to the mental activities, consciousness, thinking and emotion that are attributed to the five-*zang* organs. Among the five-*zang* organs, the brain is closely related to the Heart, Liver and Kidney.

"The place used to accept things is named the Heart." This means that the actions of the brain that accept and reflect objective things without us, and the actions of consciousness and conceptual work of the brain are called the Heart. The Heart stores the spirit, is the greater dominator of the five-*zang* organs and six-*fu* organs, and dominates mental activities, consciousness, thinking and emotion. When the action of the Heart storing the spirit is normal and the brain spirit is normal, it will manifest as refreshed spirit, consciousness, prompt thinking, rapid response, and good memory. Dysfunction of the Heart storing the spirit can result in failure of the brain in dominating mental activities and manifesting as disorders of mental, conscious and thinking activities.

The Kidney stores essence, essence generates marrow, and marrow connects upward with the brain. If the Kidney essence is sufficient, the sea of marrow is nourished, and then the brain can fully develop. It manifests as being energized, having good hearing and eyesight, and having prompt thinking and quick motion. If Kidney essence is insufficient and the sea of marrow is not nourished, the brain marrow will be empty. It manifests as dizziness, tinnitus, amnesia, blunt thinking, vague expressions, and staggering. Thus, the brain is closely related to the Kidney.

The Liver governs free coursing, and dominates emotion and consideration, and it can regulate mental and emotional activities.

The physiology and pathology of the brain is related to the five-*zang* organs. When the physiological activity of the five-*zang* organs is normal, then the actions of the brain can be exerted normally. If the brain is sick, it will manifest as disorders of the five-*zang* organs. Therefore, the pathological changes of the brain, in Chinese medicine, are treated according to the syndrome differentiation and treatment of the five-*zang* organs.

Plain Questions: *Chapter Discussion on the Elucidation of Five-Qi* (*Sù Wèn*: *Xuān Míng Wǔ Qì Piān*, 素问·宣明五气篇) says: "*Among the five storages of the five-zang organs, the Heart stores spirit, the Lung stores the interior spirit, the Liver stores the soul, the Spleen stores idea, and the Kidney stores will.*"

Plain Questions: *Chapter Major Discussion on the Theory of Yin and Yang and the Corresponding Relationships Among All the Things in Nature* (*Sù Wèn*: *Yīn Yáng Yìng Xiàng Dà Lùn*, 素问·阴阳应象大论) says: "*People have five-zang organs to transform and generate five qi, and then happiness, anger, sadness, worry and fear are generated accordingly by the five qi.*"

The Uterus

The uterus (女子胞), also called the womb, is located in the lower abdomen, behind the Bladder and in front of the rectum. Its lower port connects with the vagina and its shape looks like an inverted pear.

The uterus is one of the female internal genitals, and has the function of controlling menstruation and gestation.

① Physiological Functions of the Uterus

(1) Controlling menstruation

The uterus is the site of menstruation, which occurs at the beginning of sexual maturation. Menstruation refers to the physiological phenomenon of the periodic vaginal discharge of blood from a woman's uterus after the maturation of the female reproductive organs. When a female is about 14 years old, because of the sufficiency of Kidney essence, by the action of *tian gui*, the uterus maturates, the Ren Channel is free and the *Penetrating vessel* is filled with qi and blood, and then the menses start regularly. When one reaches his or her fifties (menopause), because of the decline and insufficiency of the Kidney essence, exhaustion of *tian gui*, and insufficiency of qi and blood in the Chong and Ren Channels, the menstruation stops (menopause).

(2) Gestation of the fetus

The uterus is the organ of becoming pregnant and is where the fetus is cultivated. After sexual maturation, women will start menstruating regularly and has the capability of pregnancy and reproduction. In this time, female and male have sexual intercourse, the two essences combine with each other, and then gestation starts and a fetus is formed. When the gestation starts, the menses stops, and the qi and blood pour into the uterus to nourish and cultivate the fetus via the Chong and Ren Channels. The womb is the location where the fetus develops in the body of the mother.

② Relationship of the Uterus to the *Zang-fu* Organs and Channels

Menstruation and the gestation of a fetus in women is an intricate physiological action, it is closely related to the Liver and the Kidney and the Chong and Ren Channels.

The actions of the Kidney (Fig. 2-18): the Kidney stores essence and dominates reproduction; this is closely related to the actions of the uterus that take charge of the menstruation and gestation of the fetus. When the essence qi in the Kidney is filled to a certain degree, it will generate *tian gui* that promotes the maturation of reproductive organs and maintains reproductive functions. Through the action of *tian gui*, the

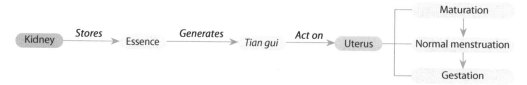

Fig. 2-18   Actions of the Kidney on the uterus

uterus maturates and the menses starts and is capable of gestating a fetus. When a woman reaches senility, the essence qi in the Kidney is insufficient and declined, the menses stops, and she is incapable of gestation.

The function of the Liver (Fig. 2-19): The

liver governs storing blood. If the Liver blood is sufficient, the blood can fill the uterus, and then the menstruation will be regular, and the blood can nourish and cultivate the fetus during gestation. Thus, it is known that "The female takes the Liver as the innate root."

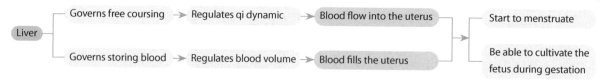

Fig. 2-19   Actions of the Liver on the uterus

The actions of the Penetrating and Ren Channels: likewise, the Penetrating and Ren Channels originate from the uterus. The Penetrating *vessel* can regulate the qi and blood of the twelve regular channels, and so the Penetrating *vessel* is named as "the sea of the blood". The Ren Channel is related to gestation, so it is said "The Ren Channel dominates the fetus in the uterus." The qi and blood of the human body pours in to

the uterus via the Chong and Ren Channels, and then the uterus menstruates at ordinary times and nourishes and cultivates the fetus during gestation.

Furthermore, the actions of the uterus are also related to the Heart and Spleen. The Heart governs blood circulation, and the Spleen controls blood, dominates transportation and transformation, and is the source of generation and transformation of qi and blood. The Heart and the Spleen are related to the generation and circulation of the blood in the human body and influence menstruation and the gestation of the fetus in women.

Plain Questions: Chapter Ancient Ideas on Flow to Preserve Natural Healthy Energy (Sù Wèn: Shàng Gǔ Tiān Zhēn Lùn, 素问·上古天真论) says: "*For a woman,...At the age of fourteen, Tian gui begins to appear, and the Ren Channel and Penetrating vessel are vigorous in function. Then a woman begins to have menstruation and is able to conceive a baby... At the age of forty-nine, as both the Ren Channel and Penetrating vessel become deficient and menstruation stops, she becomes physically feeble and is no longer able to conceive a baby.*"

Classified Classic: Chapter Class of Visceral Manifestations (Lèi Jīng: Zàng Xiàng Lèi, 类经·藏象类) says: "*When the yin and yang combine, the fetus is formed, and where it is stored is called the uterus.*"

Succinct Contentions and Principles of Medical Classics of Integration of Traditional Chinese and Western Medicine (Zhōng Xī Huì Tōng Yī Jīng Jīng Yì, 中西汇通医经精义) says: "*The womb of female is also called the uterus and is where the baby is conceived.*"

Section 4   Relationship between *Zang-Fu* Organs

The relationship between *zang-fu* organs is the primary content of holistic linkage in the theory of visceral manifestations. Although each organ of the human body has different actions, they are an intimate and organic whole. Besides the structural linkage, the linking mode primarily refers to the mutual restriction, interdependence, and mutual cooperation in the aspect of physiological functions. Therefore, in pathologic conditions, the sickness of each organ can interplay on each other.

Relationship between the *Zang* Organs

① Relationship between the Heart and Lung

The relationshiop between the Heart and Lung primarily refers to the interactive relationship between the action of the Heart governing blood and the action of the Lung dominating qi. (Fig. 2-20)

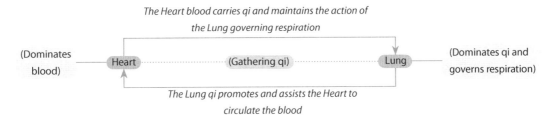

Fig. 2-20   Interactive relationship of the Heart governing blood to the Lung dominating qi

The function of the Heart governing blood promotes blood circulation. Blood can carry qi and maintain the action of the Lung governing respiration, therefore, it is conducive to the normal action of the Lung dominating qi and governing respiration.

The Lung dominates qi, governs respiration, and is the organ where all the vessels converge. It promotes and assists the Heart to drive the blood circulation, and is the requirement in guaranteeing normal circulation of the Heart blood.

The Heart and the Lung are located in the chest cavity. The gathering qi is located in the chest too, and has the function of passing through the Heart channel, bypassing the respiratory tract and governing breathing. Therefore, gathering qi also strengthens the coupling action between the Lung and Heart.

The pathological changes of the Heart and Lung can affect each other.

Lung qi insufficiency results in weak

circulation of the blood; or failure of the Lung in dispersing and descending results in obstruction of blood circulation, which may manifest as cough with dyspnea, shortness of breath, an oppressed feeling in the chest, palpitations, and cyanotic lips and tongue.

Insufficiency of the Heart qi, lack of vigor of the Heart yang, and obstruction of blood circulation can affect the respiratory action of the lungs and result in palpitation and cyanotic lips and tongue, as well as cough with dyspnea and an oppressed feeling in the chest.

② Relationship between the Heart and Spleen

The relationship between the Heart and Spleen mainly finds expression in two aspects: the interactive relationship in the aspect of the generation of blood, and the cooperative relationship in the aspect of blood circulation.

Regarding the aspect of the generation of blood (Fig. 2-21): the Heart governs blood and the Heart blood nourishes the Spleen maintain the

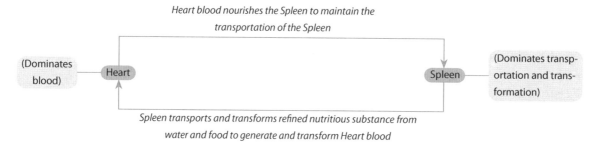

Fig. 2-21　Interactive relationship of the Heart governing blood with the Spleen dominating transformation and transportation

normal transportation and transformation of the Spleen. The Spleen dominates transportation and transformation and is the source of generation and transformation of qi and blood. The normal transportation and transformation of the Spleen can guarantee the sufficiency of Heart blood.

Regarding the aspect of blood circulation (Fig. 2-22), the Heart governs blood and continually drives blood circulation. The Spleen controls blood and keeps the blood circulating inside the vessels instead of overflowing. When the Heart and Spleen cooperate, the blood circulation will be normal.

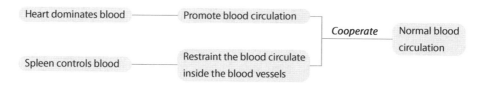

Fig. 2-22　Cooperative relationship between the Heart and Spleen in blood circulation

The pathological changes of the Heart and Lung can affect each other.

The diseases of the Heart involve the Spleen: if the Heart blood is insufficient and is incapable of maintaining the Spleen, or if over-thinking results in the dysfunction of the Spleen in transporting, it will result in pathological changes of palpitations, insomnia, poor appetite, abdominal fullness and loose stool etc.

The diseases of the Spleen involve the Heart:

dysfunction of the Spleen in transporting results in the insufficient source for transformation and generation, or failure of the Spleen in controlling the blood results in profuse blood loss. It can result in Heart blood insufficiency and manifest as poor appetite and loose stool or symptoms of chronic hemorrhage, as well as a lusterless complexion, palpitations, insomnia and dreamfulness etc. The above symptoms are the interplay of the pathological changes of the Heart and Spleen that result in the deficiency of both Spleen and blood.

③ Relationship between the Heart and Liver

The relationship between the Heart and Liver mainly finds expression in aspects of blood circulation and mental and emotional activities. Their relations are interactive and mutually cooperative.

In the aspect of blood circulation (Fig. 2-23), the Heart governs blood and the Liver stores blood. If the Heart blood is sufficient and the Heart qi is vigorous, the blood circulation will be normal, and then the Liver will have blood to store. If the Liver stores sufficient blood and regulates the blood flow normally, it is conducive to the Heart in promoting blood circulation.

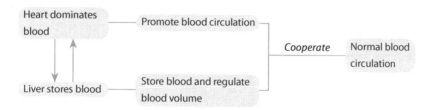

Fig. 2-23　The Chart of the interactive relationship of the Heart governing blood to the Liver storing blood

In the aspect of mental and emotional activities (Fig. 2-24), the Heart stores the spirit and dominates mental and emotional activities. The Liver dominates free coursing and regulates mental and emotional activities. Normal Heart spirit can be conducive to the free coursing of the Liver qi. The normal free coursing of the Liver can regulate the mental and emotional activities, and is conducive to the action of the Heart dominating the mind. The Heart and Liver are mutually interactive and cooperative, and maintain normal mental and emotional activities.

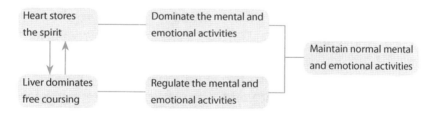

Fig. 2-24　The Chart of correlation of the Heart dominating mental activities to the Liver regulating emotions

Regarding the pathological changes of blood and mind, the Heart and Liver mutually interact on each other.

Insufficiency of Heart blood can result in insufficiency of Liver blood. Contrarily, insufficient Liver blood can result in insufficiency of the Heart blood, since they are interactive. From that, the symptoms of the syndrome of deficiency of the Heart and Liver blood will occur in terms of lusterless expression, palpitations, dizziness, vertigo and scanty menstruation with light color.

Discomposure of the Heart spirit can result in the failure of the Liver in free coursing; or impairment of the emotions always relates to the discomposure of the Heart spirit. From there, pathological changes of mind imbalance can be seen in terms of vexation, palpitations, insomnia, impatience, testiness or unhappiness due to depression.

④ Relationship between the Heart and Kidney

The physiological relationship between the Heart and Kidney is known as "the communication between the Heart and the Kidney". This is a generalization of the mutual interactive restrictive relationship between the Heart and the Kidney. They find their expression in the mutual assistance of the fire and water, mutual supplementation of yin and yang, mutual transformation of essence and blood, and mutual interaction of essence and spirit of the Heart and Kidney. (Fig. 2-25)

Mutual assistance of water and fire: the Heart resides in the upper *Jiao* and belongs to yang, and it belongs to fire among the five phases. The Kidney resides in the lower *Jiao* and belongs to yin, and it belongs to water among the five phases. Regarding the ascent and descent of water and fire, the Heart fire must descend to the Kidney to warm the Kidney yang and keep the Kidney water away from cold. The Kidney water must ascend to the Heart to nourish the Heart yin and restrain the Heart fire and keep it from being hyperactive. The ascent and descent, as well as mutual assistance of the Heart fire and Kidney water maintain the harmony and balance between the physiological functions of the two *zang* organs. The ancients called the relationship between the ascent and descent of fire and water the communication between the Heart and the Kidney.

Mutual supplementation of yin and yang: in physiological status, the yin and yang of each *zang* organ interacts on and roots in each other to keep balance and harmony between them. The yin and yang of the two correlative *zang* organs also mutually interact and root. The yin and yang of the Heart supplement the yin and yang of the Kidney, and the yin and yang of the Kidney also supplement the yin and yang of the Heart, therefore, the yin and yang of the Heart and Kidney are kept in harmony and equilibrium.

Mutual generation of essence and blood: essence and blood are the requisite substances that maintain the life activity of the human body, and essence and blood can mutually generate and transform each other. The Heart governs blood and the Kidney stores essence, so, there exists a mutual generation and transformation relationship between the Heart blood and the Kidney essence. This sets the material basis for

the communication between the Heart and the Kidney.

Mutual interaction of spirit and essence: the Heart stores spirit and is the dominator of the life activity of the human body, therefore, the spirit can supplement essence, and then the essence will not discharge unreservedly. The Kidney stores essence, the essence generates marrow to fill the brain, the brain dominates the original spirit, and so the accumulation of the essence can nourish the spirit and then the spirit can be guarded internally. Essence can generate spirit, and the spirit can drive essence. Thus the mental activities of humans are closely related to the Heart and Kidney.

The pathological changes of the Heart and Kidney can affect each other.

For instance: yin deficiency of the Heart and Kidney can interact upon each other and can also result in hyperactivity of fire due to yin deficiency, manifesting as symptoms of the syndrome of yin deficiency of the Heart and Kidney and hyperactivity of fire in terms of palpitations, vexation, insomnia, dreamfulness, tinnitus, aching in the waist and knees, or wet dream in males and females, known as the disharmony of the Heart and Kidney.

If the deficient Kidney yang fails to warm up water and fluids and results in the invasion of the Heart by water due to yang deficiency, manifesting as aversion to cold, pale complexion, oliguria, edema, palpitation etc., it is known as "attack of the Heart by the water qi".

If insufficient Heart blood fails to nourish the spirit, and deficient Kidney essence results in emptiness of the brain marrow, it can result in essence and blood deficiency of the Heart and Kidney and lack of nourishment of the spirit, manifesting as amnesia, dizziness, tinnitus, insomnia and dreamfullness etc.

Recipes Worth a Thousand Gold: *Chapter Recipes for Heart Diseases* (Qiān Jīn Fāng: Xīn Zàng Fāng, 千金方·心脏方) says: "*The Heart belongs to fire and the Kidney belongs to water, the Kidney water and the Heart fire communicate with each other.*"

Posthumous Manuscript of Shenzhai: *Yin and Yang of Zang-fu Organs* (Shèn Zhāi Yí Shū: Yīn

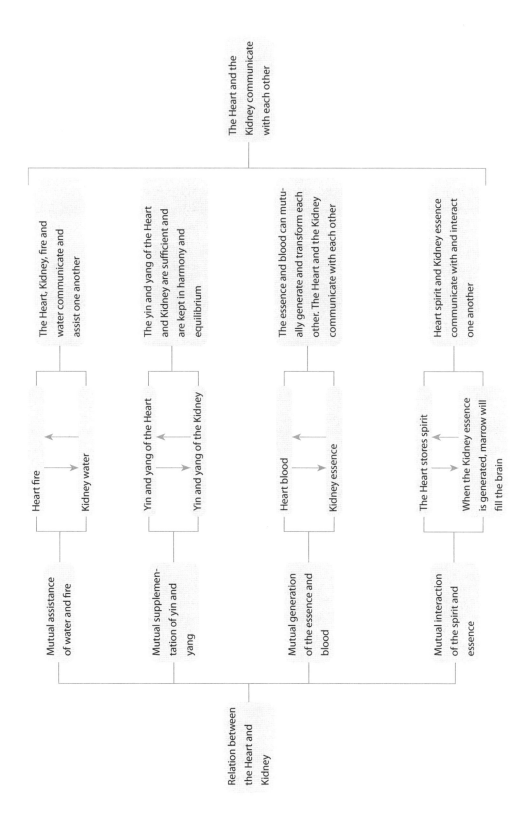

Fig. 2-25 The communication between the Heart and the Kidney

Yáng Zàng Fǔ, 慎斋遗书·阴阳脏腑) says: *"The communication of the Heart and Kidney depends on the movements of ascent and descent…The Heart fire descends and the Kidney water ascends."*

Seek the Meaning of the Master by Deduction: Section Fear, Chapter Miscellaneous Diseases, (*Tuī Shī Qiú Yì: Bù, Zá Bìng Mén,* 推师求意·杂病门·怖) says: *"The Heart takes spirit as its dominance and yang as its action; the Kidney takes will as its dominance and yin as its action. Qi and fire belong to yang; essence and water belong to yin. All conditions where the Kidney water and Heart fire communicate with each other depend on the ascent of the Kidney yin essence to control the Heart spirit; the descent and the storage of Heart yang qi will control the will of the Kidney. Otherwise, the Heart spirit will move and can not stay in the body, and the Heart yang qi will diffuse outside, the will of the Kidney will be confused inside, and the Kidney yin essence goes downwards."*

⑤ Relationship between the Lung and Spleen

The relationship between the Lung and Spleen mostly find their expression in the generation of qi and the metabolism of water.

In the aspect of qi generation (Fig. 2-26), it primarily refers to the generation of gathering qi. The Lung governs respiration and inhales the clear qi from nature. The Spleen dominates transformation and transportation and absorbs the essence qi from water and food. The clear qi and the essence qi converge in the chest and generate gathering qi. After birth, the gathering qi is formed and become the primary source of qi for the whole body. The Spleen dominates transformation and transportation and is the source of generation and transformation of qi and blood. The Spleen absorbs the essence qi of water and food, which depends on the dispersing and descending actions of the Lung to distribute the essence qi to the whole body. Therefore, it is known that "the Spleen is the source that generates qi, and the Lung is the pivot that dominates qi."

Regarding the aspect of water metabolism

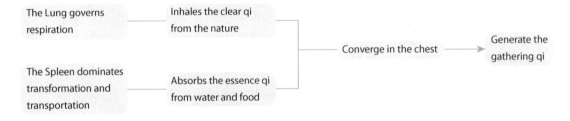

Fig. 2-26 Chart of the actions of the Lung and Spleen on the generation of gathering qi

(Fig. 2-27): the water and fluid metabolism is the combined action of several *zang-fu* organs. Regarding the Lung and Spleen, the normal distribution and discharge of water and fluid requires the dispersing and descending action of the Lung to clear and regulate the water passage. It also requires the transporting and transforming actions of the Spleen to absorb and distribute the water and fluid, so that the fluids can be normally generated and distributed. The mutual cooperation and interaction of the Spleen and Lung is the key section of the normal generation, distribution and discharge of water and fluids.

The pathological changes of the Spleen and Lung can affect each other.

For instance: Spleen qi deficiency and insufficient generation of qi can result in Lung qi deficiency or chronic Lung disease which results in the exhaustion of qi and affects the Spleen. This can result in poor appetite, abdominal fullness, loose stools, fatigue, cough with dyspnea, and shortness of breath, which are the symptoms of qi deficiency of the Lung and Spleen.

If the deficient Spleen qi is incapable of transporting and transforming the water dampness, water dampness will stop internally, form the retention of phlegm and fluid and affect the Lung, and then the Lung will fail to disperse and descend. After that it will result in

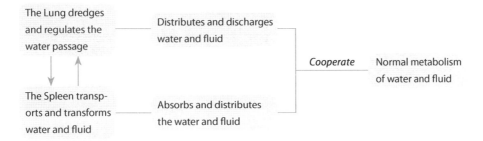

Fig. 2-27   Actions of the Lung and Spleen on water and fluid metabolism

poor appetite, abdominal fullness, cough with dyspnea, and abundant expectoration, which are symptoms of the syndromes of deficiency of the Lung qi and the internal retention of phlegm dampness. Therefore, it is known that "the Spleen is the source that generates phlegm, and the Lung is the container that stores phlegm."

⑥ Relationship between the Lung and Liver

The relationship between the Lung and Liver mostly finds expression in the aspect of the regulation of the ascent and descent of the qi dynamic of the human body. (Fig. 2-28)

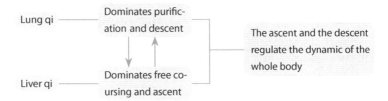

Fig. 2-28   Chart of the actions of the Lung and Liver on the qi dynamic regulation

The Lung qi is in favor of purification and descent and the Liver qi is in favor of ascending and dispersing. If the purification and descent of the Lung qi is normal, it is beneficial to the ascending and dispersing of the Liver qi; and the normal ascending and dispersing of Liver qi is beneficial to the purification and descent of the Lung qi. The ascent of the Liver and the descent of the Lung mutually restrict and interact on each other. The close coordination of the Liver and Lung, one ascending and another descending, plays a key role in regulating the qi dynamic of the whole body.

The pathological changes of the imbalance of the qi dynamic of the Spleen and Lung can affect each other.

If the stagnation of the Liver qi transforms into fire, the qi and fire will adversely invade the Lung. Then the Lung will fail to disperse and descend, or fail to clear and purify, which will result in internal excessive dry-heat and affect the Liver. As well, the Liver will fail to ascend and disperse. All of these can result in the symptoms of the diseases of both Liver and Lung in terms of headache, flushed face, red eyes, chest and hypochondrium pain, cough and emptysis. The pathogenesis of the invasion of the Lung by the Liver fire is always summarized by the theory of five phases as "wood-fire impairs metal "or "vigorous wood insults metal."

⑦ Relationship between the Lung and Kidney

The relationship between the Lung and Kidney mainly finds expression in the mutual cooperation and interaction in the aspects of water and fluid metabolism and respiratory movement, and in the mutual generation of the Lung and Kidney yin.

In the aspect of water metabolism (Fig. 2-29), the Lung dominates purifying and regulating the water passage, and is the upper source of water. The descent and purification of the Lung qi

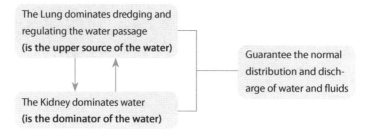

Fig. 2-29   Chart of actions of the Lung and Kidney on water and fluid metabolism

lowers the water and fluids down to the Kidney and is conducive to the action of the Kidney to dominate water. The Kidney is the dominator of water, Kidney qi moves, and Kidney yang steams, which is beneficial to the dispersion, purification and descent of the Lung. The mutual cooperation and interaction of the Kidney and Lung guarantees the normal distribution and discharge of water and fluids.

In the aspect of respiratory movement (Fig. 2-30), the Lung dominates qi and governs respiration, and then it can dominate the qi of respiration and be the dominator of qi. The Kidney governs the reception of qi to keep the depth of respiration, and is the root of qi. The Lung qi purifies and descends in its function of governing respiration; it is conducive to the action of the Kidney receiving qi. The Kidney qi is sufficient and is powerful in receiving qi. It is beneficial to the purification and descent of the Lung qi. Therefore, the Kidney and Lung mutually cooperate and interact with each other and complete the work of breathing together.

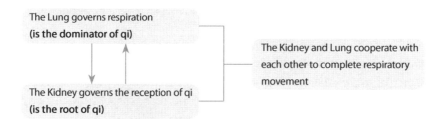

Fig. 2-30   Chart of actions of the Lung and Kidney on respiratory movement

In mutual generation of Lung yin and Kidney yin, the lung belongs to Metal and the Kidney belongs to Water; Metal can generate water and Water can moisten metal. If the Lung yin is sufficient and is transported down to the Kidney, the Kidney yin will be sufficient. The Kidney yin is the root of yin fluid of the whole body, so if the Kidney yin is sufficient, it can nourish the Lung and suffuse the Lung yin. The mutual generation of the Lung yin and the Kidney yin maintains the yin sufficiency of the two *zang* organs and keeps the equilibrium between the Lung yin and Kidney yin.

The following three aspects mainly embody the mutual pathological influence of the Lung and

Kidney.

a. The metabolic disturbance of water and fluids: the Lung fails to diffuse and descend and clear and regulate the water passage, or the Kidney qi fails to transform water and fluids, which can result in disorders of the distribution and discharge of water and fluids. Therefore, symptoms of cough with dyspnea, oliguria and edema will occur.

b. Abnormal respiration: long-term Lung qi deficiency can result in failure of the Lung in purifying and descending, interplaying with the insufficiency of the Kidney qi that fails to receive qi. It can result in the pathological changes of the syndrome of the Kidney failing to grasp qi in terms of shortness of breath, asthma, shallow breathing, or more expiration with less inspiration.

c. Yin deficiency of both the Lung and Kidney: deficiency of the Kidney yin becomes incapable of nourishing the Lung yin, or deficiency of the Lung yin involves the Kidney yin. These can result in yin deficiency of both the Lung and Kidney, which manifest as the symptoms of the syndrome of endogenous heat due to yin deficiency of the Lung and Kidney in terms of steaming bones, tidal fever, night sweats, zygomatic flushing, dry cough, hoarse throat, and aching waist and knees.

Plain Questions: *Chapter Discussion on Water and Heat Diseases* (*Sù Wèn: Shuǐ Rè Xuè Lùn,* 素问·水热穴论) says: "*The root of edema is in the Kidney, the branch of edema is in the Lung. If the the Lung or Kidney are not sound, fluid retention will occur.*"

Treatment of Different Kinds of Diseases: Chapter Panting Syndrome (*Lèi Zhèng Zhì Cái: Chuǎn Zhèng,* 类证治裁·喘证) says: "*The Lung is the dominator*

of qi, the Kidney is the root of qi. The Lung governs exhalation, and the Kidney governs inhalation and receiving qi. Yin and yang communicate, and then breathing will be harmonious and normal."

⑧ Relationship between the Liver and Spleen

The relationship between the Liver and Kidney mainly finds expression in the aspects of digestion and blood circulation.

In the aspect of digestion (Fig. 2-31), the Liver dominates free coursing and regulates the ascent and descent of the qi dynamic of the Spleen and Stomach, and promotes the excretion of bile to assist the digestion and absorption of water and food. The Spleen dominates transformation and transportation, so if the Spleen qi is vigorous, the actions of transportation and transformation of the Spleen will be normal. Then the essence of water and food can transform and generate qi and blood to nourish the Liver, which is conducive to the free coursing of the Liver. When the Liver and Spleen interact with each other, digestion will be normal.

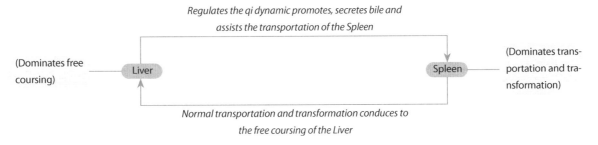

Fig. 2-31 The interactive relationship of the Liver governing free coursing to the Spleen dominating transformation and transportation

In the aspect of blood circulation (Fig. 2-32), the Heart governs normal blood circulation, but it is also closely related to the Liver and Spleen. The Liver stores blood and regulates blood flow. The Spleen transforms, generates and controls blood, and keeps the blood circulating inside the vessels instead of overflowing. The Liver and Spleen cooperate with each other to maintain the normal

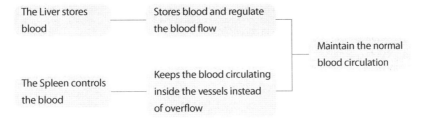

Fig. 2-32 The cooperative relationship between the action of the Liver storing blood and the action of the Spleen controlling blood

circulation of blood.

The pathological changes of the Spleen and Liver can affect each other.

For instance: failure of the Liver in free coursing and invasion of the Spleen by Liver qi depression can result in dysfunction of the Spleen in transporting, which manifests as mental depression, oppressed feeling in the chest, deep sighing, loss of appetite, abdominal fullness, diarrhea, etc. all symptoms of the syndrome of disharmony between the Liver and Spleen. The dysfunction of the Spleen in transporting can result in the generation of damp-heat which can stagnate in the Liver and Gallbladder and result in the pathological changes of poor appetite and jaundice etc.

Prolonged dysfunction of the Spleen in transportation can result in the lack of source for the generation of blood, or the deficient Spleen failing to control blood and resulting in bleeding. These factors can result in deficiency of Liver blood and result in poor appetite, fatigue, dizziness, vertigo, and scanty menstruation with light color. Various hemorrhagic diseases can also be caused by the Liver failing to store blood and the Spleen failing to control blood simultaneously.

⑨ Relationship between the Liver and Kidney

The relationship between the Liver and Kidney, in the ancient Chinese medical works, is described by saying that "the Liver and the Kidney share the common source" or "*Yi* and *Gui* share the same source." This primarily finds expression in three aspects in terms of the following: that the essence and blood have a common source; the action of free coursing of the Liver and the action of sealing and storing of the Kidney interact; and that yin and yang mutually generate and restrict each other.

Regarding the idea that essence and blood have a common source (Fig. 2-33): the Liver stores blood, and the Kidney stores essence, and essence and blood are both transformed and generated by the essence from water and food. Essence and blood can also nourish and transform each other, namely, the Kidney essence can transform and generate Liver blood, and Liver blood can suffuse and nourish Kidney essence. Therefore, it is said of the Liver and the Kidney that "essence and blood have common source".

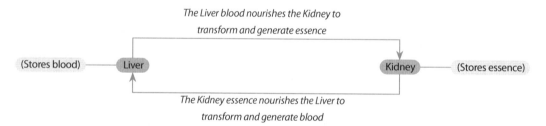

The Liver blood nourishes the Kidney to transform and generate essence

(Stores blood) — Liver   Kidney — (Stores essence)

The Kidney essence nourishes the Liver to transform and generate blood

Fig. 2-33   Relationship between the Liver blood and Kidney essence that transform and generate each other

The free coursing of the Liver and the storing and sealing of the Kidney interact on each other (Fig. 2-34): the Liver dominates free coursing and the Kidney governs sealing and storing, which mutually interact with and restrict one another. The normal free coursing of the Liver qi

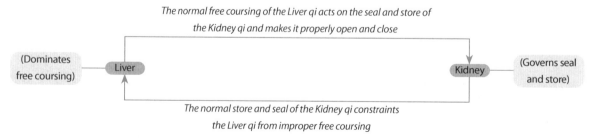

The normal free coursing of the Liver qi acts on the seal and store of the Kidney qi and makes it properly open and close

(Dominates free coursing) — Liver   Kidney — (Governs seal and store)

The normal store and seal of the Kidney qi constraints the Liver qi from improper free coursing

Fig. 2-34   Correlation between the free coursing of the Liver and the storing and sealing of the Kidney

influences the sealing and storing of the Kidney qi and makes it properly open and close. The normal functions of the Kidney qi in storing and sealing constraint the Liver qi from improperly free coursing. The free coursing of the Liver and the storing and sealing of the Kidney are opposite but are helpful to each other, because they interact and restrict one another, which can help normally regulate the menstruation and ejaculation.

Regarding yin and yang mutually generating and restricting one another (Fig. 2-35): there is mutual generation and restriction between the yin and yang of the Liver and the Kidney. Vigorous and sufficient Kidney yin can nourish and generate Liver yin, and sufficient Liver yin can nourish Kidney yin. Yin can constraint yang, so sufficient yin of the Liver and Kidney can not only generate and nourish one another, but also can constraint Liver yang and inhibit Kidney fire, so that Liver yang and Kidney fire won't be hyperactive. Therefore, the sufficiency and balance of the yin and yang of the Liver and the Kidney can be kept.

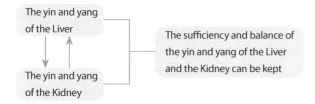

Fig. 2-35   Relationship between the yin and yang of the Liver and the Kidney, which transform and generate each other

Regarding the pathological changes of the Liver and Kidney, they interplay and are always sick simultaneously.

For instance, Kidney essence deficiency can result in insufficiency of Liver blood and in the reverse, Liver blood insufficiency can also result in Kidney essence deficiency. They manifest as symptoms of the syndrome of deficiency of Liver blood and Kidney essence.

Insufficient Kidney essence and Liver blood or hyperactivity of fire due to deficiency of Liver yin and Kidney yin can result in the imbalance of the Liver in dominating free coursing and the

Kidney in governing storing and sealing. They manifest as menstrual disorders in terms of profuse menses or amenorrhea in females, and spermatorrhea or premature ejaculation in men.

Liver yin insufficiency can result in insufficiency of Kidney yin and hyperactivity of Kidney fire. Insufficiency of Kidney yin can also cause Liver yin insufficiency and result in hyperactivity of Liver yang. This manifests as dizziness, vertigo, flushed face, red eyes, vexation, insomnia, tinnitus, spermatorrhea, low fever and night sweating, all symptoms of the syndrome of hyperactivity of fire due to deficiency of Liver yin and Kidney yin.

⑩ Relationship between the Spleen and Kidney

The relationship between the Spleen and Kidney is primarily embodied by the innate and acquired relationship and their relationship regarding water and fluid metabolism.

The innate and acquired relationship (Fig. 2-36): the Spleen transports and transforms the essence of water and food, and transforms and generates qi and blood to maintain life activities. Thus the Spleen is the acquired root of body constitution. The Kidney stores the innate essence that originates in innateness, dominates reproduction, is the root of life, and is the root of congenital constitution. The innate and acquired essences nourish and generate one another, the actions of transportation and transformation of the Spleen must depend on the warming and steaming actions of the Kidney yang, and then the Spleen can transport normally. The essence qi in the Kidney relies on the supply of the essence of water and food formed by the actions of transportation and transformation of the Spleen, so that the essence qi in the Kidney can be continually suffused. The innate essence

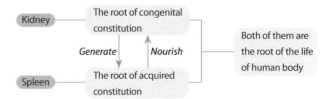

Fig. 2-36   Chart of the relationship between the Kidney, the innate root, and the Spleen, the acquired root

stimulates and nourishes the acquired essence, and the acquired supplies and nourishes the innate. They nourish and generate one another, as well as promote each other. Both of them are the roots of the life of the human body.

In the aspect of water metabolism (Fig. 2-37), the spleen transports and transforms water and fluids, and relates to the generation and distribution of the water and fluids of the

human body, which need the warming and steaming action of the Kidney yang. The Kidney stores water and presides over the metabolic balance of water and fluids of the whole body, and also needs restriction by the Spleen qi. The mutual cooperation and interaction of the Kidney and Spleen guarantee the normal generation, distribution and discharge of water and fluids.

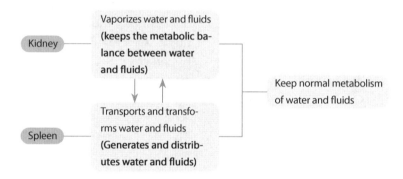

Fig. 2-37　Chart of the relationship of the Spleen and Kidney in metabolism of water and fluids

The pathological changes of the Spleen and Kidney can affect each other.

For instance: insufficiency of Spleen qi that fails in transportation can result in insufficiency of Kidney essence, and may manifest as poor appetite, abdominal fullness, loose stools, emaciation, soreness of waist, tinnitus, or delayed growth and development or maldevelopment in adolescence caused by deficiency of both the Spleen and Kidney essences.

If insufficiency of Kidney yang fails to warm the Spleen yang or prolonged deficiency of Spleen yang impairs the Kidney yang, they may manifest as cold pain in the abdomen, diarrhea with undigested food in the stool, aching and cold waist and knees, and diarrhea before dawn, symptoms belonging to the syndrome of insufficiency of both the Spleen and Kidney yang.

If Spleen deficiency fails to transport and transform the water and fluids, and Kidney deficiency fails to vaporizing water and fluids, it may result in the disorder of distribution and excretion of water and fluids and manifest as oliguria, edema, abdominal fullness, loose stools, waist and knees being achy and limp,

intolerance of cold, and cold limbs, symptoms of the syndrome of insufficiency of both the Spleen and Kidney yang, with internal retention of water and fluids.

Jing-yue's Complete Works: Chapter Discussion on Spleen and Stomach (Jǐng Yuè Quán Shū: Lùn Pí Wèi, 景岳全书·论脾胃) says: *"Before a baby is born, they depend on essence and blood; after a baby is born, they are supported and nourished by water and food. The foundation of the human body can't be set without essence and blood; the body won't be strong and grow up without water and food...So, the sea of water and food depends on the dominance of the congenital essence, and the sea of essence and blood must depend on the support of the acquired root."*

Golden Mirror of Medicine: Chapter in Abridged and Supplemented Discussion on Formulae of Famous Physicians (Yī Zōng Jīn Jiàn: Shān Bǔ Míng Yī Fāng Lùn, 医宗金鉴·删补名医方论) says: *"The acquired qi will cycle vigorously when it wins the congenital qi; the congenital qi will start to change endlessly when it gets acquired qi."*

Discussion of Blood Syndromes: Chapter Discussion on Yin Water and Yang Fire (Xuè Zhèng Lùn: Yīn Yáng Shuǐ Huǒ Lùn, 血证论·阴阳水火论)

says: "*At the beginning of the formation of the fetus, the innate essence generates the acquired essence. After birth, the acquired essence supports and generates the acquired essence.*"

Relationship between the *Fu*-Organs

The physiological features of the six *fu*-organs are to transport and transform water and food, which is embodied by the digestion, absorption and discharge of water and food. Thus, the relationships between the six *fu*-organs mainly find their expression in their intimate cooperation in the course of the digestion, absorption and discharge of water and food. (Fig. 2-38)

The Stomach dominates receiving, containing, rotting, and ripening water and food, which

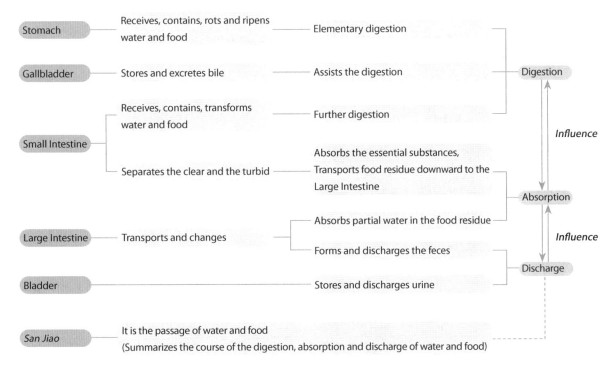

Fig. 2-38   The sketch of the actions of transporting and transforming water and food by the six *fu*-organs and their relationships

means that the Stomach elementarily digests the water and food. The Gallbladder stores and excretes bile to assist with the digestion of water and food. The Small Intestine receives, contains, transforms and further digests water and food. It separates the clear and the turbid, absorbs the essential substances, and by the action of being unobstructed and with the descent of the Stomach, it transports food residue downward to the Large Intestine. The Large Intestine transports and changes water and food, absorb partial water in the food residue, and forms and discharges the feces. The Bladder stores urine, and by its qi transformation, the urine is discharged outside the body. The *San Jiao* is the passage of water

and food, and of water and fluid circulation. It attends to the whole course of the digestion, absorption and discharge of water and food. The digestion of the six *fu* organs is related to the actions of the Stomach, Gallbladder and Small Intestine. The action of absorption relates to the actions of the small and Large Intestines. The action of discharge relates to the actions of the Large Intestine and Bladder. Thus, in the course of transporting and digesting water and food by the six *fu*-organs, they cooperatively complete the task of the digestion of water and food, the absorption of refined nutritious substances and water and fluids, and the discharge of draff.

Thus, the pathological changes of the six *fu*-

organs can affect each other, and dysfunction of any *fu*-organs can affect the actions of digestion or absorption or discharge of water and food.

Plain Questions: Chapter Discussion on the Secret Classics Stored in Royal Library (Sù Wèn: Líng Lán Mì Diǎn Lùn, 素问·灵兰秘典论) says: *"The Spleen and Stomach are the like the officials of a granary and are responsible for the five flavors of food. The Large Intestine is like the official in charge of transmitting dregs, and is responsible for the change and transformation of water and food…The San Jiao is like the official in charge of dredging and is responsible for the waterway. The Bladder is like the official in charge of the reservoir where the body fluids are stored and are responsible for qi transformation."*

Classic of Questioning: The Thirty-first Question (Nàn Jīng: Sān Shí Yī Nàn, 难经·三十一难) says: *"The San Jiao is the passage of water and food and is where qi starts and stops."*

Plain Questions: Chapter Different Discussion on the Five-zang Organs (Sù Wèn: Wǔ Zàng Bié Lùn, 素问·五脏别论) says: *"The six-fu organs transport and transform water and food but do not store them, so the six-fu organs can be filled but not substantialized. Why it is so? That's because after the water and food are taken into the mouth, the Stomach is filled but the intestine is empty. When food enters the intestine, the intestine is filled but the Stomach is empty."*

Relationship between *Zang* Organs and *Fu* Organs

The relationship between *zang*-organs and *fu*-organs, chiefly, is that the relationship of the five *zang*-organs matches the six *fu*-organs. *Zang* belong to yin and *fu* belong to yang. Yin dominates the interior, and yang dominates the exterior. The *zang*, *fu*, yin, yang, exterior and interior cooperate and form the exterior and interior relationship of the *zang-fu* organs in terms of the Heart cooperating with the Small Intestine, the Lung cooperating with the Large Intestine, the Spleen cooperating with the Stomach, the Liver cooperating with the Gallbladder, and the Kidney cooperating with the Bladder, which is also known as the relationship of "the exterior

cooperating with the interior".

The exterior and interior cooperation of each *zang* organ and the correspondent *fu* organ mainly finds its expression in three aspects:

a. Structurally, they connect with each other by channels and collaterals. Specifically, the channel of each *zang* organ pertains to the *fu* organ that has an exterior-interior relationship with it; the channel of each *fu* organ pertains to the *zang* organ that has an exterior-interior relationship with it.

b. Physiologically, they cooperate with each other. The correspondent *zang* organ and *fu* organ mutually interplay and cooperate to complete one function together.

c. Pathologically, they affect each other. The pathological changes of the correspondent *zang* organ and *fu* organ can affect each other. The disease of the *zang* organ can involve the *fu* organ, and the disease of the *fu* organ can affect the *zang* organ. Thus the *zang* and the related *fu* organ can be sick simultaneously. Therefore regarding the therapeutic methods, accordingly, there are methods of treating the *fu* organ when the correspondent *zang* organ is sick, treating the *zang* organ when the correspondent *fu* organ is sick, or treating the *zang* and *fu* organs simultaneously. Thus the theory of *zang* organs cooperating with their correspondent *fu* organs possesses important significance in guiding clinical practices.

Miraculous Pivot: Chapter On Acupoints (Líng Shū: Běn Shū, 灵枢·本输): *"The Lung cooperates with the Large Intestine"*, *"The Spleen cooperates with the Stomach"*, *"The Liver cooperates with the Gallbladder"* and *"The Kidney cooperates with the Bladder."*

Classic of Questioning: The Thirty-five Question (Nàn Jīng: Sān Shí Wǔ Nàn, 难经·三十五难) says: *"The Small Intestine is the residence of the Heart; the Large Intestine is the residence of the Lung; the Gallbladder is the residence of the Liver; th Stomach is the residence of the Spleen; and the Bladder is the residence of the Kidney."*

① Relationship between the Heart and Small Intestine

Structurally, the Heart channel belongs to the

Heart and connects with the Small Intestine. The Small Intestine channel belongs to the Small Intestine and connects with the Heart. The two organs connect via channels and form the exterior and interior relationship.

Physiologically, the Heart belongs to fire and dominates blood. The warming action of the Heart fire and the nourishing function of the Heart blood are helpful to the digestion and transformation of water and food by the Small Intestine. The Small Intestine dominates transformation and digestion of water and food, separates the clear and the turbid from each other, and absorbs refined nutritious substances to generate the Heart blood.

Pathologically, there is the theory of the Heart fire spreading heat to the Small Intestine. On one hand, hyperactive Heart fire spreads downward to the Small Intestine via the channels, and then produces heat in the Small Intestine. On the other hand, the exuberant heat in the Small Intestine can also flame upward via the channels to the Heart and result in hyperactive Heart fire. Both conditions manifest as vexation, a red tongue, oral sores and painful urination with a burning sensation.

To Know Medicine: Section The Six Fu-Organs (*Yī Xué Jiàn Néng: Liù Fǔ*, 医学见能·六腑) says: *"The Small Intestine is the residence of the Heart, belongs to fire, and dominates digesting water and food into fluid that is distributed upward and forms the Heart blood."*

Golden Mirror of Medicine: Chapter in Abridged and Supplemented Discussion on Formulae of Famous Physicians (*Yī Zōng Jīn Jiàn: Shān Bǔ Míng Yī Fāng Lùn*, 医宗金鉴·删补名医方论) says: *"Oral and glossal ulceration, yellow urine, pain in penis and stranguria are the symptoms of the syndrome of Heart heat spreading into the Small Intestine."*

② Relationship between the Lung and Large Intestine

Structurally, the Lung and Large Intestine connect with each other via channels and form an exterior and interior relationship.

Physiologically, the relationship is embodied by the mutual interaction of the purification and descending function of the Lung qi, and conveyance and transportation of the Large Intestine. The purification and descent of the Lung and the conveyance and transportation of the Large Intestine can affect the qi dynamic of the *zang-fu* organs. Thus if the action of purification and descent of Lung qi is normal and the Lung qi goes downward, the qi dynamic will be free and harmonious, can distribute fluids and promote the conveyance and transportation of the Large Intestine, which is conducive to the discharge of dregs. The Large Intestine normally conveys and transports the dregs downward, and is conducive to the purification and descent of Lung qi. When the purification and descent of the Lung and the conveyance and transportation of the Large Intestine cooperate, the qi dynamics of the Lung and Large Intestine will be free and harmonious to influence both respiratory movement and defecation. (Fig. 2-39)

Pathologically, the diseases of the Lung and Large Intestine can affect each other. For instance: If the Lung qi fails to purify, descend and go downward and the body fluid can't be distributed to the Large Intestine, then the Large Intestine will be obstructed. It may manifest as constipation due to dry intestines as well as cough and asthma. If excessive heat of the Large Intestine results in failure of it to convey

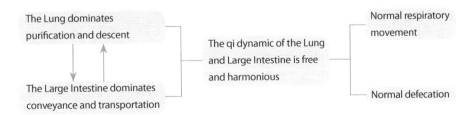

Fig 2-39　Relationship between the purification and descent of the Lung qi and the conveyance and transportation of the Large Intestine

and transport, and obstructed qi of the *fu* organ, the diffusion and descent function of the Lung would be affected. Besides constipation, it can also manifest as a fullness sensation in the chest, cough and asthma.

③ Relationship between Spleen and Stomach

Structurally, both the Spleen and Stomach are located in the middle *Jiao* and connect with each other by a membrane; they also connect with each other via channels and form an exterior and interior relationship.

Physiologically, both the Spleen and Stomach are the source of the generation and transformation of qi and blood, and are the root of acquired constitution. They cooperate to accomplish the digestion of water and food and the absorption and distribution of the refined nutritious substances. Their relationship is mainly embodied by cooperative transportation and reception, mutual dependence of ascent and descent, and mutual assistance of dryness and moistness. (Fig. 2-40)

Cooperative transportation and reception: the Spleen dominates transportation and transformation, and the Stomach dominates reception, containment and digestion of water and food. The reception, containment and digestion of the Stomach are the preparation for the transportation and transformation of the Spleen. The transportation and transformation of the Spleen are the command for the Stomach to continue its action of reception and containment. The Spleen would have no water and food to transport and transform without the reception, containment and digestion of the Stomach. Similarly, the Stomach can't receive and contain water and food without the transportation and transformation of the Spleen. Therefore, if the Stomach is harmonious, the Spleen will be fit in transportation; if the Spleen is healthy in transportation, the Stomach will be harmonious. The transportation of the Spleen and the reception of the Stomach cooperate mutually and intimately, and then the Spleen and Stomach can complete the physiological functions of reception, digestion, absorption, conveyance and distribution of water and food.

Mutual dependence of ascent and descent: the movement features of the qi of the Spleen and Stomach are as follows: Spleen qi dominates ascent and Stomach qi dominates descent. The ascent of the Spleen qi and the descent of the Stomach qi are opposite and are also supplementary to each other. The Spleen qi ascends to distribute the refined nutritious substances of water and food being digested and absorbed upward, which is conducive to the descent of the Stomach qi. The Stomach qi descends to transport water and food being elementarily digested, which is conducive to the ascent and transportation of the Spleen qi. In this way the ascent of the Spleen qi and the descent of the Stomach qi interact. If the Stomach fails to descend, the Spleen will fail to ascend. If the Spleen fails to ascend, the Stomach will fail to descend. Thu, the Spleen qi and the Stomach qi, one ascends and one descends, they depend on each other, and this guarantees the normal reception of the Stomach and the normal transportation of the Spleen.

Mutual assistance of dryness and moistness: the Spleen is a yin *zang*-organ, its normal transportation and transportation need the warmth of yang qi, so, it likes dryness and dislikes dampness; the Stomach is a yang *fu*-organ, its normal reception and containment need the nourishment of the yin fluids, so it likes moistness and dislikes dryness. What the Spleen and Stomach like or dislike are different, and the properties of dry and moist are opposite to each other, but they are also mutually restrictive and interact with one another. The Spleen is easy to be affected by damp and needs the Stomach yang to restrict dampness, so that the Spleen will not be affected by damp evil. The Stomach easily affected by dryness and needs the Spleen yin to restrict dryness, and then the Stomach will not be affected by dry evil. The moistness and dryness of the Spleen and Stomach assist each other, which is the requirement for guaranteeing the cooperation of the transportation and ascent of the Spleen and the reception and descent of the Stomach.

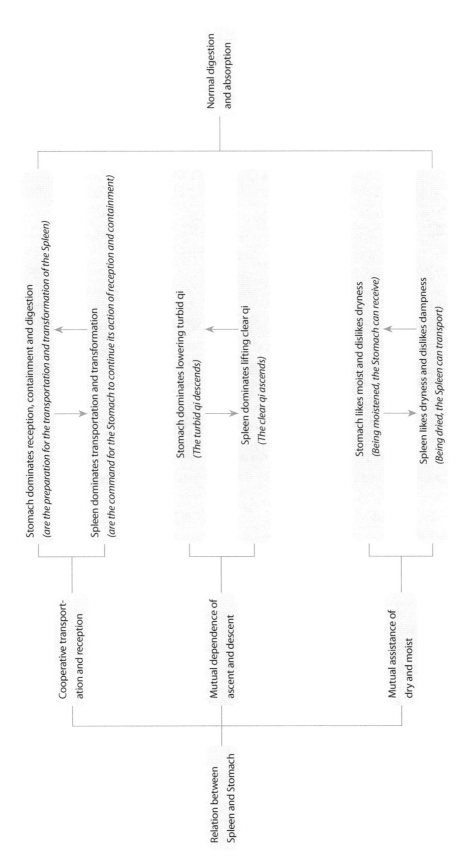

Fig. 2-40   Relationship between the Spleen and Stomach

Pathologically, although the clinical manifestations of the Spleen diseases and Stomach diseases are different, they always affect each other and are represented as a dual disease of the Spleen and Stomach.

Imbalance between transportation of the Spleen and reception of the Stomach: failure of the Spleen in transportation can result in lack of vigor of the reception and containment of the Stomach and disharmony of the Stomach qi. It manifests as poor appetite, Stomach fullness, abdominal flatulence and diarrhea, symptoms of disharmony of the Spleen in transportation and the Stomach in containment.

Abnormal ascent and descent of the Spleen and Stomach qi: qi falling due to Spleen qi deficiency can result in failure of the Stomach to be harmonious and descend, and affect the ascent and transportation of the Spleen qi. The above pathological changes may manifest as distension and a downbearing feeling in the epigastrium and abdomen, diarrhea, vomiting, regurgitation, dizziness, vertigo or prolapse of internal organs, symptoms of imbalance between the ascent and descent of the Spleen qi and Stomach qi.

Imbalance between the dryness and the moistness in the Spleen and Stomach: Dampness encumbering the transportation of the Spleen can result in lack of vigor of the reception of the Stomach and Stomach yin deficiency, which can also affect the transformation and transportation of the Spleen. It may manifest as poor appetite, distention and a downbearing feeling in the epigastrium and abdomen, constipation or diarrhea, symptoms of indigestion.

General Treatise on Causes and Manifestations of All Diseases: *Chapter Spleen and Stomach Diseases* (*Zhū Bìng Yuán Hòu Lùn: Pí Wèi Zhū Bìng Hòu*, 诸病源候论·脾胃诸病候) says: *"The Spleen qi and the Stomach qi have the exterior and interior relationship: the Stomach receives water and food, the Spleen digests them. When the qi of the Spleen and Stomach are harmonious, water and food can be digested, and then one will have a good Stomach."*

Jing-yue's Complete Works: *Chapter Discussion on Spleen and Stomach* (*Jǐng Yuè Quán Shū: Lùn*

Pí Wèi, 景岳全书·论脾胃) says: *"The Stomach dominates reception and containment, the Spleen dominates transportation and transformation. When transportation and reception is normal, the essence qi will be transformed and generated."*

Plain Questions: *Chapter Major Discussion on the Theory of Yin and Yang and the Corresponding Relationships Among All the Things in Nature* (*Sù Wèn: Yīn Yáng Yìng Xiàng Dà Lùn*, 素问·阴阳应象大论) says: *"If the clear qi stays in the lower Jiao, diarrhea will occur; if the turbid qi stays in the upper Jiao, flatulence will occur."*

Guide to Clinical Practice with Medical Records: *Chapter Spleen and Stomach* (*Lín Zhèng Zhǐ Nán Yī Àn: Pǐ Wèi*, 临证指南医案·脾胃) says: *"The Stomach dominates receiving water and food, and the Spleen dominates transportation and transformation. If the Spleen normally ascends, it will be healthy. If the Stomach normally descends, it will be harmonious. It is also said that, the taiyin wet earth can transport when it gets yang qi; the yangming yang (dry) earth can calm down when it gets yin. That's because the Spleen likes strong dryness and the Stomach likes soft moistness."*

Guide to Clinical Practice with Medical Records: *Chapter Stomach Upsetting* (*Lín Zhèng Zhǐ Nán Yī Àn: Cáo*, 临证指南医案·嘈) says: *"The Spleen belongs to yin and is dominated by blood; the Stomach belongs to yang and is dominated by qi. The Stomach is apt to be disturbed by the dry pathogen and depends on the Spleen yin to be harmonized; the Spleen is apt to be disturbed by the damp pathogen and depends on the Stomach yang to transport. Thus, the yang and the yin have an exterior and interior relationship and have the nature of being harmonious and balanced, and are the source of generation and transformation of the acquired constitution."*

Treatise on Spleen and Stomach: *Chapter Discussion on the Excess and Decline of the Spleen and Stomach* (*Pí Wèi Lùn: Pí Wèi Shèng Shuāi Lùn*, 脾胃论·脾胃胜衰论) says: *"If both the Spleen and the Stomach are vigorous, one will have a good Stomach and be strong; if both the Spleen and Stomach are declined, one will have poor appetite and be emaciated."*

Further Discussions in Medicine: *Chapter Supplementary to Discussion on the Spleen and*

Stomach (*Yī Jīng Yú Lùn: Xù Pí Wèi Lùn*, 医经余论·续脾胃论) says: *"The Spleen belongs to Ji (己, the sixth of the ten Heaven-Stems) earth, its form is in favor of dampness, so its action uses yang, just like the wet earth, and without the light by the sun, it can't generate all the creatures in the world; the Stomach belongs to Wu (戊, the fifth of the ten Heaven-Stems) earth, its form is in favor of dryness, so its action uses yin, just like the dry earth, and without the nourishment by the rain and dew, it can't generate all the creatures in the world. The Spleen dampness always depends on the Stomach yang to be transported; the Stomach dryness depends on the Spleen yin to be harmonized. They interact and help each other. However, the Stomach dominates reception and containment and the Spleen dominates digestion and absorption. Thus, the Spleen is responsible for indigestion; and the Stomach is responsible for poor appetite. The Spleen takes transportation as its strengthening method; the Stomach takes the dredging method as tonifying. To strengthen the Spleen one needs to use the method of ascent; to dredge the Stomach, one needs to use the method of descent. Therefore use the drugs with dry nature to lift the Spleen, which is the so-called light by the sun; and use the drugs with moist nature to lower the Stomach, which is the so-called nourishment by the rain and dew."*

④ Relationship between the Liver and Gallbladder

Structurally, both the Liver and Gallbladder are located at the right hypochondrium, and the Gallbladder is attached to the region between the two Liver lobes. The Liver and Gallbladder connect with each other via channels and have the exterior and interior relationship.

Physiologically, both the Liver and Gallbladder belong to wood and dominate free coursing, which is embodied by the action of digestion and mental and emotional activities.

The action of digestion: The free coursing action of the Liver secretes and excretes bile and that of the Gallbladder stores and excretes bile. Thus, if the Liver and Gallbladder cooperate, the secretion, storage and excretion of the bile will be normal, which can promote the digestion and absorption of water and food. (Fig 2-41)

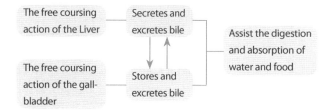

Fig.2-41 Relationship of the Liver and Gallbladder dominating free coursing for the digestion of water and food

Mental and emotional activities: the Liver dominates planning and consideration, which relates to emotional activities. The Gallbladder dominates decisions, which relates to courage. Good judgment and decisions need both the planning and consideration of the Liver and the decisions of the Gallbladder. If the Liver and Gallbladder cooperate, the mental and emotional activities will be normal, and then one can make correct resolutions when encountering different matters.

The pathological changes of the Liver and Gallbladder can affect each other. If the Liver fails in free coursing, it will affect the secretion and excretion of bile. Furthermore, if the excretion of the bile is not free it can affect the free coursing of the Liver. Then the syndromes of damp-heat retention in the Liver and Gallbladder and the blazing of the Liver and Gallbladder fire will occur. If the Liver and the Gallbladder are stagnated and phlegm-turbidity disturbs internally, it can result in the symptoms of depression, fear, timidity, insomnia and dreamfulness.

Plain Questions: Chapter Discussion on the Secret Classics Stored in Royal Library (*Sù Wèn: Líng Lán Mì Diǎn Lùn*, 素问·灵兰秘典论) says: *"The Liver is like the general and is responsible for planning and consideration. The Gallbladder is like the official of rightness and is responsible for determination."*

Classified Classic: Chapter Class of Visceral Manifestations (*Lèi Jīng: Zàng Xiàng Lèi*, 类经·藏象类) says: *"The Gallbladder attaches to the Liver and has an exterior and interior relationship with the Liver. Even if the Liver qi is strong, it can't determine without the Gallbladder. The Liver and the Gallbladder help each other, and then courage of the human is formed."*

⑤ Relationship between the Kidney and Bladder

Structurally, the Kidney and Bladder connect with each other via channels and have an exterior and interior relationship.

Physiologically, this finds expression in the aspect of urination. The Kidney dominates water, and by the qi transformation of the Kidney, the turbid part of water and fluids descends to the Bladder and forms urine that is stored in and discharged by the Bladder. The storing and discharging actions of the Bladder depend on the consolidating and qi transforming actions of the Kidney that keep the opening and closing of the Bladder working properly. The normal storage and discharge of the urine by the Bladder is beneficial to the actions of the Kidney dominating water. Thereby, the Kidney and Bladder interact and cooperate with each other and complete the generation, storage and excretion of the urine together. (Fig. 2-42)

In the aspect of pathology, the Kidney and Bladder always affects each other. The deficiency of Kidney qi, failure of the qi transformation, or weak consolidation can affect the storage and discharge of urine by the Bladder and result in a urinary disorder, difficulty in urination or urinary incontinence. Damp-heat in the urinary Bladder can affect the Kidney and cause frequent urination, red urine, dysuria and lumbago.

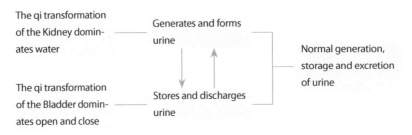

Fig. 2-42   The actions of the Kidney and Bladder on urination

Chapter 3
Essence, Qi, Blood and Fluid

Essence, qi, blood and fluid are the fundamental substances forming the human body and maintaining its vital activities. Tissues and organs of the body such as the *zang-fu* organs, channels and collaterals, body parts, sense organs, and orifices are all composed of these substances, and depend on their nourishment so that normal functional activities can proceed. At the same time, the generation and metabolism of these substances also depends on the physiological activities of these tissues and organs. Hence, there exists a close relationship between them.

Section 1   Essence

Fundamental Concept of Essence

① Concept of Essence (Fig. 3-1)

Essence (精), meaning extract or cream, is an essential substance. It is the most fundamental substance constituting the human body and maintaining its vital activities.

② Distributions and Classification of Essence (Fig. 3-1)

Essence is stored in the Kidneys, and is also stored separately in tissues and organs such as the five *zang* organs, the six *fu* organs, body parts, sense organs and orifices.

Essence, in Chinese medicine, has various names and meanings according to its different origins, distributions and functions. They mainly include:

(1) Congenital essence   It is inherited from a person's parents and originates from their reproductive essence. It is the primordial matter to form embryos and is the origin of life.

(2) Reproductive essence   It is stored in the Kidneys and originates from Kidney essence, which is transformed by congenital essence and replenished with acquired essence, and has the function of producing offspring. The reproductive essence of males and females combines with each other to form embryos and produce offspring.

(3) Essence from water and food   This is also called acquired essence, and is transformed from the water and food absorbed by the Spleen and the Stomach on a continual basis. It is an important substance in maintaining the vital activities of the human body.

(4) Visceral essence   This is the essence stored in the five *zang* organs and six *fu* organs, or viscera, hence the name. The functional activities of visceral essence need not only the activation and promotion of congenital essence but also the replenishment of acquired essence. Therefore, visceral essence embraces congenital essence as well as acquired essence. It plays a part in maintaining the functional activities of *zang-fu* organs.

In addition, essence is also defined in a broad sense and a narrow sense. Essence in

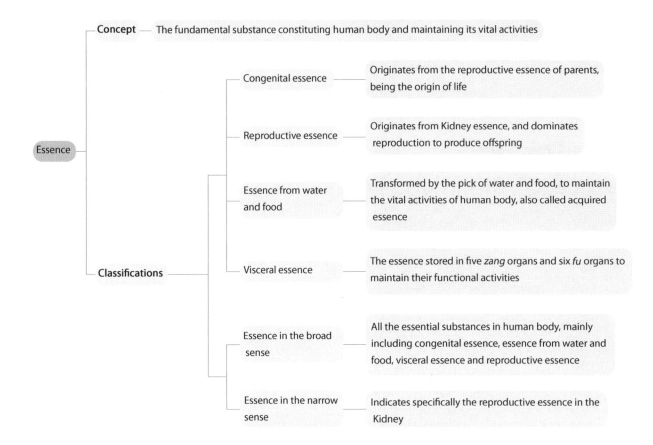

Fig. 3-1 Chart of the concept and classification of essence

the narrow sense indicates specifically the reproductive essence in the Kidney, which carries on reproductive functions. Essence in the broad sense indicates all the essential substances in human body, mainly congenital essence, essence from water and food, visceral essence and reproductive essence.

Plain Questions: Chapter Discussion on Important Ideas in the Golden Chamber (Sù Wèn: Jīn Guì Zhēn Yán Lùn, 素问·金匮真言论) says: "*The essence is the root of life."*

Generation of Essence

Generally speaking, essence is inherited from parents and replenished by water and food. As far as the source of essence is concerned, it can be divided into congenital essence and acquired essence. (Fig. 3-2)

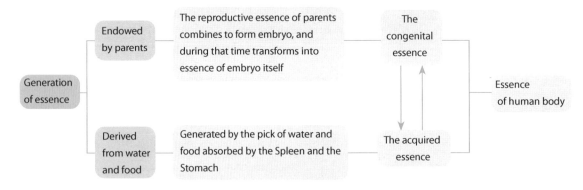

Fig. 3-2 Summary of the Generation of Essence

Congenital essence is inherited from parents. The reproductive essence of the parents combines to form an embryo, and then transforms into the essence of the embryo itself (the next generation). The fetus in utero depends on nourishment from the mother's qi and blood. This means that congenital essence is also dependent upon the nutrients absorbed from the mother by the fetus.

Acquired essence is derived from water and food. After birth, the Spleen and Stomach absorb, transport and transform the essence from water and food, and distribute it to the five *zang* organs and six *fu* organs to turn it into visceral essence, maintaining the physiological functions of the *zang-fu* organs. The surplus is stored in the Kidneys to maintain the abundance of Kidney essence.

Therefore, the essence of the human body is based on congenital essence and is constantly replenished by acquired essence. Congenital and acquired essence both promote and assist each other to maintain the abundance of essence in the human body.

Miraculous Pivot: Chapter On Channels (Líng Shū: Jīng Mài, 灵枢·经脉) says: *"The initiation of human life begins with the formation of essence."*

Miraculous Pivot: Chapter The Diseases Caused by Spiritual Activities (Líng Shū: Běn Shén, 灵枢·本神) says: *"The origin of life is essence."*

Miraculous Pivot: Chapter The Dredge of Qi (Líng Shū: Jué Qì, 灵枢·决气) says: *"The substance from both parents, which is generated before birth, combines to form the body, and this is known as essence."*

Plain Questions: Chapter Ancient Ideas on Flow to Preserve Natural Healthy Energy (Sù Wèn: Shàng Gǔ Tiān Zhēn Lùn, 素问·上古天真论) says: *"The Kidney dominates water, takes in the essence of the five zang organs and six fu organs and stores it; only when the five zang organs are excess can they be discharged."*

Functions of Essence

Essence is the fundamental substance creating the human body and maintaining its vital activities. The functions of essence mainly include (Fig. 3-3):

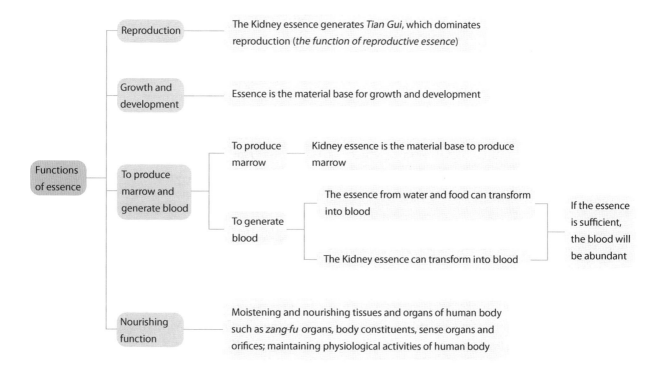

Fig. 3-3 Summary of the Functions of Essence

① Reproduction

Reproductive essence is the primordial matter of life, possessing the function of generating to breed offspring. This kind of essence that possesses reproductive abilities is known as *Tian Gui* (天癸). *Tiangui* comes into being when Kidney essence is abundant to a certain degree and has the ability to dominate reproduction.

② Growth and Development

Essence is the material base for growth and development of the human body. The formation of the embryo, and fetal growth and development, are the functional outcome of congenital essence. After birth, a person depends on both their congenital essence and the nourishment of acquired essence, so that the process of growth and development can continue normally. Following the up and down of essential qi, the human body progresses through the path of birth, growth, prime, senility and death. Hence, insufficiency of congenital and acquired essence will affect the growth and development of human body.

③ To Produce Marrow and Generate Blood

The Kidney stores essence and essence can produce marrow. Marrow in Chinese medicine includes cerebral marrow, spinal cord and bone marrow, all taking Kidney essence as their material base. Essence is also the most important substance to generate blood. On one hand, essence from water and food can transform into blood; on the other hand, Kidney essence (which can produce marrow) can transform into blood. Therefore, if essence is sufficient, blood will be abundant.

④ Nourishing Function

Essence has the function of moistening and nourishing the tissues and organs of the human body such as the *zang-fu* organs, body parts, sense organs and orifices. If the congenital and acquired essence is abundant, the essence of the five *zang* organs and six *fu* organs as well as Kidney essence will also be sufficient, thus the tissues and organs of the whole body can be nourished by essence, and all physiological functions can progress normally. If essence is deficient, body tissues and the *zang-fu* organs will present a state of hypo-function.

Section 2　Qi

Concept of Qi

Qi (气) is an essential substance with strong energy and constant movement, which is the most fundamental substance to constitute the human body and maintain its vital activities.

Qi is a philosophical idea of ancient China; a kind of perspective and methodology of ancient people to understand the world and explain its various changes. The philosophy is that everything in the world consists of qi, and various changes in the world are the effect of qi. Ancient doctors introduced qi into medicine to explain vital phenomena. Human beings are a product of nature, and the human body is composed of the qi found between heaven and earth. Human vital activities need to absorb nutrients from the qi between heaven and earth to maintain physiological activities of the body.

Various physiological functions in vital activities occur due to the constant movement of qi. In Chinese medicine, qi is also used to explain the physiological functions of the *zang-fu* organs and the tissues of the human body. For instance, when referring to the idea that the Heart governs blood and the Spleen governs transformation and transportation, the functions of Heart qi and Spleen qi are being discussed. Therefore, qi in Chinese medicine indicates both the fundamental substance to constitute human body and the summary of the substance and its functions in human vital activities.

Plain Questions: Chapter Discussion on Preserving Health and Protecting Life (Sù Wèn: Bǎo Mìng Qáun Xíng Lùn, 素问·宝命全形论) says: "Humans are generated by qi of heaven and earth." "The combination of qi between heaven and earth is called humanity."

Plain Questions: Discussion on Six-Plus-Six System and the Manifestations of the Viscera (Sù Wèn: Liù Jié Zàng Xiàng Lùn, 素问·六节藏象论) says: "The heavens feed people with five qi, and the earth feeds people with five flavors. The five qi enter the nose and are stored in the Heart and Lung, making the five complexions good-looking and bright, and the voice sonorous in the upper part of the body. The five flavors enter the mouth and are stored in the intestines and Stomach to nourish the five qi. Qi generated due to harmony, and accompanied by fluid, produces spirit spontaneously."

Miraculous Pivot: Chapter The Dredge of Qi (Líng Shū: Jué Qì, 灵枢·决气) says: "The upper Jiao activates and distributes the five flavors of food to warm the skin, replenish the body and moisten the hair like mist and dew. This is known as qi."

Principle and Prohibition for Medical Profession: Chapter Discussion on Great Qi (Yī Mén Fǎ Lù: Dà Qì Lùn, 医门法律·大气论) says: "As qi gathers, the body exists, and as qi scatters, the body disappears."

Generation of Qi

① Source of Qi

The generating source of qi mainly includes two aspects: the innate and the acquired.

The innate source is the essence inherited from parents, which is also called "congenital qi", transformed from the parents' congenital essence, which is also known as "genuine qi" or "source qi", and is the root of qi in human body.

The acquired source is the essential qi garnered from water and food combined with the clear qi in nature. Since it is acquired after birth, it is called "acquired qi".

② The Effects of the *Zang-fu* Organs on Qi (Fig. 3-4)

Both congenital qi and acquired qi are transformed into the qi of the human body by the effects of the *zang-fu* organs involved. Most important are the physiological functions of the

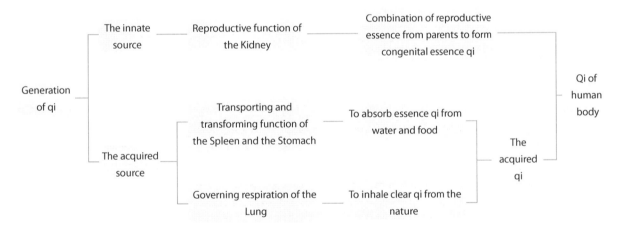

Fig. 3-4　Summary of the relationship between qi generation and *zang-fu* organs

Kidneys, Spleen, Stomach, and Lungs.

The reproductive function of the Kidneys: congenital qi combines the reproductive essence of both parents through the reproductive function of the Kidney to form embryos, which are the primordial and root qi of every human body.

The transporting and transforming function of the Spleen and Stomach: the Stomach controls the intake and digestion of water and food, and the Spleen is in charge of transporting and

transforming water and food. Together they control the digestion of food and the absorption of essential substances. The absorbed essence from water and food, also called "qi from water and food" or "food essence", distributes upward to the Heart and the Spleen in order to generate qi and blood, and then distributes to the whole body, being the main source of qi in the body. Hence, the Spleen and Stomach together are called the "source of qi".

The function of controlling respiration of the Lung: the Lung controlling respiration essentially starts with inhaling fresh air. The fresh air combines with food essence to produce "gathering qi", which is a part of acquired qi and is the fundamental substance maintaining vital human activities.

To sum up, under the effects of the Kidneys, Spleen, Stomach, and Lungs, inherited parental essence, essence qi from water and food, and clear qi from nature are transformed into the qi of human body. That is to say, there are two basic conditions of the generation of qi in human body: one is that the physiological functions of the Kidney, the Lung, the Spleen and the Stomach are normal; the other is that the sources of the congenital essence, essence qi from water and food, and clear qi in nature are abundant. If the functions of *zang-fu* organs are abnormal or their substantial sources are insufficient, qi generation will be affected.

Miraculous Pivot: Chapter The Criterions of Pricking and the Difference between Healthy Qi and the Evil Qi (Líng Shū: Cì Jié Zhēn Xié, 灵枢·刺节真邪) *says: "The genuine qi is endowed by the heavens and replenishes the body together with food essence."*

Principle and Prohibition for Medical Profession: Chapter Discussion on Five Important Methods to Differentiating Syndrome of Direct Cold Attack (Yī Mén Fǎ Lù: Lùn Biàn Zhòng Hán Zhèng Yào Fǎ Wǔ Tiáo, 医门法律·论辨中寒证要法五条) *says: "Flesh and blood of the human body pertains to yin. As the combination of essence from parents, a bit of genuine yang, which is generated before life, is stored in the two Kidneys, thus the original qi of the whole body is produced. Thus it is called the source of life qi."*

Miraculous Pivot: Chapter The Issue of Distribution and Operation of The Defensive Qi and Nutritive Qi (Líng Shū: Yíng Wèi Shēng Huì, 灵枢·营卫生会) *says: "Qi in the human body is gained from food. Food enters the Stomach and then qi is transported to the Lung, and ultimately the five zang organs and six fu organs."*

Plain Questions: Chapter Major Discussion on the Theory of Yin and Yang and the Corresponding Relationships Among All the Things in Nature (Sù Wèn: Yīn Yáng Yìng Xiàng Dà Lùn, 素问·阴阳应象大论) *says: "The heaven qi communicates with the Lung."*

Golden Mirror of Medicine: Chapter in Abridged and Supplemented Discussion on Formulae of Famous Physicians (Yī Zōng Jīn Jiàn: Shān Bǔ Míng Yī Fāng Lùn, 医宗金鉴·删补名医方论) *says: "The acquired qi will be generated constantly if it gets the congenital qi; and the congenital qi will transform unceasingly if it gets the acquired qi."*

Miraculous Pivot: Chapter The Five Flavors (Líng Shū: Wǔ Wèi, 灵枢·五味) *says: "Therefore, if no food is taken in, qi will decline for half a day and will be deficient in a day."*

Movement of Qi

① Mutual interaction of spirit and essence

The movement of qi is called the qi dynamic (气机). Qi has the property of movement, and qi of the human body is an essential substance with strong energy and constant movement, which flows to the whole body, exerting an activating and promoting function to the *zang-fu* organs and tissues.

② Patterns of Qi Movement (Fig. 3-5)

The patterns of qi movement are various, and they are summarized into the four basics of ascent, descent, exit and entrance in *Internal Classic* (Nèi Jīng, 内经). Ascent indicates the movement of qi from lower to the upper. Descent indicates that of qi from upper to the lower. Exit indicates that of qi from inside to outside. Entrance indicates that of qi from outside to inside. Qi movement in a normal state implies that it must be smooth and there must be a harmonious balance among those patterns. This normal state is called "harmony of the qi dynamic".

③ Location of Qi Movement

Qi movement is located in tissues and organs such as *zang-fu* organs, channels and collaterals. Only in these tissues and organs can the ascending, descending, exiting and entering movement of qi be embodied concretely. Generally speaking,

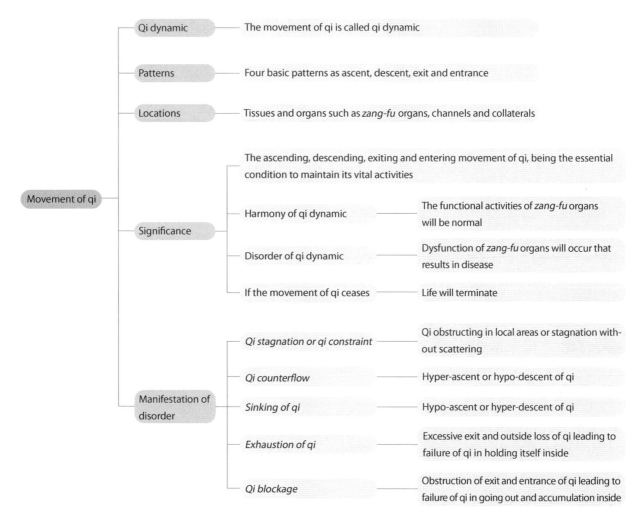

Fig. 3-5　Summary of the movement of qi

the five *zang* organs store essence qi and ought to ascend; six *fu* organs transport and transform food and ought to descend. When speaking of the five *zang* organs, the Heart and Lung, being located in the upper part of body, are in charge of descent; the Liver and Kidney, being located in the lower part, are in charge of ascent; and the Spleen and the Stomach, being located in the middle and communicating to both the upper and lower are the hinge of ascent, descent, exit and entrance. When speaking of the six *fu* organs, they do not store, but transport and transform the food, and they function normally when they are unobstructed and can send down soundly. During the process of digestion and absorption of food and discharge of waste, they dominate descent in general, as well as the ascending actions that exist within these processes. As far as the relationshipship between the *zang* and *fu* organs

is concerned, the Lung dominates exhalation while the Kidney dominates inhalation; the Liver dominates ascent and dispersion while the Lung dominates purification and descent; the Spleen governs sending up the clear while the Stomach governs sending down the turbid; and the Heart communicates with the Kidney. All these show that the functional activities of *zang-fu* organs are in a state of ascending, descending, exiting and entering movement of qi.

④ Significance of Movement of Qi

The ascending, descending, exiting and entering movement of qi, being the essential condition to maintain its vital activities, is of great importance to the human body. If the movement of qi is normal and the qi dynamic is harmonious, the functional activities of *zang-fu* organs will be normal and physiological activities of human body can be maintained. If the movement of qi is abnormal and the qi dynamic is disordered, dysfunction of *zang-fu* organs will occur that results in disease. If the movement of qi ceases, the body will lose the function of maintaining vital activities of qi, and life will terminate. Therefore, in a sense, vital activities of human body are the movement of qi.

⑤ Manifestation of Disorder of Qi Movement

The ascending, descending, exiting and entering movement of qi losing its coordination and balance is called "disorder of the qi dynamic" or "dysfunction of the qi dynamic". It mainly manifests as follows:

Abnormal qi movement obstructing local areas or causing stagnation without scattering is called "qi stagnation" or "qi constraint".

Hyper-ascent or hypo-descent of qi is called "qi counterflow".

Hypo-ascent or hyper-descent of qi is called "sinking of qi".

Excessive exit and outside loss of qi leading to failure of qi in holding itself inside is called "exhaustion of qi".

Obstruction of exit and entrance of qi leading to failure of qi in going out and accumulation inside is called "qi blockage".

(See pathological mechanism for details.)

Plain Questions: Chapter Major Discussion on the Abstruseness of the Six Kinds of Qi (Sù Wèn: Liù Wēi Zhǐ Dà Lùn, 素问·六微旨大论) says: "If exit and entrance stop, changes of all things will cease; if ascent and descent terminate, the existence of qi will be in danger. Therefore, without exit and entrance, there won't be birth, growth, prime, senility or death; without ascent and descent, there won't be generation, growth, transformation, reaping and storage. Thus nothing can go on without ascent, descent, exit and entrance. The body is the location of generation and transformation; when the body is ruined, qi will scatter, and the process of generation and transformation will cease. Thus everything must exit or enter, and everything must ascend or descend. "*

*Essays of Reading Medical Works: Chapter Discussion on Ascent, Descent, Exit and Entrance (Dú Yī Suí Bǐ: Shēng Jiàng Chū Rù Lùn, 读医随笔·*升降出入论)* says: "Therefore, the reason why eyes, ears, nose, tongue, body, consciousness, spirit and mind function is due to smooth ascent, descent, exit and entrance; if the movement is blocked, they will not function. Thus, eyes failing to see, ears failing to hear, nose failing to smell, tongue failing to taste, tendon atrophy, bone blockage, nails degenerate, decayed teeth, loss of hair, numbness of skin and failing of the intestines and the Stomach to transport and discharge, are all caused by accumulation of heat and blockage of sweat pores, leading to fluid, blood vessels, nutritive qi, defensive qi, clear qi and turbid qi failing to ascend, descend, exit and enter. … Ascent, descent, exit and entrance are the function of heaven and earth, storage of everything, the compendium of all kinds of diseases, and the hinge of life and death."*

Functions of Qi

Qi is the fundamental substance not only to constitute the human body but also to maintain its vital activities, so it has very important functions in the body.

Classic of Questioning: The Eighth Question (Nàn Jīng: Bā Nàn, 难经·八难) says: "*Qi is the root of men.*"

Principle and Prohibition for Medical Profession: Chapter Maxim of Sage (Yī Mén Fǎ Lù: Xiān Zhé Gé Yán, 医门法律·先哲格言) says: "*What a man depends on is only qi. He is alive when qi gathers, and he will die when qi scatters.*"

Investigation of Prescriptions: Chapter Category of Qi (Yī Fāng Kǎo: Qì Mén, 医方考·气门) says: "*Qi transforms along with the generation of things; qi changes along with the change of things; qi gets exuberant along with the predominance of things; qi gets weak along with the decline of things; qi is normal along with the harmony of things; qi is chaotic along with the disorder of things; qi vanishes along with the death of things.*"

The physiological functions of qi are mainly of the following aspects:(Table 3-1)

① Propelling Function

The propelling function of qi indicates that qi is of activating and promoting functions in the process of vital activities. As qi is an essential substance

Table 3-1   Table of Physiological Functions of Qi

Function	Implication	Manifestation
Propelling Function	Activating and promoting functions	The growth, development and reproduction of the human body; functional activities of all the viscera, bowels, tissues and organs; the generation and circulation of blood; and the generation, distribution and excretion of fluid
Warming Function	The function of producing heat to warm the body	Maintaining a relatively constant body temperature; functional activities of all the viscera, bowels, tissues and organs; the normal circulation of blood and fluid
Defensive Function	The function of defending muscles and skin, and resisting evil qi	Defending muscles and skin in order to resist invasion of exogenous evils; striving against evil qi in order to expel it
Consolidating Function	The function of restricting, controlling and commanding the liquid substances of the body	Controlling blood in oder to prevent it from overflowing from the vessels; controlling urine and sweat so as to prevent their leakage outside; controlling saliva, gastric, and intestinal juices to prevent loss of body fluid; controlling semen to prevent its undue excretion; consolidating internal organs to keep their locations relatively constant
Qi Transformation	Various changes caused by movement of qi	Substantial metabolism of essence, qi, blood and fluid as well as their mutual transformation; various changes produced by functional activities of tissues and organs such as bowels, viscera, channels and collaterals
Nourishing Function	Qi is an essential substance with nourishing function	Nourishing bowels, viscera, tissues, organs of the whole body to ensure their normal functional activities

with strong energy and constant movement, it can engender activating and promoting functions.

The main manifestations of the propelling functions of qi are: the growth, development and reproduction of the human body, functional activities of all the organs, bowels, tissues and organs; the generation and circulation of blood, and the generation, and distribution and excretion of fluid. All of these depend on the activating and promoting functions of qi to progress normally.

If the propelling function of qi weakens, the growth, development and reproduction of the human body will be affected, and it will also lead to pathological changes such as hypo-function of all the organs, bowels, channels, collaterals, tissues and organs, insufficient generation and sluggish circulation of blood, and metabolic obstruction of fluid.

② Warming Function

The warming function of qi indicates that qi can produce heat to warm the body, which mainly refers to the warming function of yang qi.

The main manifestations of the warming functions of qi are the relatively constant body temperature of people, functional activities of all the organs, bowels, tissues and organs, the normal circulation of blood and fluid, etc, all of which depend upon the warming function of qi to maintain their normality.

If yang qi is deficient and its warming function weakens, it will result in pathological changes with cold symptoms such as a drop in body temperature, fear of cold, cold limbs, hypo-function of *zang-fu* organs, and sluggish circulation of blood and fluid.

Classic of Questioning: The Twenty-second Question (*Nàn Jīng:* Èr Shí Èr Nàn, 难经·二十二难) says: "*Qi is in charge of warming.*"

Danger Zone of Medicine: Chapter Qi (*Yī Biān: Qì,* 医碥·气) says: "*Yang qi is a kind of warm qi.*"

Register of Questions: Chapter Discussion on

Yang Being Abundant Usually (Zhì Yí Lù: Lùn Yáng Cháng Yǒu Yú, 质疑录·论阳常有余) says: "*The warmness of whole body is due to yang qi.*"

General Treatise on Causes and Manifestations of All Diseases: Chapter Symptoms of Cold Qi (Zhū Bìng Yuán Hóu Lùn: Lěng Qì Hóu, 诸病源候论·冷气候) says: "*Qi deficiency of the zang organs will result in cold symptoms internally.*"

③ Defensive Function

The defensive function of qi indicates that qi can defend muscles and skin and resist the evil qi. Qi with this defensive function is generally called right qi (defensive qi), and this indicates the evil-resist function of right qi.

There are two main manifestations of the defensive function of qi: one is to defend the muscles and skin of the whole body in order to resist invasion of exogenous evils; the other is to strive against evil qi in order to expel it.

If right qi is deficient, with weak evil-resistant ability and decreased defensive function, exogenous evils can attack the body easily to cause onset of disease, or the disease gets worse or difficult to recover from due to right qi failing to expel evils after its onset.

Plain Questions: Chapter Discussion on Acupuncture Methods (Sù Wèn: Cì Fǎ Lùn, 素问·刺法论) says: "*When the right qi remains inside, the evil qi will be unable to attack.*"

Plain Questions: Chapter Comments on Febrile Diseases (Sù Wèn: Píng Rè Bìng Lùn, 素问·评热病论) says: "*Where there is invasion of the evil qi, there is the deficiency of the right qi.*"

Miraculous Pivot: Chapter The Treating Therapy from Oral Inquiry (Líng Shū: Kǒu Wèn, 灵枢·口问) says: "*Where there is the evil qi, there is deficiency.*"

Remainder of Medical Lemma: Chapter Gathering qi, Nutritive qi and Defensive Qi (Yī Zhǐ Xù Yú: Zōng Qì Yíng Qì Wèi Qì, 医旨绪余·宗气营气卫气) says: "*The defensive qi indicates defending the whole body, warming the muscles and fattening interstitial spaces to avoid invasion of exogenous evils.*"

④ Consolidating Function

The consolidating function indicates that qi has the function of restricting, controlling and commanding the liquid substances of the body.

The consolidating function of qi mainly manifests as follows:

Qi controls blood in order to prevent it from overflow and to keep blood flowing inside the vessels.

Qi controls urine and sweat so as to prevent their leakage outside and restrict their excretion.

Qi controls saliva, and gastric and intestinal juices to prevent loss of body fluid.

Qi controls semen to prevent its undue excretion.

Qi consolidates internal organs to keep their location relatively constant so as to prevent prolapse.

Reduced consolidating function of qi will lead to the loss of a vast amount of liquid substances of the body or prolapse of internal organs.

⑤ Qi's Transformative Function

Qi's transformative function indicates the various changes caused by the movement of qi, mainly including substantial metabolism of essence, qi, blood and fluid as well as their mutual transformation.

Qi's transformation function runs through the whole life of a person. Substantial metabolism of essence, qi, blood and fluid as well as their mutual transformation, and various changes produced by functional activities of tissues and organs such as bowels, viscera, channels and collaterals, are all the outcome of qi transformation. For instance, qi's transformation function turns food and drink into essence from water and food and waste; essence from water and food is transformed into essence, qi, blood and fluid further to supply the human body, and the wastes are excreted out of the body. Every part of this series of changes is a concrete embodiment of qi transformation. In fact, the process of qi transformation is simply that of substantial metabolism of human body, and that of substantial transformation and energetic transformation.

If qi's transformation function is disordered, it will affect digestion of food and drink and discharge of waste, generation and excretion of sweat, urine and feces, and functional activities of *zang-fu* organs, leading to all sorts of pathological changes. Therefore, it is obvious that qi transformation exists in the whole course of human life, and there will not be vital activities without it.

Plain Questions: Chapter Major Discussion on the Theory of Yin and Yang and the Corresponding Relationships Among All the Things in Nature (Sù Wèn: Yīn Yáng Yìng Xiàng Dà Lùn, 素问·阴阳应象大论) says: "Foods nourish the body, and the body produces qi; qi turns into essence, and essence generates the transformation function; essence relies on qi and the body needs foods; transformation produces essence, and qi nourishes the body. Essence transforms into qi."

Plain Questions: Chapter Major Discussion on the Abstruseness of the Six Kinds of Qi (Sù Wèn: Liù Wēi Zhǐ Dà Lùn, 素问·六微旨大论) says: "The generation of things is due to transformation; the termination of things is caused by change; the interaction of transformation and change is the reason of birth and death."

Plain Questions: Chapter Discussion on the Secret Classics Stored in Royal Library (Sù Wèn: Líng Lán Mì Diǎn Lùn, 素问·灵兰秘典论) says: "The urinary Bladder is a reservoir in which fluid is stored, and urine is discharged by its function of qi transformation."

Preserved Medical Manuscript of Jingjingshi (Jǐng Jǐng Shì Yī Gǎo Zá Cún, 景景室医稿杂存) says: "Human beings in their beginning are transformed by qi. Human beings living between heaven and earth are transformed by qi and then the body is generated. Essence and blood from both parents gives birth to children and grandchildren, but it must last ten months and experience yin qi and yang qi of four seasons, and then the fetus can be deLivered. So the formation and development of the fetus are related to qi transformation. After birth, the nose accepts qi from the heavens and the mouth accepts flavors from the earth. Gathering qi, defensive qi and nutritive qi are generated by qi transformation, and these three forms of qi will further transform into Jin, Ye, essence and blood; and then essence transforms into qi again to nourish the body. When it says 'foods nourish the body, and the body produces qi; qi turns into essence,

and essence generates the transformation function; the transformation produces essence, and qi generates the body; essence transforms into qi' in Internal Classic (Nèi Jīng), it indicates that preserving health to enjoy the natural lifespan depends on qi transformation."

⑥ Nourishing Function

This function indicates that qi is an essential substance with a nourishing function in the human body. Qi with nourishing function mainly indicates essence qi from water and food. Essence qi from water and food combines with clear qi in nature to generate gathering qi; essence qi combines with fluid to produce blood, which is distributed to the whole body by the functions of the Heart and the Lung to provide *zang-fu* organs and tissues with nutrients to maintain their physiological activities.

Miraculous Pivot: Chapter The Length of Channels (Líng Shū: Mài Dù, 灵枢·脉度) says: "The flowing qi irrigates zang-fu organs interiorly and nourishes interstitial spaces exteriorly."

Miraculous Pivot: Chapter The Five Flavors (Líng Shū: Wǔ Wèi, 灵枢·五味) says: "Therefore, if no food is taken in, qi will decline for half a day and will be deficient in one day."

Classification of Qi

Due to various sources, distributive locations, and functional characteristics of qi, it has different names. In Chinese medicine, qi is mainly classified as original qi, gathering qi, nutritive qi, or defensive qi, as well as qi of zang-fu organs and qi of channels and collaterals. (Fig. 3-6)

Principles and Prohibitions for the Medical Profession: Chapter Law of Pinpointing Great Qi in the Chest (Yī Mén Fǎ Lǜ: Míng Xiōng Zhōng Dà Qì Zhī Fǎ, 医门法律·明胸中大气之法) says: "In the body, there exists nutritive qi, defensive qi, and gathering qi as well as qi of zang-fu organs and qi of channels and collaterals; and they should be distinguished."

Principle and Prohibition for Medical Profession: Chapter Maxim of Sage (Yī Mén Fǎ Lǜ: Xiān Zhé Gé

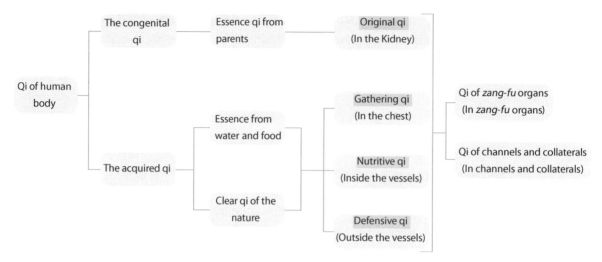

Fig. 3-6 Chart of names, classification and distribution of qi

Yán, 医门法律·先哲格言) says: "*Qi is of the external, indicating the six climatic agents between heaven and earth; and it is of the internal, indicating original qi of human body. Disordered qi is known as evil qi, and harmonious qi is known as right qi or genuine qi. The location of genuine qi is in three places: the upper, the middle and the lower. The upper, endowed by the heavens, maintains respiration; the middle, generated from water and food, replenishes the nutritive qi and defensive qi; the lower transforms into essence and is stored in the life gate. … What a man depends on is only qi.*"

Danger Zone of Medicine: Chapter Qi (Yī Biān: Qì, 医碥·气) says: "*Qi is only of one. When it goes outside the vessels, it is called defensive qi; when circulating inside the vessels, it is called nutritive qi; when accumulating in the chest, it is called gathering qi. Though it has three names, they are not different in essence.*"

① Original Qi, 元气 (Fig. 3-7)

Original qi, also called source qi, is the primordial and root qi to form the human body, as well as the movement of vital activities.

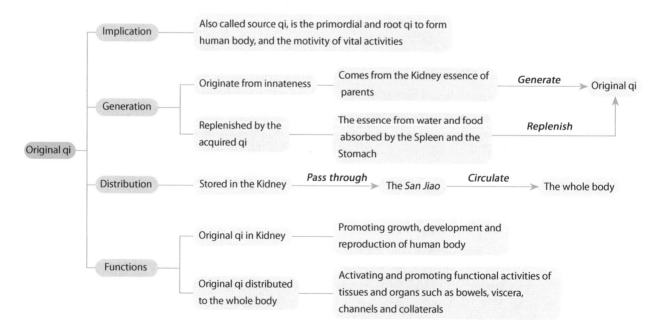

Fig. 3-7 Summary of generation, distribution and functions of original qi

(1) Generation

Original qi is an innate substance, which comes from the Kidney essence of the parents during the formation of embryos. After birth, it is replenished by the essence from water and food absorbed by the Spleen and the Stomach so as to maintain its sufficiency. So, whether original qi is sufficient or not depends on both congenital constitution and the function of absorbing acquired essence from water and food through the Spleen and the Stomach.

(2) Distribution

Original qi is stored in the Kidneys and circulates in the whole body through the *San Jiao*. The *San Jiao* has the function of carrying original qi and is the pathway of it. Therefore, original qi circulates ubiquitously to the *zang-fu* organs interiorly and to muscles, skin, and interstitial spaces exteriorly.

(3) Main Functions

Original qi is stored in the Kidneys and distributed to the whole body. There are two aspects to its main functions, as follows:

First, original qi in the Kidneys, i.e. Kidney qi, has the functions of activating and promoting growth, controlling the development and reproduction of human body, and consolidating semen and urine, as well as receiving qi.

Secondly, original qi after it has been distributed to the whole body has the functions of activating and promoting functional activities of tissues and organs such as bowels, viscera, channels and collaterals.

Hence, original qi is the root qi of the human body and the energy for vital activities. Deficiency of original qi will lead to pathological changes such as slow development and hypo-function of *zang-fu* organs and tissues.

Notes of Medical Readings: Chapter Discrimination of Tongyizi's Essay (Yī Xué Dú Shū Jì: Tōng Yī Zǐ Zá Lùn Biàn, 医学读书记·通一子杂论辨) says: "*Original qi is inherent, and it wanes and waxes gradually, being the basis of exuberance and decline over the entire course of a person's life.*"

Treatise on the Headstream of Medicine (Yī Xué Yuán Liú Lùn, 医学源流论) says: "*When the embryo forms, there already exists a form of original qi.*"

Treatise on Spleen and Stomach: Chapter

Discussion on Deficiency of the Spleen Leading to Obstruction of Nine Orifices (Pí Wèi Lùn: Pí Wèi Xū Zé Jiǔ Qiào Bù Tōng Lùn, 脾胃论·脾胃虚则九窍不通论) says: "*Genuine qi, also known as original qi, is the essence generated before life, and nothing but Stomach qi can nourish it.*"

Jing-yue's Complete Works: Chapter Discussion on Spleen and Stomach (Jǐng Yuè Quán Shū: Lùn Pí Wèi, 景岳全书·论脾胃) says: "*So, from birth to old age, the majority of people with congenital deficiency can be treated by reinforcing the acquired qi to engender notable effects. Qi of the Spleen and the Stomach is of great value to life.*"

Classic of Questioning: The Thirty-sixth Question (Nàn Jīng: Sān Shí Liù Nàn, 难经·三十六难) says: "*The life gate… to which original qi adheres.*"

Classic of Questioning: The Sixty-sixth Question (Nàn Jīng: Liù Shí Liù Nàn, 难经·六十六难) says: "*San Jiao… is the ambassador of original qi; it dominates circulating three kind of qi throughout five zang organs and six fu organs.*"

Origin of Medicine: Chapter Discussion on Key Methods Based on Yin-Yang (Yī Yuán: Yīng Yáng Zhì Fǎ Dà Yào Lùn, 医原·阴阳治法大要论) says: "*The congenital genuine qi is generated by going from the lower to the upper to meet with the acquired Stomach qi, becoming the most valuable substance of the human body.*"

Jing-yue's Complete Works: Section Supplementary Discussion on the Life Gate, Chapter Chuan Zhong Lu (Jǐng Yuè Quán Shū: Chuán Zhōng Lù, Mìng Mén Yú Yì, 景岳全书·传忠录·命门余义), says: "*The life gate is the root of original qi, the residence of water and fire; the yin qi of the five zang organs can't be nourished without it, and the yang qi of th five zang organs can't disperse without it.*"

② Gathering Qi, 宗气 (Fig. 3-8)

Gathering qi, also called great qi, indicates qi accumulated in the chest, being an Chinese medicine.

(1) Generation

The generation of gathering qi is the combination in the chest of the clear qi in nature inhaled by the Lung and the essence qi from water and food absorbed and transported by the Spleen and

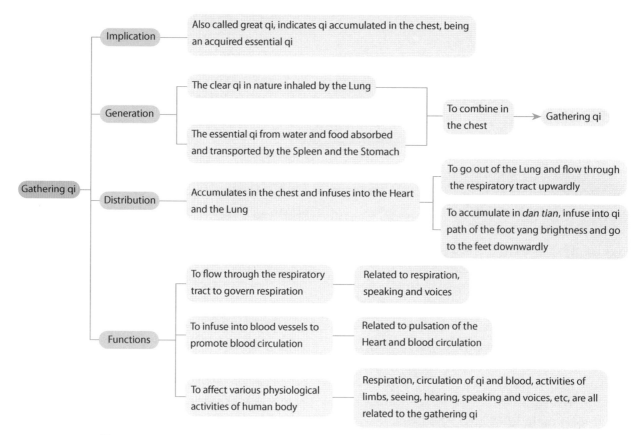

Fig. 3-8 Summary of generation, distribution and functions of the gathering qi

the Stomach. Hence, whether the gathering qi is sufficient or not has a direct relationship with the functions of the Lung, the Spleen and the Stomach.

(2) Distribution

The gathering qi accumulates in the chest and infuses into the Heart and the Lung. It goes out of the Lung and flows through the respiratory tract to govern respiration; and it goes out of the Heart and infuses into blood vessels to promote blood circulation. Since the chest is the location where gathering qi accumulates, it is called "the upper sea of qi", or "*Shanzhong, 膻中*".

(3) Main functions

The gathering qi accumulates in the chest, and the Heart and the Lung are also in the chest. Thus the gathering qi is related to the functions of the Heart governing blood and the Lung controlling respiration. The physiological functions of gathering qi have the following aspects:

First, the gathering qi goes out of the Lung and flows through the respiratory tract along the throat to assist the Lung in governing respiration. Therefore, respiration, speaking and the voice are all related to gathering qi. If the gathering qi is sufficient, respiration will be regular and forceful, and the voice will be resonant; if the gathering qi is deficient, respiration will be short and weak, and the voice will be low and feeble.

Second, the gathering qi goes out of the Heart and infuses into the Heart vessels to promote blood circulation. Therefore, blood circulation, the beating of the Heart and Heart's rhythm are related to gathering qi. If gathering qi is sufficient, the beating of Heart will be forceful and the rhythm will be regular; if the gathering qi is deficient, the he beating of Heart will be weak and the rhythm will be irregular. Thus exuberance and decline of gathering qi can be examined through he beating of Heart.

Third, the gathering qi can affect various physiological activities. Since the gathering qi is acquired essence qi with functions of assisting the Lung with respiration and the Heart with circulating blood, it can affect various physiological activities. Such as respiration, the circulation of qi and blood, activities of the limbs, and seeing, hearing, speaking, etc., they are all related to the exuberance or decline of gathering qi. Thus it is said that gathering qi is the "driving qi" of the human body.

Miraculous Pivot: Chapter The Five Flavors (*Líng Shū: Wǔ Wèi,* 灵枢·五味) says: "*The great qi gathers and stores in the chest, which is known as the sea of qi. It goes out of the Lung and follows the throat, and exits and enters the body along with inhalation and exhalation.*"

Discussion on Medicine by Jing'an (*Jìng Ān Shuō Yī,* 靖盦说医) says: "*Dàn Zhōng (RN 17 or the center of the chest) is the location where the great qi stays. The great qi is also called gathering qi.*"

Miraculous Pivot: Chapter Retention of the Evil Qi (*Líng Shū: Xié Kè,* 灵枢·邪客) says: "*The gathering qi accumulates in the chest, goes out of the throat, and infuses into the Heart and vessels to promote respiration.*"

Miraculous Pivot: Chapter The Criteria of Pricking and the Difference between Healthy Qi and Evil Qi (*Líng Shū: Cì Jié Zhēn Xié,* 灵枢·刺节真邪) says: "*The gathering qi stays in the sea of qi, infuses into the pathways of qi downwards and flows through the respiratory tract upwards.*"

Classified Classic: Chapter Category of Acupuncture (*Lèi Jīng: Zhēn Cì Lèi,* 类经·针刺类) says: "*(The gathering qi) accumulates in the dantian (丹田), infuses into the qi path of the foot yang brightness and goes downward to the feet.*"

Essays of Reading Medical Works: Chapter Discussion on Qi, Blood, Essence and Spirit (*Dú Yī Suí Bǐ: Qì Xuè Jīng Shén Lùn,* 读医随笔·气血精神论) says: "*The gathering qi is an driving qi. Respiration, speech capabilities and volume as well as the activities of limbs and the strength of tendons are all related to the functions of gathering qi.*"

Plain Questions: Chapter Discussion on the Pulse Condition of Healthy People (*Sù Wèn: Píng Rén Qì Xiàng Lùn,* 素问·平人气象论) says: "*The large collateral of the Stomach channel is called Xuli (虚里). It penetrates the diaphragm, connects with the Lung and goes out below the left breast. The pulsation can be felt with hand, and this is the location where the gathering qi is examined.*"

③ Nutritive Qi, 营气 (Fig. 3-9)

Nutritive qi indicates qi circulating in vessels with a nourishing function. Since it has the function to nourish, it is also called "flourishing qi". Since nutritive qi moves in vessels as an important component of blood, nutritive qi has a close relationship with blood and they cannot be separated. Thus, they are also grouped together as "nutrient blood".

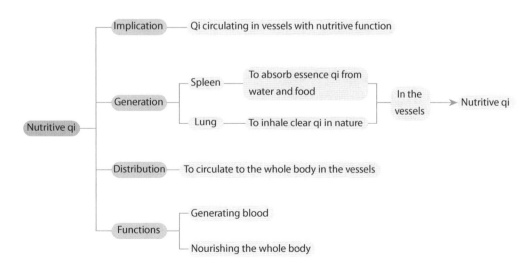

Fig. 3-9   Summary of generation, distribution and functions of the nutritive qi

(1) Generation

The essence qi from water and food that is absorbed and transformed by the Spleen and Stomach combines with clear qi in nature inhaled by the Lung to produce nutritive qi circulating in the vessels.

The essence qi from water and food that is absorbed by the Spleen and Stomach in the middle *Jiao* must be transported upwards to the Lung to generate gathering qi, defensive qi and nutritive qi. After its generation, the gathering qi goes out of the Heart and the Lung, then circulates separately along the pathway of nutritive qi inside the vessels and that of defensive qi outside the vessels, and finally distributes to the whole body. That is to say, nutritive qi and defensive qi are two kinds of qi that the gathering qi distributes to the whole body. Therefore, the generation of nutritive qi and defensive qi needs the clear qi inhaled by the Lung as well as the essential qi from water and food absorbed by the Spleen and the Stomach.

(2) Distribution

After its generation, the nutritive qi circulates to the whole body through the channels. Through the twelve channels, *Du* meridian and *Ren* meridian, nutritive qi circulates to the *zang-fu* organs interiorly and the limbs and joints exteriorly, going round and round endlessly.

(3) Main functions

The physiological functions of nutritive qi have the following aspects:

The first is generating blood. The nutritive qi infuses into the vessels and combines with fluid, being an important component of blood. Thus they are also grouped together as "nutrient blood".

The second is nourishing the whole body. Nutritive qi has a nourishing function and circulates in the vessels to the whole body, so it can exert a nourishing function to all the *zang-fu* organs and tissues.

If the nutritive qi is insufficient, it will cause pathological changes such as deficiency of blood and hypo-function of tissues and organs due to a lack of nutrients.

Miraculous Pivot: Chapter The Issue of Distribution and Operation of The Defensive Qi and Nutritive Qi (Líng Shū: Yíng Wèi Shēng Huì, 灵枢·营卫生会) says: "*The human body distills essence qi from food. When food enters the Stomach, it is transformed into qi, and is then distributed to the Lung as well as the five zang organs and six fu organs. The clear portion is the nutritive qi circulating in the vessels, and the turbid portion is the defensive qi going outside of the vessels. The nutritive qi circulates fifty cycles over the course of a day and a night and then meets with the defensive qi. Thus, yin and yang connect with each other to form a circular course, like a loop without a starting point... The process of distilling the essence qi is excreting waste, vaporizing fluid, transforming essence and infusing into the Lung meridian to generate blood and nourish the body. It travels in the channels solely and nothing is more valuable than it is, so it is called nutritive qi.*"

Plain Questions: Chapter Discussion on Bi-Syndrome (Sù Wèn: Bì Lùn, 素问·痹论) says: "*Nutritive qi is the essence qi from water and food. It circulates harmoniously in the five zang organs, scatters in the six fu organs and enters the vessels. Therefore, it has the functions of circulating along the vessels, linking up the five zang organs and connecting the six fu organs.*"

Miraculous Pivot: Chapter Retention of the Evil Qi (Líng Shū: Xié Kè, 灵枢·邪客) says: "*Nutritive qi is distilled from water and food, and then infused into vessels to generate blood so as to nourish the four limbs and internally permeate into the five zang and six fu organs.*"

Miraculous Pivot: Chapter The Nutritive qi (Líng Shū: Yíng Qì, 灵枢·营气) says: "*The law of nutritive qi considers taking in food important. After the food enters the Stomach, its essence is distributed to the Lungs, flows inside the body and scatters to the exterior. Its essential part travels in the channels, circulates unceasingly, goes round and round, and this is the principle of heaven and earth.*"

Essays of Reading Medical Works: Chapter Discussion on Qi, Blood, Essence and Spirit (Dú Yī Suí Bǐ: Qì Xuè Jīng Shén Lùn, 读医随笔·气血精神论) says: "*Smoothness of channels and nourishment of the hair and skin are all the effects of nutritive qi."*

④ Defensive qi, 위기 (Fig. 3-10)

Defensive qi travels outside the vessels and has a defensive function. It can defend the body against the invasion of exogenous evils, hence the name. Compared with the nutritive qi circulating in the vessels, which pertains to yin, the defensive qi pertains to yang, and so they are also called "nutrient yin" and "defensive yang".

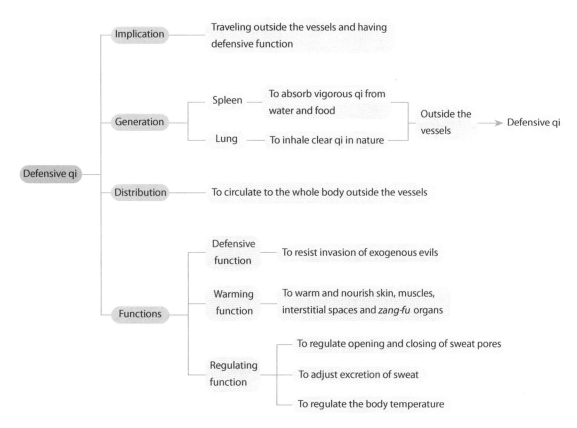

Fig. 3-10   Summary of generation, distribution and functions of the defensive qi

(1) Generation

The generation of defensive qi is the same as that of nutritive qi. Qi from water and food is absorbed and transformed by the Spleen and the Stomach and combines with the clear qi in nature inhaled by the Lung to produce defensive qi circulating outside the vessels. As to the generating source of defensive qi and nutritive qi, the clear qi inhaled by the Lung is the same, but qi from water and food absorbed and transported by Spleen and Stomach is different: the one generating nutritive qi is the essential part of water and food, while the one generating defensive qi is the vigorous part of qi from water and food.

(2) Distribution

After its generation, the defensive qi circulates to the whole body outside the vessels. The defensive qi is the vigorous qi of water and food which is not restricted by the vessels, so it travels outside the vessels along with the nutritive qi to the skin, muscles and interstitial spaces exteriorly, and the chest, abdomen and *zang-fu* organs interiorly, and scatters to the whole body.

In addition, the defensive qi circulates in the whole body through both channels and collaterals with the characteristic of traveling the yang part of the body in the daytime and the yin part at night.

(3) Main functions

The physiological functions of defensive qi are of the following three aspects:

The first is a defensive function. The skin and

interstitial spaces in the body surface constitute a barrier to resist the invasion of exogenous evils. The defensive qi has the functions of warming muscles, skin and interstitial spaces, and controlling the opening and closing of sweat pores, making them dense and maintaining their normal functions so as to resist exogenous evils.

The second is a warming function. Defensive qi belongs to yang qi with its warming and nourishing functions. The chest, the abdomen and the *zang-fu* organs of the interior, as well as the skin, muscles and interstitial spaces of the exterior are all warmed and nourished by the defensive qi so as to maintain a relatively constant body temperature, as well as the density of the muscles, skin and interstitial spaces, and normal functional activities of *zang-fu* organs.

The third is a regulating function. Defensive qi can affect the body surface to regulate the opening and closing of skin, hair and sweat pores, and adjust the excretion of sweat so that the body temperature can be regulated.

If the defensive qi is deficient, leading to a decrease of the warming, nourishing and regulating functions, the patient will be easily affected by exogenous evils.

Plain Questions: Chapter Discussion on Bi-Syndrome (Sù Wèn: Bì Lùn, 素问·痹论) say: *"The defensive qi is the vigorous qi of water and food. It is rapid and slippery and cannot enter the vessels, so it circulates to skin and muscles, vaporizes on the Huang membrane* (肓膜) *and scatters in the chest and abdomen."*

Miraculous Pivot: Chapter Retention of the Evil Qi (Líng Shū: Xié Kè, 灵枢·邪客) says: *"The defensive qi, due to its vigorousness and rapidness, travels first to the four limbs, muscles and skin ceaselessly. It travels the yang part of body in the daytime and the yin part at night."*

Miraculous Pivot: Chapter The Defensive Qi (Líng Shū: Wèi Qì, 灵枢·卫气) says: *"The floating qi that does not circulate in the vessels is the defensive qi; the essence qi circulating inside the vessels is the nutritive qi. The defensive qi and the nutritive qi circulate together, connecting with each other just like*

a loop without a starting point."

Classic of Questioning: The Thirtieth Question (Nàn Jīng: Sān Shí Nàn, 难经·三十难) says: *"The nutritive qi travels inside the vessels while the defensive qi travels outside the vessels. The nutritive qi circulates fifty cycles for every day and night and then meets with defensive qi. Thus, yin and yang connect with each other to form a circular course, like a loop without a starting point. Hence, the defensive qi and the nutritive qi accompany each other."*

Miraculous Pivot: Chapter The Various Conditions of Internal Organs Relating Different Diseases (Líng Shū: Běn Zàng, 灵枢·本脏) says: *"Defensive qi has the functions of warming muscles, nourishing skin, fattening interstitial spaces and governing opening and closing (of sweat pores)."*

Miraculous Pivot: Chapter The Dredge of Qi (Líng Shū: Jué Qì, 灵枢·决气) says: *"The upper Jiao activates and distributes the five flavors of food to warm the skin, replenish the body and moisten the hair like mist and dew. This is known as qi."*

Essays of Reading Medical Works: Chapter Discussion on Qi, Blood, Essence and Spirit (Dú Yī Suí Bǐ: Qì Xuè Jīng Shén Lùn, 读医随笔·气血精神论) says: *"Defensive qi is a kind of hot qi. Warming muscles and digesting water and food are its functions."*

Remainder of Medical Lemma: Chapter Gathering qi, Nutritive qi and Defensive Qi (Yī Zhǐ Xù Yú: Zōng Qì Yíng Qì Wèi Qì, 医旨绪余·宗气营气卫气) says: *"Defensive qi indicates that it can defend the whole body, warm muscles and fatten the interstitial spaces in order to avoid the invasion of exogenous evils."*

A. Comparison of generation and distribution between gathering qi, nutritive qi and defensive qi (Fig. 3-11)

Generation: Generation of gathering qi, nutritive qi and defensive qi are the same, i.e. they are all produced by the combination of clear qi in nature inhaled by the Lungs with qi from water and food absorbed and transported by the Spleen and Stomach. As for their generation, the essence of these three types of qi is the same. Therein, the qi from water and food generating nutritive qi is different from that generating the defensive qi,

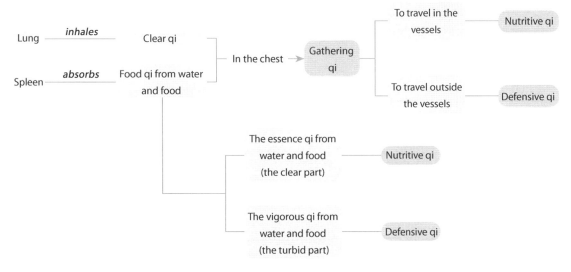

Fig. 3-11　Chart of comparisons of generation and distribution between gathering qi, nutritive qi and defensive qi

i.e. that generating the nutritive qi is the essence qi from water and food (the clear part), while that generating the defensive qi is the vigorous qi from water and food (the turbid part).

Distribution: The distributive locations and circulating paths of the above-mentioned three types of qi are different. Gathering qi accumulates in the chest and infuses into the Heart and Lung, while nutritive qi and defensive qi are two kinds of qi that the gathering qi transports from the chest to the whole body. The nutritive qi circulates in the vessels to the whole body while the defensive qi circulates outside the vessels.

B. Comparison between nutritive qi and defensive qi (Table 3-2)

Points in Common: The generating sources of nutritive qi and defensive qi are the same, i.e. they are both produced by the combination of qi from water and food absorbed and transported by the Spleen and Stomach with the clear qi in nature inhaled by the Lung, and they both circulate through the whole body.

Difference: There are differences in characteristics, distribution and function between nutritive qi and defensive qi. Nutritive qi is the essential part of qi from water and food, which is pure in characteristic; while defensive qi is the

Table 3-2　Comparison of the nutritive qi and the defensive qi

		Nutritive qi	Defensive Qi
Commonness		The generating sources of nutritive qi and defensive qi are the same, i.e. they are both produced by the combination of the qi from water and food absorbed and transported by the Spleen and the Stomach with the clear qi in nature inhaled by the Lung	
Differences	Characteristic	The essential qi from water and food (the clear part)	The vigorous qi from water and food (the turbid part)
	Distribution	Circulating in the vessels	Circulating outside the vessels
	Functions	Generating blood; nourishing the whole body	Resistance against invasion of exogenous evils; warming the zang-fu organs, muscles and body surface; controlling the opening and closing of sweat pores; controlling the excretion of sweat
	Attributed to Yin or Yang	Yin	Yang

vigorous part of qi from water and food, with rapid and slippery characteristics. Nutritive qi travels inside the vessels while defensive qi travels outside the vessels. Nutritive qi has the function of generating blood to nourish the whole body; while defensive qi has the functions of resisting invasion of exogenous evils, warming the *zang-fu* organs, muscles and body surface, controlling the opening and closing of sweat pores as well as controlling the excretion of sweat. The nutritive qi belongs to yin while the defensive qi belongs to yang.

Plain Questions: Chapter Discussion on Bi-Syndrome (Sù Wèn: Bì Lùn, 素问·痹论) says: "*Nutritive qi is the essence qi of water and food, while defensive qi is the vigorous qi of them.*"

Miraculous Pivot: Chapter The Five Flavors (Líng Shū: Wǔ Wèi, 灵枢·五味) says: "*The nutritive qi and the defensive qi go out of the chest and circulate in two different paths.*"

Posthumous Manuscript of Shenzhai (Shèn Zhāi Yí Shū, 慎斋遗书) says: "*The Spleen scatters the essence and sends it up to the Heart, and then the Heart to the Lung; the Lung distributes the essence to the skin, hair, and body hair. The light and clear enters the channels and collaterals, becoming the nutritive qi; the rapid enters the skin, becoming the defensive qi.*"

Essays of Reading Medical Works: Chapter Discussion on Qi, Blood, Essence and Spirit (Dú Yī Suí Bǐ: Qì Xuè Jīng Shén Lùn, 读医随笔·气血精神论) says: "*The gathering qi is the combination of the nutritive qi and the defensive qi, which goes out of the Lung and stores in the sea of qi.*"

Danger Zone of Medicine: Chapter Qi (Yī Biān: Qì, 医碥·气) says: "*Qi is only of one. When it goes outside the vessels, it is called defensive qi; when circulating inside the vessels, it is called nutritive qi; when accumulating in the chest, it is called gathering qi. Though it has three names, they are not different in essence.*"

In addition, there are still the forms of qi of the *zang-fu* organs, and the qi of channels and collaterals. They are the original qi, gathering qi, nutritive qi and defensive qi that distribute and function in the *zang-fu* organs, channel and collaterals as the energy of their functional activities. For example, there is the Heart qi, the Lung qi, the Spleen qi, the Stomach qi, the channel qi and the collateral qi, etc.

Section 3　Blood

Concept of Blood

Blood (血) is a red liquid with abundant nutrients circulating in the vessels. It is one of the basic substances constituting the human body and maintaining its vital activities. Its main components are the nutritive qi and fluid.

Blood circulates in the vessels. The vessels can restrict blood circulation, so they are called "blood houses". If blood extravasates out of the vessels, this is bleeding, and it is called "extravasated blood". If the blood circulation is sluggish or stagnant, it will lead to blood stasis.

Blood is an important nutritive substance in vital human activities. If blood is deficient, it will affect the function of the bowels, viscera, tissues and organs, and lead to various diseases.

Nutritive qi can generate blood. If fluid is harmonized and permeates into the vessels, it can also generate blood. Therefore, the nutritive qi and fluid in the vessels are the main components of blood.

Plain Questions: Chapter Discussion on the Regulation of Channels (Sù Wèn: Tiáo Jīng Lùn, 素问·调经论) says: "*What a man has is only blood and qi.*"

Plain Questions: Chapter Discussion on the Essentials of Pulse (Sù Wèn: Mài Yào Jīng Wēi Lùn, 素问·脉要精微论) says: "*The vessels are the houses of blood.*"

Generation of Blood

The main substance to generate blood is the essence from water and food and Kidney essence, transformed into blood under the joint action of the Spleen and Stomach, as well as the Heart, the Lung, the Liver and the Kidney.

① The Essence from Water and Food Transforms into Blood (Fig. 3-12)

The essence from water and food transforming into blood is accomplished with the action of the Spleen, the Stomach, the Heart and the Lung, etc.

Food and drink is transported and transformed by the Spleen and the Stomach; the essence from water and food (including the nutritive qi and the defensive qi) is absorbed and transported to the Heart and the Lung, combining with the clear qi inhaled by the Lung, via the "red-transforming function" of Heart fire (i.e. the qi-transforming function of the Heart and the Lung), and turns into red liquid and enters the vessels to become blood.

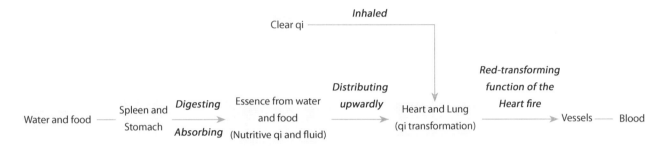

Fig. 3-12 Chart of the essence from water and food transforming into blood

The essence from water and food embraces the nutritive qi and fluid, which are the main substances to generate blood. Hence, there are sayings about "the nutritive qi transforming into blood" and "fluid transforming into blood".

The essence from water and food absorbed by the Spleen and the Stomach transforms into blood, so it is said that the Spleen and the Stomach are the source of blood generation. Dysfunction of the Spleen and the Stomach failing to generate essence from water and food will lead to the pathological change of insufficient blood generation.

Miraculous Pivot: Chapter The Dredge of Qi (*Líng Shū: Jué Qì,* 灵枢·决气) says: "The middle Jiao absorbs the essence qi from water and food and turns it into red liquid, and this is known as blood."

Miraculous Pivot: Chapter The Issue of Distribution and Operation of The Defensive Qi and Nutritive Qi (*Líng Shū: Yíng Wèi Shēng Huì,* 灵枢·营卫生会) says: "The middle Jiao... absorbs the essence qi from water and food, excretes the waste, vaporizes the fluid, transforms the essence and infuses it into the Lung vessels to generate blood."

Miraculous Pivot: Chapter On Carbuncle and Deep-rooted Carbuncle (*Líng Shū: Yōng Jū,* 灵枢·痈疽) says: "The middle Jiao disperses the essence qi like dew... Thus fluid is harmonized and turns into red liquid which is known as blood."

Remainder of Medical Lemma: Chapter Gathering qi, Nutritive qi and Defensive Qi (*Yī Zhǐ Xù Yú: Zōng Qì Yíng Qì Wèi Qì,* 医旨绪余·宗气营气卫气) says: "Common people take the nutritive qi as blood, and this is wrong. It is that the nutritive qi turns into blood."

Classified Differentiation of Lushantang: Chapter Differentiation of Blood (*Lǔ Shān Táng Lèi Biàn: Biàn Xuè,* 侣山堂类辨·辨血) says: "Blood is the juice generated by the middle Jiao. The juice flowing inside the body is called essence, and that which is sent to the Heart and transformed into red liquid is called blood."

Danger Zone of Medicine: Chapter Blood (*Yī Biān: Xuè,* 医碥·血) says: "The reason why only blood is red is that it is transformed via the function of Heart fire."

Discussion of Blood Syndromes: Chapter Discussion on Yin, Yang, Water, Fire, Qi and Blood (*Xuè Zhèng Lùn: Yīn Yáng Shuǐ Huǒ Qì Xuè Lùn,* 血证论·阴阳水火气血论) says: "The color of blood is the red of fire. Fire is governed by the Heart and generates blood to nourish the whole body. Fire pertains to yang while it can generate the yin of blood."

Arcanum of Physicians (Yī Jiā Mì Ao, 医家秘奥) says: *"The middle qi ascends to the Lung and then descends from it to generate blood."*

② The Kidney Essence Transforms into Blood (Fig. 3-13)

The Kidney essence generating blood is mainly related to the functions of the Liver and the Kidney.

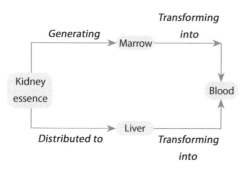

Fig. 3-13　Demonstration of the Kidney essence transforming into blood

The Kidney stores essence that can generate marrow, and marrow is the fundamental substance to generate blood. Hence, it is said that essence and marrow can transform into blood.

The Kidney stores essence and the Liver stores blood; Liver blood can nourish Kidney essence while Kidney essence can generate Liver blood. Their mutual transformation is the implication of Liver blood and Kidney essence sharing the same source.

Moreover, the warming function of Kidney yang can promote the Spleen and the Stomach in generating essence from water and food, and then send it up to the Heart to transform into blood.

In summary, the generation of blood takes the essence from water and food and Kidney essence as its substantial basis. Therefore, as essence is sufficient, blood is sufficient; as essence is deficient, blood is insufficient. The generation of blood is accomplished with the functional activities of the Spleen, the Stomach, the Heart, the Lung, the Liver and the Kidney. Dysfunction of any internal organ will engender insufficiency of blood generation leading to the pathological condition of blood deficiency.

Plain Questions: Chapter Discussion on the Interrelationship between Life and Nature (Sù Wèn: Shēng Qì Tōng Tiān Lùn, 素问·生气通天论) says: *"If marrow and bones are solid, qi and blood flow smoothly."*

Zhang's Treatise on Medicine: Section All Syndromes of Bleeding, Category of All Blood Syndromes (Zhāng Shì Yī Tōng: Zhū Xuè Mén, Zhū Jiàn Xuè Zhèng, 张氏医通·诸血门·诸见血证) says: *"It is said in Internal Classic (Nèi Jīng) that blood and qi are of the same source with different names. Although they have differences in the nature of yin, yang, clearness and turbidity, they are all generated by essence from water and food. At the beginning they are one integrated mass without distinction of clearness or turbidity. It is activated and transported by the Spleen qi, vaporized upwards to the Lung like mist to turn into qi; qi tends to the Kidney without dissipation to become essence; essence tends to the Liver with no leakage to generate the clear blood; the clear blood tends to the Heart with no effusion to produce the genuine blood by the action of fire."*

Essays of Reading Medical Works: Chapter Discussion on Qi, Blood, Essence and Spirit (Dú Yī Suí Bǐ: Qì Xuè Jīng Shén Lùn, 读医随笔·气血精神论) says: *"The blood, being the essence of water and food, is vaporized by the genuine fire of the life gate to generate muscles, skin and all types of hair."*

Circulation of Blood

① Direction of Blood Circulation

Blood circulates in the vessels to the whole body unceasingly. This is called "like a loop without starting point", or "to travel circularly and ceaselessly" in *Internal Classic (Nèi Jīng, 内经)*.

The Heart governs blood and the vessels, which is the energy of blood circulation. The vessels (channels and collaterals) are the pathways of blood circulation, which constitutes a relatively independent cardiovascular system together with the Heart. Blood circulation starts from the Heart, travels via the channels to collaterals and minute collaterals, and then goes to all the tissues of the body, exerting its nutritive function. After blood is utilized, it will return to the Heart via the minute collaterals, collaterals and channels. Blood starts from the Heart and then returns to it, taking on a centrifugal or centripetal circulation ceaselessly. (Fig. 3-14)

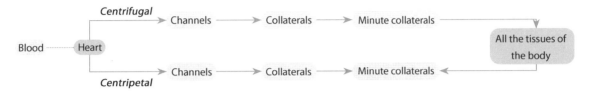

Fig. 3-14   Demonstration of blood circulation "like a loop without starting point"

Plain Questions: Chapter Special Discussion on Channels and Vessels (*Sù Wèn: Jīng Mài Bié Lùn Piān*, 素问·经脉别论) first put forward blood circulation and its route concerning the Heart, the Lung, channels, collaterals and four *zang* organs (the whole body), and pointed out the essence from water and food transforming into blood and the rough circulating directions. (Fig. 3-15)

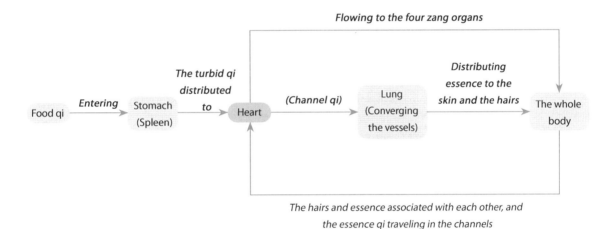

Fig. 3-15   Demonstration of blood circulation put forward by *special discussion on channels and vessels* (*jīng mài bié lùn*, 经脉别论)

2 Factors Affecting Blood Circulation

The function of the *zang-fu* organs, actions of qi, heat and cold, as well as smoothness of vessels, etc, all affect blood circulation.

(1) Functions of zang-fu organs

The normal circulation of blood is closely related to the functions of the Heart, the Lung, the Liver and the Spleen.

The Heart governs blood and the vessels, and Heart qi is the basic energy propelling blood circulation. The Lung converges vessels and governs qi to assist in the circulation of blood.

The Liver governs free coursing and regulates the qi dynamic so as to promote blood circulation; the Liver stores blood and regulates blood volume in accordance with the requirement of the body. The Spleen controls blood. The actions of the Spleen qi can prevent blood from overflowing out of the vessels. These four organs function with each other to ensure the normal circulation of blood. (Fig. 3-16)

(2) Functions of qi

Qi and blood circulate with each other. The propelling function of qi is the fundamental energy of blood circulation. The consolidating

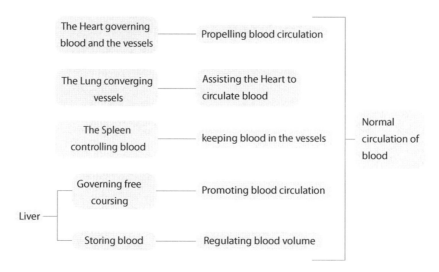

Fig. 3-16　Summary of the relationship between blood circulation and internal organs

function of qi can control blood circulating within the vessels and prevent it from overflowing. The warming function of qi can produce heat to keep blood circulating smoothly and avoid stagnancy due to cold.

(3) Heat and cold

Blood circulation requires a certain temperature to warm blood so that it can circulate smoothly in the vessels. Excessive cold will cause stagnancy of blood leading to a pathological change of blood stasis. Excessive heat will cause acceleration of blood circulation or even force blood to go out of its normal passage leading to hemorrhage. Therefore, it is said that blood circulates smoothly when it is warm, coagulates when cold, and goes out of its normal passage when hot.

Besides this, the smoothness of the vessels is also the fundamental condition to ensure its normal circulation. If the vessels are obstructed by phlegm or stagnated blood, it will lead to pathological changes of sluggish circulation or obstruction.

Plain Questions: Chapter Discussion on Flaccidity (Sù Wèn: Wěi Lùn, 素问·痿论) says: "The Heart governs blood and the vessels of the body."

Plain Questions: Chapter Special Discussion on Channels and Vessels (Sù Wèn: Jīng Mài Bié Lùn Piān, 素问·经脉别论) says: "After food gets into the Stomach, the turbid qi is distributed to the Heart and the pure essence infuses into the vessels

in which it is transformed into channel qi. The channel qi goes up to the Lungs, which converge all the vessels and distribute the essence to the skin and hair. There the hair, body hair, and essence are associated with each other, and the essence qi travels in the channels smoothly and regularly. Then it goes to the four organs, and finally returns to the Lungs." (Fig. 3-15)

Miraculous Pivot: Chapter On Carbuncle and Deep-rooted Carbuncle (Líng Shū: Yōng Jū, 灵枢·痈疽) says: "If blood is harmonized, the minute collaterals will overflow first, and then infuse into collaterals; when they are all full, blood will infuse into channels."

Miraculous Pivot: Chapter The Issue of Distribution and Operation of The Defensive Qi and Nutritive Qi (Líng Shū: Yíng Wèi Shēng Huì, 灵枢·营卫生会) (when discussing the circulation of the nutritive qi and the defensive qi) says: "Like a loop without a starting point," and "The nutritive qi circulates unceasingly."

Essay of Reading Medical Works: Chapter Patient becomes Conscious after Maculation of Warm-Heat Disease (Dú Yī Suí Bǐ: Wēn Rè Bìng Fā Bān Qí Rén Fǎn Qīng, 读医随笔·温热发斑其人反清) says: "Blood in all the vessels of the whole body starts from the Heart and returns to it, circulating unceasingly."

Subtle Implications of Plain Questions and Miraculous Pivot: Chapter Explanation of Visceral Manifestations (Sù Líng Wēi Yùn: Zàng Xiàng Jiě,

素灵微蕴·藏象解) says: *"After water and food gets into the Stomach, the Spleen digests them, discharges the waste downwards and sends the essence upwards to transform into mist… The mist spreads via the zang organs to the collaterals, then from the collaterals to the skin and interstitial spaces to nourish the skin, replenish the body and moisten hair… Since yin tends toward the interior; from skin to collaterals, then collaterals to channels, it returns to the zang-fu organs."*

Plain Questions: Chapter Discussion on the Regulation of Channels (Sù Wèn: Tiáo Jīng Lùn, 素问·调经论) says: *"Blood and qi have a property of preference for warmness and aversion to cold. If they are cold, they will coagulate and cannot flow; if warm, they will thaw and flow."*

Functions of Blood

Blood can nourish and moisten the whole body, and it is the substantial basis for mental activities.

① To Nourish and Moisten the Whole Body

The main ingredients of blood are the nutritive qi and fluid, so blood has nourishing and moistening functions. Blood circulates in the whole body through the vessels to nourish the zang-fu organs, channels and collaterals, body constituents, and sense organs and orifices to maintain their normal physiological functions.

The nourishing function of blood can be reflected by the complexion, muscles, hair, senses motions, etc. If blood is sufficient and its nourishing function is normal, the complexion will be reddish and moist, the muscles strong, skin dense, hair lustrous, senses sharp and motions free. If blood is deficient and its nourishing function decreased, the complexion will be lusterless or sallow, muscles emaciated, skin dry, hair lack luster, limbs numb and motions inflexible, etc.

Classic of Questioning: The Twenty-second Question (Nàn Jīng: Èr Shí Èr Nàn, 难经·二十二难) says: *"Blood dominates nourishing."*

Plain Questions: Chapter Discussion on Various Relationships Concerning the Five Zang-Organs (Sù

Wèn: Wǔ Zàng Shēng Chéng Piān, 素问·五脏生成篇) says: *"When the Liver is nourished by blood, the eyesight will be normal; when feet are nourished by blood, they can walk; when hands are nourished by blood, they can grasp; when fingers are nourished by blood, they can hold."*

② Being the Substantial Basis of Mental Activities

The mental and emotional activities are the external manifestations of zang-fu organs, which take qi and blood as their substantial activities. Only if the zang-fu organs dominating the mind are nourished by blood, can the mental and emotional activities be normal. If blood is sufficient and the mind is nourished, it will manifest as consciousness, and agility in response and thinking. If blood is deficient and fails to nourish the mind, it will manifest as exhaustion, insomnia, amnesia, dreaminess, restlessness, palpations, or even trance, delirium and coma, etc.

Miraculous Pivot: Chapter The Fast of an Ordinary Man (Líng Shū: Píng Rén Jué Gǔ, 灵枢·平人绝谷) says: *"Only if blood is harmonized and the vessels are smooth, can the mind reside."*

Miraculous Pivot: Chapter The Issue of Distribution and Operation of The Defensive Qi and Nutritive Qi (Líng Shū: Yíng Wèi Shēng Huì, 灵枢·营卫生会) says: *"Blood, generated from essence qi, is the substantial basis of the mind."*

Plain Questions: Chapter Discussion on the Elucidation of Influence of the Eight Directions on Acupuncture (Sù Wèn: Bā Zhèng Shén Míng Lùn, 素问·八正神明论) says: *"Blood is the substantial basis of the mind, so it should be taken good care of."*

Section 4   Fluid

Fundamental Concept of Fluid

Fluid (津液) is a general term for all normal liquids in the body, including the interstitial fluid of the bowels, viscera, tissues and organs, and their normal secretions, which is one of the fundamental substances to constitute the human body and maintain vital activities. (Fig. 3-17)

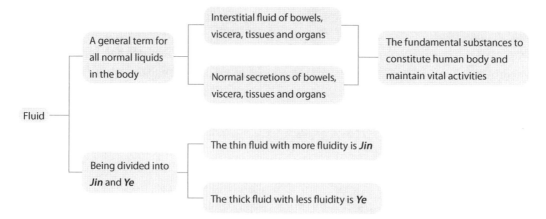

Fig. 3-17   Summary of fundamental concept of fluid

It is divided into *Jin* (津) and *Ye* (液) in *Internal Classic* (*Nèi Jīng*). There are some differences in property, distributive locations and functions between them. In general, thin fluid with more fluidity, which is distributed to skin, muscles and orifices to play a moistening role, is called *Jin*; the thick fluid with less fluidity, which infuses into articular cavities, *zang-fu* organs, brain, and marrow to play a nourishing role, is called *Ye*. (Table 3-3)

Table 3-3   Difference between *Jin* and *Ye*

	Jin	Ye
Property	Thin, with more fluidity	Thick, with less fluidity
Distribution	Distributed to skin, muscles and orifices	Articular cavities, *zang-fu* organs, brain and marrow
Function	Moistening	Nourishing

Although there are some differences between them, they both originate from water and food, their generation both depends on the transporting and transforming function of the Spleen and the Stomach, they can turn into each other during the course of circulation and metabolism, and they can affect each other in pathological processes. Therefore, they are usually not strictly differentiated in physiology, and are collectively termed "fluid". However, they must be differentiated when pathological changes of "injury of *Jin*" and "exhaustion of *Ye*" occur. Injury of *Jin* is a slight case while exhaustion of *Ye* is a severe one.

Miraculous Pivot: Chapter The Five Kinds of Body Fluids (*Líng Shū: Wǔ Lóng Jīn Yè Bié*, 灵枢·五癃津液别) says: "*Jin and Ye circulate in their individual paths. The essence qi dispersed by the San Jiao to warm muscles and replenish skin is Jin; while*

the retained qi is Ye."

Miraculous Pivot: Chapter The Dredge of Qi (*Líng Shū: Jué Qì*, 灵枢·决气) says: "*The interstitial space open, and skin perspires moistly. This is called Jin... After food enters the Stomach, the body is filled with qi generated by food. The thick fluids infuse into bones, thus the joints bend and extend flexibly; it is also distributed to the brain and marrow to nourish them, and skin to moisten it. This is called Ye.*"

Plain Questions: Chapter Discussion on the Secret Classics Stored in Royal Library (*Sù Wèn: Líng Lán Mì Diǎn Lùn*, 素问·灵兰秘典论) says: "*The urinary Bladder is a reservoir in which fluid is stored, and urine is discharged by its function of qi transformation.*"

Essays of Reading Medical Works: Chapter Treating Phlegm and Fluid Retention Separately (*Dú Yī Suí Bǐ: Tán Yǐn Fēn Zhì*, 读医随笔·痰饮分

治) says: "*Sweat and urine can both be called fluid; actually they are both water.*"

Classified Classic: Chapter Class of Visceral Manifestations (Lèi Jīng: Zàng Xiàng Lèi, 类经·藏象类) says: "*Jin and Ye are of the same source, but they are different in yin-yang attribute. Jin is the clear Ye, and Ye is the turbid Jin. Jin circulates to the interstitial spaces to generate sweat, so it belongs to yang; while Ye infuses into bones to nourish the brain and marrow, so it belongs to yin.*"

Metabolism of Fluid

Metabolism of fluid includes its generation, distribution, and excretion, which is a complicated physiological process involving various *zang-fu* organs. (Fig. 3-18)

1 Generation of Fluid

Fluid originates from water and food, and is generated by the absorbing and digestive functions of the Spleen, Stomach, Small Intestine and large intestine.

The Stomach dominates receiving and digesting water and food. When the Stomach is full of fluid, it will distribute the floating qi upwards to the Spleen. The Spleen governs transportation and transformation, digesting and absorbing liquids and the essence of water and food to generate fluid. The Small Intestine is in charge of *Ye*, separates the clear from the turbid and absorbs essence and liquids. The Large Intestine is in charge of *Jin*, and it can absorb fluid from the waste of food in process of passing. The essence and fluid absorbed by the Small Intestine and Large Intestine will be distributed to the Spleen. "The Spleen scatters the essence qi"; it can transport the essence and fluid to the Heart and the Lung and then distribute it to the whole body. Therefore, the generation of fluid is accomplished by the physiological functions of the Spleen, the Stomach, the Small Intestine and the large intestine. If their function of absorbing liquids is interrupted, the generation of fluid will be affected, leading to a pathological change of deficiency of fluid

generation.

2 Distribution of Fluid

The collective effects from the Spleen, the Lung, the Kidney, the Heart, the Liver and the *San Jiao* accomplish distribution of fluid.

The Spleen dominates transporting and transforming fluid by "scatting the essence qi". On one hand, it sends fluid up to the Lung; on the other hand, it distributes fluid throughout the body.

The Lung dominates diffusion and descent; and it smooths the waterways. Fluid is distributed to the body surface by diffusion of Lung qi, and to internal organs by its descending function. The fluid will be transported to the Kidney and urinary Bladder after the *zang-fu* organs and tissues utilize it.

The Kidney governs water. The qi-transforming action of the Kidney on fluid has two aspects: one is to govern the water metabolism of the whole body; the other is the Kidney separating the clear from the turbid, sending up the clear fluid and holding it inside the body, and distributing the turbid fluid to the urinary Bladder to generate urine.

The Heart governs blood, and promotes its circulation. Fluid is a main ingredient of blood, so distribution of fluid is related to blood circulation.

The Liver governs free movement and regulating of the qi dynamic. Fluid will circulate smoothly if the qi dynamic is normal, so the smoothing function of the Liver qi can promote fluid circulation.

The *San Jiao* is viewed as an officer in charge of water passage dredging, being the pathway of fluid circulation. By the qi-transforming function of the *San Jiao*, fluid can be distributed throughout the body.

3 Excretion of Fluid

The excretion of fluid depends on the collective functions of the Lung, the Kidney, the urinary Bladder, the Large Intestine and the *San Jiao*, and is accomplished through the respiratory tract, sweat, urine and feces.

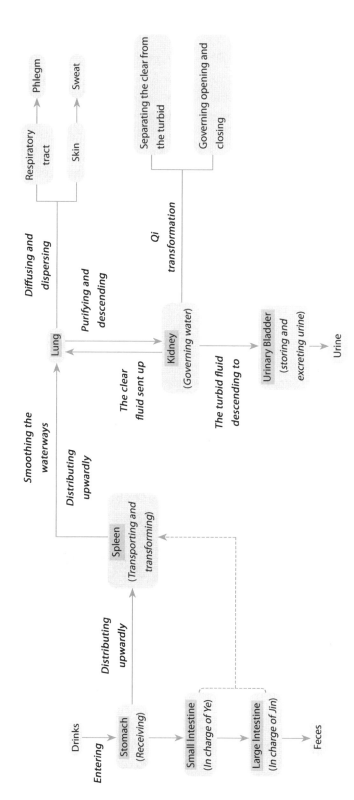

Fig. 3-18   Demonstration of relationship between fluid metabolism and major internal organs

The Lung qi disperses fluid to the respiratory tract upwardly, and to the skin and hairs of the body surface exteriorly. After being utilized, the waste liquid will be discharged either through the respiratory tract (phlegm or exhaled air) or sweat pores (sweat).

The Kidney governs water. Through the qi-transforming function of the Kidney, the turbid fluid turns into urine after being metabolized, and is distributed to the urinary Bladder, which possessing the function of storing and excreting urine. The urine is excreted outside the body by the collective function of the Kidney and the urinary Bladder.

The Large Intestine transports the waste and excretes feces. During this course, it will take away some surplus water.

The *San Jiao* circulates fluid. The lower *Jiao* serves as a drain. Through the qi-transforming function of the *San Jiao*, the turbid fluid, once metabolized, turns into urine to be excreted outside the body.

Dysfunction of the above-mentioned *zang-fu* organs will result in retention of fluid leading to phlegm and rheum, edema, etc, or over-excretion leading to deficiency of fluid.

In general, the process of the generation, distribution and excretion of fluid needs the collective functions of various *zang-fu* organs to accomplish. Therein, the Spleen, the Lung and the Kidney are of special importance. Hence, it is said, "the root of fluid metabolism rests with the Kidney, the branch rests with the Lung, and the regulation rests with the Spleen."

Plain Questions: Chapter Special Discussion on Channels and Vessels (Sù Wèn: Jīng Mài Bié Lùn Piān, 素问·经脉别论) says: "*After drink gets into the Stomach, the floating essence qi is distributed to the Spleen upwardly; the Spleen again scatters it upwardly to the Lung, which smoothes the water passages and distributes it downwardly to the urinary Bladder. Thus, the essence of water is spread throughout the body and the channels of the five zang organs.*"

Plain Questions: Chapter Discussion on Disharmony (Sù Wèn: Nì Tiáo Lùn, 素问·逆调论) says: "*The Kidney is a water organ that governs fluid.*"

*Plain Questions: Chapter Discussion on Genuine-Zang Pulses (Sù Wèn: Yù Jī Zhēn Zàng Lùn,*素问·玉机真脏论) says: "*The channel of the Spleen belongs to earth, being a solitary zang organ to irrigate its surrounding adjacencies.*" Notation by Wang Bing (王冰) says: "*To take in water and food, transform fluid and irrigate the Liver, the Heart, the Lung and the Kidney.*"

Plain Questions: Chapter Discussion on the Secret Classics Stored in Royal Library (Sù Wèn: Líng Lán Mì Diǎn Lùn, 素问·灵兰秘典论) says: "*The San Jiao is like an Official for water passage dredging who is responsible for water-ways. The urinary Bladder is the reservoir in which fluid is stored, and urine is discharged by its function of qi transformation.*"

Miraculous Pivot: Chapter The Issue of Distribution and Operation of The Defensive Qi and Nutritive Qi (Líng Shū: Yíng Wèi Shēng Huì, 灵枢·营卫生会) says: "*The lower Jiao serves as a drain.*"

Treatise on Spleen and Stomach: Chapter Discussion on Large Intestine, Small Intestine and Five Zang Organs All Belonging to the Stomach, With Deficiency of the Stomach Leading to Disorders of All These Organs (Pí Wèi Lùn: Dà Cháng Xiǎo Cháng Wǔ Zàng Jiē Shǔ Yú Wèi Wèi Xū Zé Jù Bìng Lùn, 脾胃论·大肠小肠五脏皆属于胃胃虚则俱病论) says: "*The Large Intestine is in charge of Jin while the Small Intestine is in charge of Ye.*"

Jing-yue's Complete Work: Section Treatment of Edema, Chapter Swelling and Distention, Volume 22, (*Jǐng Yuè Quán Shū: Shuǐ Zhǒng Lùn Zhì, Zhǒng Zhàng,* 景岳全书·二十二卷·肿胀·水肿论治) says: "*Edema is due to the mutual affection of the Spleen, the Lung and the Kidney. Water pertains to extreme yin, so its root rests with the Kidney; water is transformed by qi, so its branch rests on the Lung; water is afraid of earth only, so its governance rests on the Spleen.*"

Functions of Fluid

1 Moistening and Nourishing

Fluid is the liquid substance containing abundant water and nutrients, so it is of moistening and nourishing functions. Fluid distributed to the body surface can moisten skin and muscles, making skin and hair lustrous and muscles plump; fluid permeating into the interior can nourish *zang-fu* organs and maintain their normal functions; fluid flowing into orifices can moisten the mouth, nose, ears and eyes; fluid infusing into bone joints can lubricate them; fluid infusing into marrow can replenish bone, spinal cord and cerebral marrow. By comparison, *Jin* is clear and thin in property, and takes moistening as its major function; while *Ye* is thick in property, and takes nourishing as its major function.

② Generating Blood

Fluid permeates into vessels via minute collaterals to generate blood and circulate to the whole body, exerting a moistening and nourishing function. Fluid can also regulate the concentration and volume of blood. When blood concentration is high or blood volume is insufficient, fluid will permeate into vessels to dilute it and supplement the volume.

In addition, fluid metabolism can play a regulating role to environmental changes inside and outside the body. Take the changes of heat and cold for example. When it is cold or the body temperature drops, the skin, hairs and sweat pores will close with no perspiration. Thus fluid will not excrete outside so as to maintain a relatively constant body temperature, while the surplus water will be excreted by urine. When it is hot or the patient has a fever, fluid will transform into sweat and excrete outside to scatter heat in order to regulate body temperature. At that time the volume of urine decreases to avoid excessive loss of fluid.

Miraculous Pivot: Chapter On Carbuncle and Deep-rooted Carbuncle (Líng Shū: Yōng Jū, 灵枢·痈疽) says: *"The middle Jiao disperses the essence qi like dew, infuses it into stream and valley and permeates into minute collaterals. Thus fluid is harmonized and turns into the red liquid which is known as blood."*

Section 5   Relationship among Essence, Qi, Blood and Fluid

Essence, qi, blood and fluid are all the fundamental substances constituting the human body as well as maintaining its vital activities. There exists a relationship of interdependence, inter-restriction and interaction. In this section, we will mainly discuss the relationship between qi and blood, qi and fluid, and blood and fluid.

Relationship between Qi and Blood

Qi dominates movement, belongs to yang and has a warming function; blood dominates stillness, belongs to yin and has a nourishing function. These are the main differences between qi and blood in property and physiological functions. However, they are closely connected in respect to generation and circulation (distribution). Qi is the energy of blood generation and circulation, while blood is the generating basis and carrier. Therefore, they can affect each other in pathology.

The relationship between qi and blood is usually generalized by saying that "qi is the commander of blood" and "blood is the mother of qi". Qi being the commander of blood indicates that the effect of qi on blood includes three aspects: qi generating blood, qi promoting blood circulation and qi controlling blood. Blood being the mother of qi indicates that the effect of blood on qi includes two aspects: blood generating qi and blood carrying qi.

Classic of Questioning: The Twenty-second Question (Nàn Jīng: Èr Shí Èr Nàn, 难经·二十二难) says: *"Qi dominates warming while blood dominates nourishing."*

Collection of Buju (Bù Jū Jí, 不居集) says: *"In the human body, qi and blood can't be independent of each other. Qi contains blood and blood contains qi. Qi and blood depend on each other and circulate ceaselessly."*

① The Effect of Qi on Blood (Fig. 3-19)

(1) Qi generating blood

Qi generating blood indicates that blood generation depends on the function of qi. First, as for the composition of blood, nutritive qi is a main ingredient of blood, since the nutritive

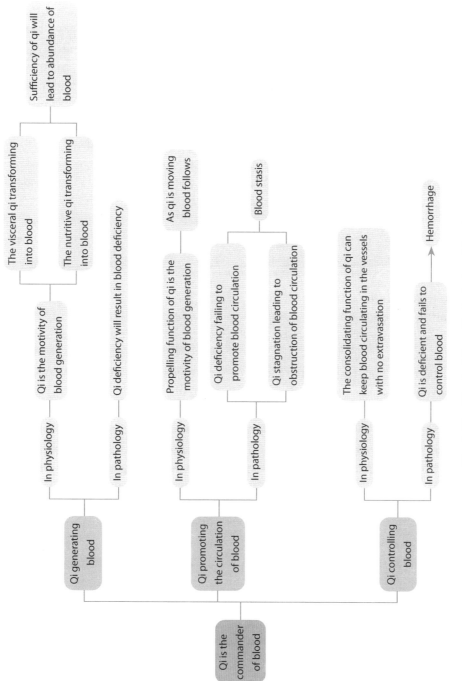

Fig. 3-19　Chart of the effect of qi on blood

qi can infuse into the vessels to generate blood. Second, as for the generating process of blood, its generation depends on the qi-transforming function of *zang-fu* organs. For instance, food and drink transforming into essence, as well as essence from water, food, and Kidney essence transforming into red blood, are completed through the movements and changes of the qi of the Spleen, the Stomach, the Heart, the Lung, the Liver and the Kidney. Therefore, qi can generate blood, and sufficiency of qi will lead to abundance of blood.

If qi is deficient and its blood-generating function decreased, it will result in blood deficiency, i.e. qi fails to generate blood. According to this theory, one often combines a blood tonic with qi-replenishing herbs when treating the syndrome of blood deficiency. Thus there is a saying that *"the corporeal blood can not grow alone, while the insubstantial qi can promote its generation."*

(2) Qi promoting the circulation of blood

Qi promoting the circulation of blood indicates that blood circulation depends on the propelling function of qi. In terms of visceral functions, it mainly indicates Heart qi, Lung qi and Liver qi. Heart qi is the fundamental energy to drive blood circulation, Lung qi can assist it, and the free coursing function of Liver qi can promote it. The propelling function of qi is the energy of blood circulation, so it is said: "as qi is moving blood follows, and as qi gets stagnant blood follows, too".

Qi deficiency failing to promote blood circulation, and qi stagnation leading to obstruction of blood circulation will both result in sluggish circulation of blood or even stagnant blood. When applying methods of activating blood and removing stasis to treat stagnant blood, one often simultaneously uses qi-replenishing or qi-activating drugs. Qi counterflow will cause blood to rush upwards due to the adverse flow of qi, and leading to hemorrhage. Clinically, the method of sending qi down in order to arrest bleeding is often adopted, and this is the practical application of this theory.

(3) Qi controlling blood

Qi controlling blood indicates that blood circu-

lating in the vessels with no overflow depends on the consolidating function of qi. This is mainly the blood-controlling function of Spleen qi.

If qi is deficient and fails to control blood, it will lead to hemorrhage. Clinically, the method of replenishing qi is adopted to control blood. As for a severe case of massive hemorrhage, a large dosage of qi-replenishing drugs should be used to consolidate collapse. This is why it is said "The corporeal blood can't be generated in short time, while the insubstantial qi should be consolidated immediately". This is also based on the principle of qi controlling blood.

Essays of Reading Medical Works: Chapter Qi Generating Blood and Blood Carrying Qi (Dú Yī Suí Bǐ: Qì Néng Shēng Xuè Xuè Néng Zài Qì, 读医随笔·气能生血血能载气) says: "*Qi which can generate blood is the nutritive qi. As the nutritive qi is exuberant blood is exuberant, and as qi declines blood declines. They depend on each other and cannot separate.*"

Classic of Questioning: The Forty-second Question (Nàn Jīng: Sì Shí Èr Nàn, 难经·四十二难) says: "*The Spleen… dominates wrapping qi.*"

Key Link of Medicine: Chapter Discussion Yin and Yang (Yǐ Guàn: Yīn Yáng Lùn, 医贯·阴阳论) says: "*A sudden and massive hemorrhage with fainting can be treated by Dú Shēn Tāng (Ginseng Decoction,* 独参汤), one liang, taken at a draught, using qi-replenishing drug only. At that moment, the corporeal blood can't be generated in a short time, while the feeble qi should be consolidated immediately, making the insubstantial produce the corporeal.*"

Discussion of Blood Syndrome: Chapter Hematemesis (Xuè Zhèng Lùn: Tù Xuè, 血证论·吐血) says: "*Qi is the commander of blood and blood follows qi; blood is the guard of qi, and qi will be calm when it is accompanied by blood. As qi is stagnant blood is coagulated, as qi is deficient blood is lost, and as qi propels blood travels. If qi does not stop, blood will not halt.*"

Plain Questions: Chapter Discussion on the Regulation of Channels (Sù Wèn: Tiáo Jīng Lùn, 素问·调经论) says: "*Disharmony of blood and qi will result in the occurrence of various diseases.*"

② The Effect of Blood on Qi (Fig. 3-20)

(1) Blood generating qi

It indicates that the generation of qi and the exertion of its functions depend on the nourishment of blood. Blood is liquid with a nourishing function, providing nutrients for the generation of the qi of the bowels, viscera, channels and collaterals and their functional activities. Hence, as blood is sufficient qi is abundant, and blood deficiency can lead to qi deficiency.

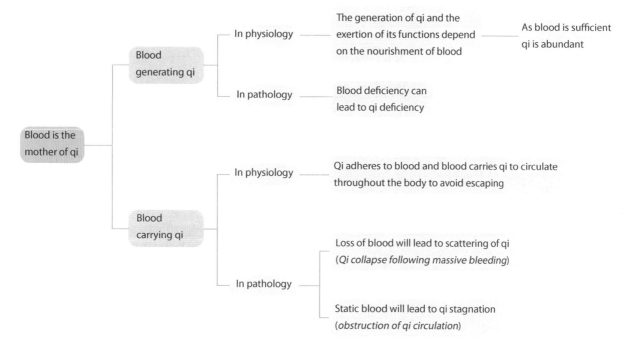

Fig. 3-20   Chart of the effect of blood on qi

(2) Blood carrying qi

It indicates that qi exists in blood and attaches itself to it so as to avoid escaping. Qi adheres to blood, and blood carries qi to circulate throughout the body. Without blood, qi would have nothing to adhere to and would be easy to dissipate. For instance, a case of massive hemorrhage will cause a massive loss of qi, leading to the pathological change of "loss of blood and scattering of qi" (qi collapse following massive bleeding). Because blood can carry qi, when blood is stagnant, it will also lead to obstruction of qi circulation.

Zhang's Treatise on Medicine: Category of All Blood Syndromes (Zhāng Shì Yī Tōng:Zhū Xuè Mén, 张氏医通·诸血门) says: *"Without blood, qi will scatter without control."*

Essays of Reading Medical Works: Chapter Qi Generating Blood and Blood Carrying Qi (Dú Yī Suí Bǐ: Qì Néng Shēng Xuè Xuè Néng Zài Qì, 读医随笔·气能生血血能载气*)* says: *"Blood storing qi indicates that qi has a rapid and vigorous property, travels ceaselessly and scatters diffusely, and if there is nothing to hold it, won't it be traveling and scattering all the time? Blood is the only thing in which qi can reside, so take blood as the house of qi, then they associate with each other to avoid scattering of qi."*

Relationship between Qi and Fluid

By comparison, qi pertains to yang while fluid to yin. Since fluid is the component part of blood in the vessels, the relationship between qi and fluid and that between qi and blood are of similarity. The generation, distribution and excretion depend on the propelling and consolidating functions of qi, and movement and changes of qi cannot go without moistening and carrying of fluid.

① The Effect of Qi on Fluid (Table 3-4)

(1) *Qi generating fluid*

It indicates that movements and changes of qi is the energy of fluid generation. Fluid originates from water and food, and is produced by the effect of the visceral qi of the Spleen and Stomach. Therefore, if the visceral qi of the Spleen and Stomach is abundant and functions soundly, fluid will be sufficient. If visceral qi is feeble and its function is weak, generation of fluid will be insufficient. Clinically, the method of reinforcing qi to generate fluid can be adopted.

Table 3-4   Table of the effect of qi on fluid

Effect	Physiology	Pathology	Treatment
Qi generating fluid	Movement and changes o f qi is the energy of fluid generation; if the visceral qi of the Spleen and Stomach is abundant, fluid will be sufficient	If visceral qi is feeble, generation of fluid will be deficient	Reinforcing qi to generate fluid
Qi promoting the circulation of fluid	Movement and changes of qi is the energy of distribution and excretion of fluid (as qi moves, water moves)	If qi is deficient or stagnant, it will lead to dysfunction of the distribution and excretion of fluid to form pathological products such as phlegm, rheum, water and dampness, etc	Reinforcing qi to excrete water, or activating qi combined with excreting water
Qi controlling fluid	The consolidating function of qi can prevent fluid from unnecessary loss, and control the normal excretion of sweat and urine	If the consolidating function of qi is decreased due to qi deficiency, polyhidrosis, spontaneous sweating, polyuria and enuresis will occur	Reinforcing qi to control fluid

(2) *Qi promoting the circulation of fluid*

It indicates that movement of qi and changes of qi are the energy of distribution and excretion of fluid. After being generated, fluid is distributed to every parts of the body through the propelling function of the visceral qi of the Spleen, the Lung, the Kidney and the *San Jiao*. After being utilized, the waste fluid and surplus water, again by the qi transforming function of the Lung, the Kidney, the urinary Bladder and *San Jiao*, is transformed into sweat and urine to excrete out of the body. Hence, the succession of distribution and excretion of fluid is accomplished through movement and changes of qi (qi transformation). So it is said, "*as qi moves, water moves*". If qi deficiency or qi stagnation occurs, its propelling function decreases, and qi transformation is obstructed, it will lead to dysfunction of distribution and excretion of fluid, producing pathological products such as phlegm, rheum, water and dampness, etc. This is called "qi failing to drive water" or "qi failing to transform water". Clinically, the method of reinforcing and activating qi is usually adopted combined with that of excreting water and resolving phlegm. This is the concrete application of the theory of qi promoting the circulation of fluid.

(3) *Qi controlling fluid*

It indicates that the consolidating function of qi can prevent fluid from unnecessary loss. The consolidating function of qi can control the normal excretion of sweat and urine to maintain a relatively constant volume of body fluid. If the consolidating function of qi decreases due to qi deficiency, polyhidrosis, spontaneous sweating, polyuria or enuresis will occur. Clinically, the method of reinforcing qi is adopted to control the excessive loss of fluid.

② The Effect of Fluid on Qi (Table 3-5)

(1) Fluid generating qi

Fluid distributed to the whole body can exert a moistening and nourishing function to all *zang-*

fu organs, maintaining vigorous functional activities of the Spleen, the Stomach, the Lung and the Kidney, etc, to make for the generation of qi. Therefore, deficiency of fluid can affect the functional activities of *zang-fu* organs leading to deficiency of qi generation.

Table 3-5   Table of the effect of fluid on qi

Effect	Physiology	Pathology
Fluid generating qi	Fluid can exert a moistening and nourishing function for all *zang-fu* organs, maintaining vigorous functional activites of the Spleen, the Stomach, the Lung and the Kidney, etc, to cause the generation of qi	Deficiency of fluid can affect functional activities of *zang-fu* organs leading to deficiency of qi generation
Fluid carrying qi	Fluid is one of the carriers of qi. In the vessels, qi adheres to fluid to circulate and avoid floating and scattering	As fluid loses abundance, qi follows (perspiration followed by loss of qi, loss of fluid followed by depletion of qi)

(2) Fluid carrying qi

It indicates that fluid is one of the carriers of qi. In the vessels, qi attaches itself to blood. Outside the vessels, qi adheres to fluid so as to circulate throughout the body. Otherwise, qi will float and scatter without a place to turn towards. Thus it is said that fluid can carry qi. As fluid loses in abundance, qi follows. For instance, in polyhidrosis due to summer-heat, qi will be lost along with perspiration, leading to impairment of both fluid and qi. Massive loss of fluid due to profuse sweating, violent vomiting and diarrhea will cause massive consumption of qi accordingly, which is called "loss of fluid followed by depletion of qi".

Essays of Studying Classics: Chapter Examining the Nutritive qi and the Defensive qi (Yán Jīng Yán: Yuán Yíng Wèi, 研经言·原营卫) says: "*Qi has no form, and it has to adhere to something to travel. Therefore, the nutritive qi circulating in the vessels*

adheres to blood, and the defensive qi circulating outside the vessels adheres to fluid."

The Essence of the Synopsis of the Golden Chamber: Chapter Phlegm and Rheum (Jīn Guì Yào Luè Xīn Diàn: Tán Yǐn, 金匮要略心典·痰饮) says: "*Qi won't be intact after vomiting and diarrhea.*"

Relationship between Blood and Fluid

Blood and fluid are both generated by essence from water and food, and both are liquids with a moistening and nourishing function. They can generate each other and transform into each other, so it is said, "*fluid and blood are of the same source*".

① Relationship between Blood and Fluid in Physiology

Physiologically, they can transform into and supplement each other. (Fig. 3-21, Fig. 3-22)

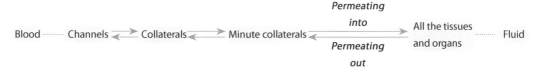

Fig. 3-21   Demonstration of circumfluence of blood and fluid

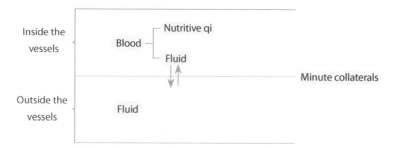

Fig. 3-22   Demonstration of mutual transformation and supplement of blood and fluid

Blood circulates in the vessels and consists of the nutritive qi and fluid. Fluid scatters to all tissues and organs of the body, and is the component of blood in the vessels. They can transform into and supplement each other in the circulating process.

Blood permeates outside the vessels through minute collaterals, and then it will transform into fluid with moistening functions, as well as supplement deficiency of fluid. Fluid can transform into sweat to be excreted out of the body, and so it is said, "blood and sweat share the same source".

Fluid outside the vessels can again permeate into the minute collaterals, thus fluid is able to generate and supplement blood, becoming its component.

Hence, there is a mutual transforming and supplementing relationship between blood and fluid.

Miraculous Pivot: Chapter On Carbuncle and Deep-rooted Carbuncle (Líng Shū: Yōng Jū, 灵枢·痈疽) say: *"The middle Jiao disperses the essence qi like dew, infuses it into stream and valley and permeates into minute collateral. Thus fluid is harmonized and turned into red liquid, which is known as blood. If blood is harmonized, the minute collaterals will overflow first, and then infuse into collaterals; when they are all full, blood will infuse into channels."*

② Relationship between Blood and Fluid in Pathology

Pathologically, pathological changes of them can affect each other.

When blood in the vessels is deficient due to massive bleeding, fluid outside the vessels will infuses into the vessels to supplement deficiency of blood volume. Thus, the fluid outside the vessels is insufficient, and pathological phenomena such as thirst, oliguria and dryness of skin will occur (Fig. 3-23). Therefore, as for patients with massive bleeding, the method of diaphoresis should not be adopted in order to avoid further impairment of blood and fluid.

When fluid outside the vessels is deficient due to massive loss, fluid inside the vessels will infuse out of the vessels to supplement depletion of fluid. Thus, it will lead to the pathological change of hollowness of blood vessels due to scantiness of fluid and dryness of blood (Fig. 3-24). Therefore, as with the case of massive loss of

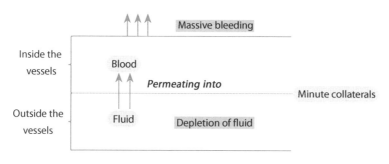

Fig. 3-23   Demonstration of depletion of fluid due to massive bleeding

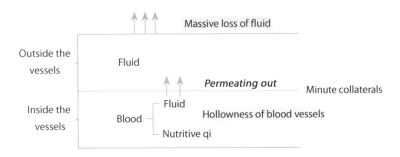

Fig. 3-24   Demonstration of hollowness of blood vessels due to massive loss of fluid

fluid, the method of phlebotomy and drastically removing blood stasis should not be adopted any more in order to avoid further impairment of blood and fluid.

Miraculous Pivot: Chapter The Issue of Distribution and Operation of The Defensive Qi and Nutritive Qi (*Líng Shū: Yíng Wèi Shēng Huì*, 灵枢·营卫生会) says: *"A patient with massive loss of blood has no sweat, and a patient with incessant profuse sweating has scanty blood volume."*

Besides this, the relationship between qi and essence mainly manifests as qi generating essence and essence transforming into qi. The relationship between blood and essence mainly manifests as essence and blood sharing the same source, and mutual generation between essence and blood. The relationship between essence and fluid is mainly that of essence from water and food and fluid; they both originate from water and food, and are both generated by the Spleen and Stomach, so they have the relationship of the same origin and generation.

Chapter 4
Channels and Collaterals

The channel-collateral doctrine is a theory that studies the composition, distribution, physiological functions, and pathological changes of the channel-collateral system of the human body and its correlation with the *zang-fu* organs, body constituents, sense organs and orifices. The channel-collateral doctrine is an important component of the theoretical system of Chinese medicine.

The channel-collateral doctrine came into being during long-term clinical practice. The ancients accumulated all kinds of experiences in acupuncture, moxibustion, *tui na* (推拿) and qi gong (气功), which were combined with the knowledge of anatomy and visceral manifestations to form the channel-collateral doctrine. It was recorded in *Miraculous Pivot* (*Líng Shū*, 灵枢) at length, which had a formed systematic theory.

The channel-collateral doctrine runs through every aspect of Chinese medicine, such as constitution, physiology, and pathology of the body, as well as diagnosis, prevention and treatment of diseases. It supplements the visceral manifestations theory and essence-qi and blood-fluid theory, profoundly expounds upon physiological activities and pathological changes of the human body, and is of great significance in guiding all clinical branches, especially acupuncture, moxibustion, *tui na*, qi gong, etc.

Miraculous Pivot: Chapter On Channels (*Líng Shū: Jīng Mài*, 灵枢·经脉) says: "*One can determine the survival or death of the patient, treat various diseases and find out whether the disease is excess or deficient according to the condition of the channels, so one must master it.*"

Miraculous Pivot: Chapter Branches of the Twelve Channels (*Líng Shū: Jīng Bié*, 灵枢·经别) says: "*The twelve channels have a close relation with the existence of man, the formation of disease, human health, and the recovery from disease. A beginner treating the disease must learn the theory of channels, and a good physician must also pay attention to it. A physician of a lower level thinks the theory of channels is easy to learn, but a physician of a higher level deems it hard to be proficient.*"

The Book about Biǎn Què's Thought (*Biǎn Què Xīn Shū*, 扁鹊心书) says: "*If a doctor does not know the channels and collaterals, he will make mistakes when inquiring about symptoms or taking pulses. The reason is as follows: if he is not clear of them, he will not realize the source of the syndrome and the transmission of yin-yang.*"

Section 1 The Concept of Channels and Collaterals and Constitution of the Channel–Collateral System

Basic Concept of Channels and Collaterals

The channel-collateral system is a generic name of all of the channels and collaterals. They are the pathways through which the human body transports qi and blood, connects the *zang-fu* organs, body constituents, sense organs and orifices, communicates with the interior, exterior, upper and lower parts, and induces and conducts messages. They are important components of the body.

Channel-collateral can be classified into two categories: channels (经) and collaterals (络). The differences between them is as follow (Table 4-1).

Channels mean paths. Channels are the trunks of the channel-collateral system. Most of them distribute interiorly and longitudinally along the depths of body and have regular courses.

Collaterals mean networks. Collaterals are small branches of channels. They distribute along the superficies crisscross and connect the whole body.

Miraculous Pivot: Chapter On Channels (Líng Shū: Jīng Mài, 灵枢·经脉) says: *"The twelve channels lie concealed and distribute deeply in the muscular layers that can hardly be seen...The floating ones which can often be seen are collaterals."*

Miraculous Pivot: Chapter The Length of Channels (Líng Shū: Mài Dù, 灵枢·脉度) says: *"The channels lie deeply inside, and the branches that separate from the channels and distribute horizontally are the collaterals, and the branches from the collaterals are the minute collaterals."*

Elementary Medicine: Chapter the Starts and Terminals of Channel Point (Yī Xué Rù Mén: Jīng Xuè Qǐ Zhǐ, 医学入门·经穴起止) says: *"Channels mean paths. Those that distribute straight are named channels; and branches of those channels are named collaterals."*

Table 4-1 The difference between channels and collaterals

	Channels	**Collaterals**
Signification	Channels mean paths; trunks of channel-collateral system	Collaterals mean networks; Small branches of the channels
Distributing Depth	Deep	Superficial
Distributing Course	Have regular distributing courses; most distribute longitudinally	Distribute crisscross and connect the whole body

The Composition of the Channel–Collateral System

The channel-collateral system is composed of channels, collaterals and their subordinates. (Fig. 4-1)

1 Channels

Channels, which are the trunks of the channel-collateral system, are classified into two categories: the primary channels and extraordinary channels. They mainly comprise the twelve channels, the eight extraordinary channels and the twelve divergent channels.

(1) The twelve channels

The twelve channels comprise the three yin channels of the hand, three yang channels of the hand, three yin channels of the foot and three yang channels of the foot. Compared to the

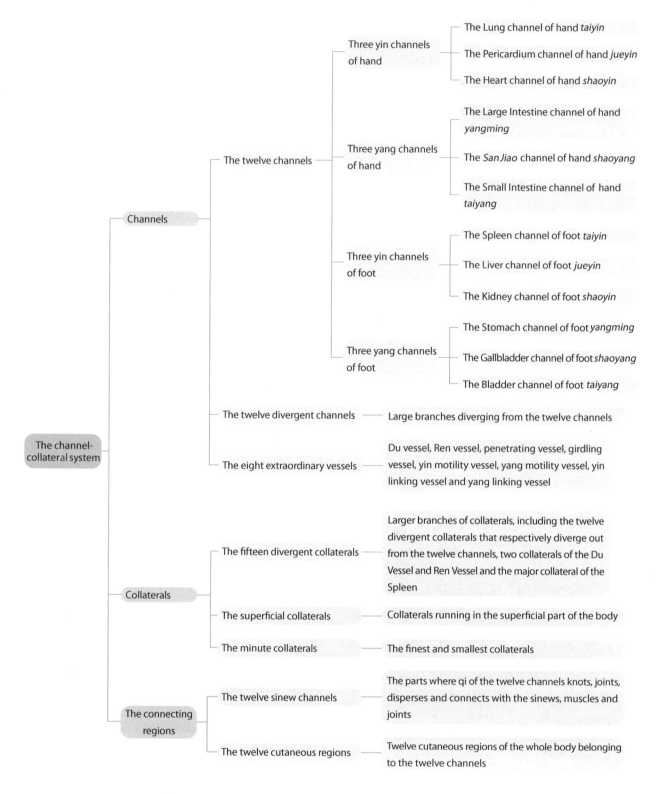

Fig. 4-1   The composition of the channel-collateral system

extraordinary vessels, they are also named the twelve primary channels. The twelve channels, as trunks of the channel-collateral system, they pertain to or connect with the *zang-fu* organs and act as the main pathways of transporting qi and blood.

(2) The Eight Extraordinary Channels

The eight extraordinary channels are comprised

of the *Du*, *Ren*, penetrating vessel, girdling vessel, yin motility vessel, yang motility vessel, yin linking vessel and yang linking vessel. Their functions are to strengthen the connection between the twelve channels and regulate the qi and blood of the twelve channels.

(3) The Twelve Divergent Channels

The twelve divergent channels are another kind of channel that diverge out from the twelve channels and have certain distributing characteristic. They diverge from the upper regions of the elbows and knees and have the function of strengthening the connection between the interiorly-exteriorly related channels and supplementing the distributions of the twelve channels. As the largest branches of the twelve channels, they still belong to the category of the primary channels.

②　Collaterals

Collaterals are the small branches of channels. They are classified into the divergent collaterals, superficial collaterals, and minute collaterals.

(1) The divergent collaterals

The divergent collaterals are the fifteen larger branches of collaterals. They are comprised of the twelve divergent collaterals that diverge out from the twelve channels, the two collaterals of the *Du* and *Ren*, and the major collateral of the Spleen. The divergent collaterals mean that they diverge out from the channels and reach other channels nearby. Their functions are to strengthen the connection between the interiorly-exteriorly related channels on the body surface and permeate them with the qi and blood of the twelve channels.

(2) The superficial collaterals

The superficial collaterals are those that distribute in the superficial part of the body.

(3) The minute collaterals

The minute collaterals are the finest and smallest collaterals, and they are also named minute channels.

③　The Connecting Regions

They mainly comprise the twelve sinew channels and twelve cutaneous regions. They are the connecting regions of the twelve channels, sinews, muscles and body surface.

(1) The twelve sinew channels

The twelve sinew channels are the parts where the qi of the twelve channels knots, joins, disperses and connects with the sinews, muscles and joints. Their function is to connect the limbs and bones, and to govern the motion of joints.

(2) The twelve cutaneous regions

The twelve cutaneous regions are the certain areas of the body surface in which the functions of the twelve channels are reflected. The entire area of the body is divided into twelve parts and pertains to the twelve channels.

Elucidation of the Fourteen Channels (Shí Sì Jīng Fā Huī, 十四经发挥) says: *"There are regular channels and extraordinary vessels. The twelve primary channels are regular; The eight extraordinary channels are not restrained, and hence they are named the extraordinary vessels. Qi and blood of the human body usually flows in the twelve channels, and when they are overflowing, they will pour into the eight extraordinary channels."*

Section 2　The Twelve Channels

The Names of The Twelve Channels

①　The Significance of the Nomenclature of the Twelve Channels (Table 4-2)

The twelve channels are symmetrically distributed on both sides of the human body. They distribute respectively on the medial or lateral side of the upper or lower limbs and pertain to a *zang* or *fu* organ, so the names of the twelve channels are different. Each name is composed of three parts: hand or foot, yin or yang, *zang* or *fu* organ. The signification of the nomenclature is as follows:

Hand-foot: Relatively, the hand is the upper and foot is the lower. Hand-foot denotes that the channels distribute along the upper or lower limbs. That is to say that the channels of the hand distribute along the upper limbs and the channels

Table 4-2   The significance of the nomenclature of the twelve channels

Content	Signification of Nomenclature
Hand, Foot	Channels of hand distribute along the upper limbs
	Channels of foot distribute along the lower limbs
Yin, Yang	Yin channels distribute along the medial aspects of the limbs
	Yang channels distribute along the lateral aspects of the limbs
Zàng organ, Fu organ	Yin channels pertain to the zang organs
	Yang channels pertain to the fu organs

of foot along the lower limbs. In addition, hand-foot also denotes the start and end points of the channels: the three yin channels of the hand terminate at the hands, the three yang channels of the hand start from the hands, the three yang channels of the foot terminate at the feet, and the three yin channels of the foot start at the feet.

Yin-yang: Relatively, the yin is the interior and yang is the exterior. Yin-yang denotes that the channels distribute along the medial or lateral aspect of the limbs. That is to say that the yin channels distribute along the medial aspect of the limbs, and the yang channels along the lateral aspect of the limbs.

Zang-fu organs: Relatively, the zang organs pertain to yin and the fu organs pertain to yang. Zang-fu organs denote the Zang or fu organs that the channels pertain to. That is to say that the yin channels pertain to the zang organs, and the yang channels pertain to the fu organs.

In addition, according to the difference of yin qi or yang qi in quantity, yin-yang is further classified into taiyin, shaoyin, jueyin, taiyang, yangming and shaoyang. It is thought that the yin qi of taiyin (three yin) is the most, shaoyin (two yin) is lesser, and the jueyin (one yin) is the least; the yang qi of taiyang (three yang) is the most, yangming (two yang) is lesser, and the shaoyang (one yang) is the least. The sequence are different from that of the three yin or yang channels of hand and foot distributing on the anterior, medial and posterior side of the limbs.

Plain Questions: Chapter Major Discussion

on the Law of Motions and Changes in Nature (Sù Wèn: Tiān Yuán Jì Dà Lùn, 素问·天元纪大论) says:"The quantity of yin qi and yang qi is different, hence there are the distinctions of three yin and three yang."

Plain Questions: Chapter Discussion on the Most Important and Abstruse Theory (Sù Wèn: Zhì Zhèn Yào Dà Lùn, 素问·至真要大论) says: "There are three yin and three yang, and what is the reason? Qi Bo (岐伯) said: This is because the yin qi and yang qi may be more or less in quantity and they are different in functions." Wang Bin (王冰) notes: "The yin qi of taiyin and the yang qi of taiyang are the most, then the yin qi of shaoyin and the yang qi of shaoyang are lesser, and the yang qi of yangming and the yin qi of jueyin are the least."

② The Classification of the Names of the Twelve Channels (Table 4-3)

The twelve channels are classified into four groups: the three yin channels of the hand (the Lung channel of hand *taiyin*, the Pericardium channel of hand *jueyin*, the Heart channel of hand *shaoyin*), the three yang channels of the hand (the Large Intestine channel of hand *yangming*, the *San Jiao* channel of hand *shaoyang*, the Small Intestine channel of hand *taiyang*), the three yin channels of the foot (the Spleen channel of foot *taiyin*, the Liver channel of foot *jueyin*, the Kidney channel of foot *shaoyin*), and the three yang channels of the foot (the Stomach channel of foot *yangming*, the Gallbladder channel of foot *shaoyang*, the Bladder channel of foot *taiyang*).

Table 4-3   The classification of the names of the twelve channels

The three yin channels of hand-foot	Names of the twelve channels		The three yang channels of hand-foot
The three yin channels of hand	The Lung channel of hand *taiyin* The Pericardium channel of hand *jueyin* The Heart channel of hand *shaoyin*	The Large Intestine channel of hand *yangming* The *San Jiao* channel of hand *shaoyang* The Small Intestine channel of hand *taiyang*	The three yang channels of the hand
The three yin channels of foot	The Spleen channel of foot *taiyin* The Liver channel of foot *jueyin* The Kidney channel of foot *shaoyin*	The Stomach channel of foot *yangming* The Gallbladder channel of foot *shaoyang* The Bladder channel of foot *taiyang*	The three yang channels of the foot

The Distributing Direction and Connecting Rule of the Twelve Channels

The Twelve Channels are classified into four groups: the three yin channels of the hand, the three yang channels of the hand, the three yin channels of the foot, and the three yang channels of the foot. The distributing direction and connecting sequence of each group are identical.

① The Distributing Direction of the Twelve Channels

The distributing direction of the twelve channels is as follows: the three yin channels of the hand distribute from the chest to the hand where they connect to the three yang channels of the hand; the three yang channels of the hand distribute from the hand to the head where they connect to the three yang channels of the foot; the three yang channels of the foot distribute from the head to the foot where they connect to the three yin channels of the foot; the three yin channels of the foot distribute from the foot to the abdomen and the chest where they connect to the three yin channels of the hand.

Miraculous Pivot: Chapter Different Acupuncture Therapies to People of Different Fat and Lean Physiques and the Adverse and Agreeable Conditions of the Twelve Channels (Líng Shū: Nì Shùn Féi Shòu,

灵枢·逆顺肥瘦) says: "*The three yin channels of the hand distribute from the chest to the hand; the three yang channels of the hand distribute from the hand to the head; the three yang channels of the foot distribute from the head to the foot; the three yin channels of the foot distribute from the foot to the abdomen.*"

② The Connecting Rule of the Twelve Channels

(1) According to the distributing direction, the connecting rule is as follows: the three yin channels of the hand distribute from the chest to the hand where they connect to the three yang channels of the hand; the three yang channels of the hand distribute from the hand to the head where they connect to the three yang channels of the foot; the three yang channels of the foot distribute from the head to the foot where they connect to the three yin channels of the foot; the three yin channels of the foot distribute from the foot to the abdomen (and the chest) where they connect to the three yin channels of the hand. (Fig. 4-2)

(2) According to the connecting regions of the twelve channels, the connecting rule is as follows: the yin channels connect with the yang channels at the terminal end of the limbs (the hand or foot), the yang channels connect with the yang channels on the head and face, and the yin channels connect with the yin channels in the chest and abdomen.

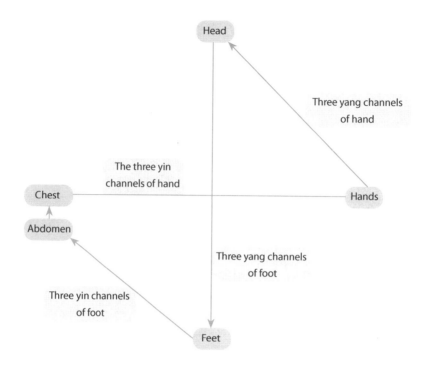

Fig. 4-2   The distributing direction and connecting rule of the twelve channels

The Body Surface Distribution of the Twelve Channels

1 Head and Face (Table 4-4)

The head-face (body-surface) distribution of the twelve channels is as follows:

Table 4-4   Distribution of the Twelve Channels in head-face

Head and face		Distribution of channels
The anterior	face and forehead	the channels of hand-foot *yangming*
	cheek	the hand *taiyang* channel
The lateral	ear and temple	the channels of hand-foot *shaoyang*
The posterior	vertex, occiput and neck	the channel of foot *taiyang*

The anterior: The channels of hand-foot *yangming*

are distributed on the face and forehead, and the channel of hand *taiyang* is distributed on the cheek.

The lateral: The channels of hand-foot *shaoyang* are distributed at the ear and temple.

The posterior: The channel of foot *taiyang* is distributed at the vertex, occiput and nape.

The three yang channels of the hand terminate on the head, the three yang channels of the foot start from the head, and the three yang channels of the hand connect with the three yang channels of the foot on the head and face, and hence it is known that "the head is the confluence of all yang channels".

Classic of Questioning: The Forty-seventh Question (Nàn Jīng: Sì Shí Qī Nàn, 难经·四十七难) says: *"Why is the face can resist cold? The answer is as follows: The head is the confluence of all the yang channels. All the yin channels reach the neck and then return, but only yang channels distribute up to the head and ear, and therefore the face is cold-resistant."*

2 Trunk (Table 4-5)

The trunk (body-surface) distribution of the twelve channels is as follows:

The anterior: from the interior to the exterior,

Table 4-5   Distribution of the twelve channels in trunk

Trunk		Distribution of channels		
		1st Lateral Line	2nd Lateral Line	3rd Lateral Line
The Anterior	Chest	The Kidney channel of foot *shaoyin* （2 *cun* lateral to the chest median line）	The Stomach channel of foot *yangming* （4 *cun* lateral to the chest median line）	The Spleen channel of foot *taiyin* （6 *cun* lateral to the chest median line）
	Abdomen	The Kidney channel of foot *shaoyin* （0.5 *cun* lateral to the abdomen median line）	The Stomach channel of foot *yangming* （2 *cun* lateral to the abdomen median line）	The Spleen channel of foot *taiyin* （4 *cun* lateral to the abdomen median line） The Liver channel of foot *jueyin* obliquely runs from the lateral side of the lower abdomen onto the lateral thorax
The Posterior	Back	The Bladder channel of foot *taiyang* （1.5 *cun* lateral to the back median line）	The Bladder channel of foot *taiyang* （3 *cun* lateral to the back median line）	
	Scapula	The three yang channels of the hand		
The Lateral	Armpit	The three yin channels of the hand		
	Lateral thorax, & the lateral side of the abdomen	The Gallbladder channel of foot *shaoyang*, the Liver channel of foot *jueyin*		

the channel of foot *shaoyin*, the channel of foot *yangming*, the channel of foot *taiyin* and the channel of foot *jueyin* are distributed on the chest and abdomen in order.

The posterior: the channel of foot *taiyang* is distributed on the back, and the three yang channels of hand on the scapula region.

The lateral: the channels of foot *shaoyang* and foot *jueyin* are distributed on the lateral thorax and the lateral side of the lower abdomen, and the three yin channels of hand emerge from the armpit.

③ Limbs (Table 4-6)

The limb distribution of the twelve channels is as follows:

The yin channels are distributed on the medial aspects of the limbs, while the yang channels on the lateral aspects of the limbs.

The medial aspects of the upper limbs: the channel of hand *taiyin* is on the anterior border, the channel of hand *jueyin* is on the medial line, and the channel of hand *shaoyin* is on the posterior border.

The lateral aspects of the upper limbs: the channel of hand *yangming* is on the anterior border, the channel of hand *shaoyang* is on the medial line, and the channel of hand *taiyang* is on the posterior border.

The medial aspects of the lower limbs: under the level of 8 *cun* above the medial malleolus, the channel of foot *jueyin* is on the anterior border, the channel of foot *taiyin* is on the medial line, and the channel of foot *shaoyin* is on the posterior border. Above the level 8 *cun* above the medial malleolus, the channel of foot *taiyin* is on the anterior border, the channel of foot *jueyin*

Table 4-6 Distribution of the twelve channels in limbs

Limbs		Distribution of the channels	
		Medial aspects（yin channels）	Lateral aspects（yang channels）
Upper limbs	Anterior line	The channel of hand *taiyin*	The channel of hand *yangming*
	Medial line	The channel of hatnd *jueyin*	The channel of hand *shaoyang*
	Posterior line	The channel of hand *shaoyin*	The channel of hand *taiyang*
Lower limbs	Anterior line	The channel of foot *taiyin*▲	The channel of foot *yangming*
	Medial line	The channel of foot *jueyin*▲	The channel of foot *shaoyang*
	Posterior line	The channel of foot *shaoyin*	The channel of foot *taiyang*

▲Commentary: Under the level of 8 *cun* above the medial malleolus, the channel of foot *jueyin* is on the anterior line and the channel of foot *taiyin* on the medial line.

Above the level of 8 *cun* above the medial malleolus, the channel of foot *taiyin* is on the anterior line and the channel of foot *jueyin* on the medial line.

is on the medial line, and the channel of foot *shaoyin* is on the posterior border.

The lateral aspects of the lower limbs: the channel of foot *yangming* is on the anterior border, the channel of foot *shaoyang* is on the medial line, and the channel of foot *taiyang* is on the posterior border.

The Exterior–Interior Relation of the Twelve Channels

The twelve channels are classified into six yin channels and six yang channels. The yin channels pertain to the interior, and the yang channels pertain to the exterior. A yin channel corresponds to the other yang channel by the communication of the divergent channel and collaterals. This is known as the exterior-interior confluent relationship of the twelve channels.

The content of the exterior-interior relation of the twelve channels is as follows: the six yin channels and the six yang channels form six pairs of exterior-interior confluent relations. The relations are as follows: the Lung channel of hand *taiyin* and the Large Intestine channel of hand *yangming*, the Pericardium channel of hand *jueyin* and the *San Jiao* channel of hand

shaoyang, the Heart channel of hand *shaoyin* and the Small Intestine channel of hand *taiyang*, the Spleen channel of foot *taiyin* and the Stomach channel of foot *yangming*, the Gallbladder channel of foot *shaoyang* and the Liver channel of foot *jueyin*, and the Kidney channel of foot *shaoyin* and the Bladder channel of foot *taiyang*.

Each of the twelve-channel pair of exterior-interior channels of has this characteristic distribution: they both connect at the terminal end of the limbs, respectively distribute along the opposite location on the medial or lateral aspect of the limbs, and respectively pertain to or connect with the interiorly-exteriorly related *zang-fu* organs (the yang channel, which pertains to the *zang* organ and connects with the *fu* organ, is the exterior; the yin channel, which pertains to the *fu* organ and connects with the *zang* organ, is interior). (Fig. 4-3)

The significance of the exterior-interior relation of the twelve channels is as follows: not only the connection between the interiorly-exteriorly related channels but also the structural connection of the interiorly-exteriorly related *zang-fu* organs is strengthened by the channels, and hence *zang-fu* organs can cooperate in physiological functions, affect each other pathologically, and interact in treatment.

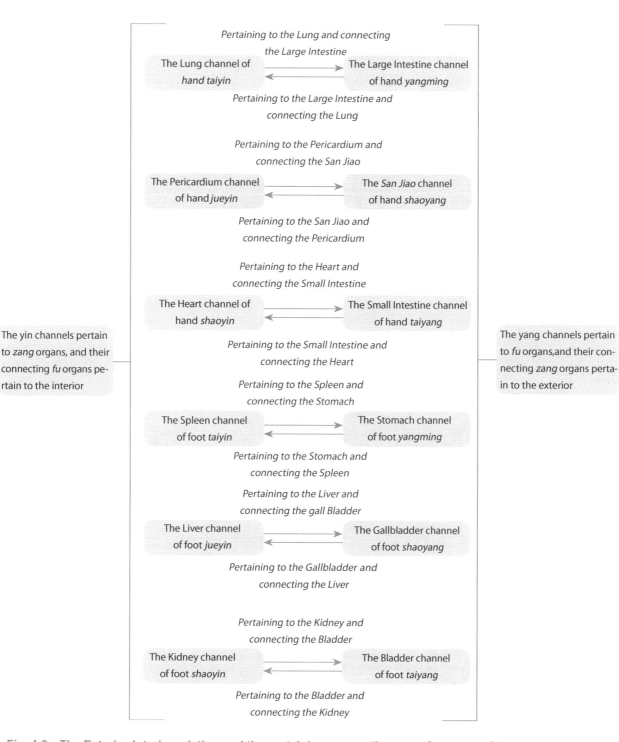

Fig. 4-3 **The Exterior-Interior relation and the pertaining-connecting *zang-fu* organs of the twelve channels**

Plain Questions: Chapter Discussion on Blood, Qi, Body and Emotions (Sù Wèn: Xuè Qì Xíng Zhì Piān, 素问·血气形志篇) says: "The channel of foot taiyang and the Channel of foot shaoyin form the exterior-interior relation, the channel of foot shaoyang and the channel of foot jueyin form the exterior-interior relation, the channel of foot yangming and* *the channel of foot taiyin form the exterior-interior relation: these are the relations between the three yin and yang channels of the foot. The channel of hand taiyang and the channel of hand shaoyin form the exterior-interior relation, the channels of hand Shaoyang and the channel of hand jueyin form the exterior-interior relation, and the channel of hand*

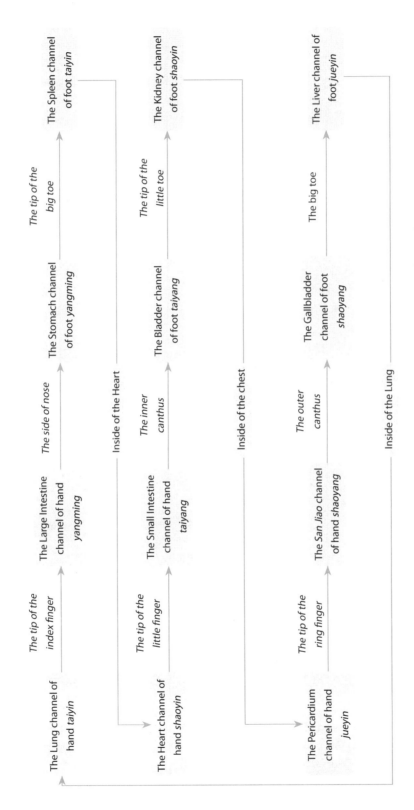

Fig. 4-4 The cyclical flow of qi and blood in the twelve channels

yangming and the channel of taiyin for the exterior-interior: these are the relations between the three yin and yang channels of the hand."

The Cyclical Flow of Qi and Blood in the Twelve Channels

The twelve channels are the main pathways to transport qi and blood, and they distribute from the beginning to the end in order and form the cyclical flow of qi and blood in the twelve channels. (Fig. 4-4)

The cyclical flow of qi and blood in the twelve channels is as follows: it originates from the Lung channel of hand *taiyin*, runs in the sequence of the twelve channels, and ends in the Liver channel of foot *jueyin*, then returns to the Lung channel of hand *taiyin*. Thus a cyclical flow of qi and blood in the twelve channels is formed. (Fig. 4-4)

Miraculous Pivot: Chapter The Nutritive qi (Líng Shū: Yíng Qì, 灵枢·营气) says: "The circulating paths of the nutritive qi: ... (nutritive qi) starts from the channel of (hand) taiyin, pours into the channel of hand yangming...pours into the channel of foot yangming...joins up with the channel of (foot) taiyin...runs along the channel of hand shaoyin channels...joins up with the channel of hand taiyang...joins up with the channel of foot taiyang...pours into the channel of foot shaoyin...runs along the Pericardium channel (the channel of hand jueyin)...joins up with the channel of hand shaoyang...pours into the channel of foot shaoyang...joins up with the channel of foot jueyin...runs through the Liver and decants into the Lung...".(The word "decant" (zhu) means to pour; the word "join" (he) means the connection regions of the yin-yang channels exterior-interior channels, and upper-lower channels.)

The Pathway of the Twelve Channels

① The Lung Channel of Hand *Taiyin*, 手太阴肺经

Miraculous Pivot: Chapter On Channels (Líng Shū: Jīng Mài, 灵枢·经脉) states, "The Lung channel

of hand taiyin originates from the middle Jiao and runs down to connect with the Large Intestine. It then returns and ascends along the cardiac orifice of the Stomach and crosses the diaphragm before connecting to the Lungs. It exits the "Lung system" (trachea and throat) and runs down along the medial side of the upper arm anterior to the Heart channel of hand shaoyin and the Pericardium channel of hand jueyin. It then passes through the cubital fossa and enters Cun Kou (on the wrist over the radial artery where a pulse can be felt, 寸口) along the radial border of the medial side of the forearm. It continues along the thenar eminence and ends at the tip of the thumb.

A branch separates from the main channel at the styloid proces, and travels directly to the radial side of the tip of the index finger." (Fig. 4-5)

Zang-fu Organ Connection: Lung, Large Intestine, Middle *Jiao* (Stomach), and diaphragm.

Organs Passed Through: Lung system.

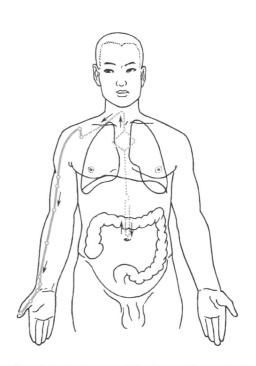

Fig. 4-5　Pathway of the Lung Channel of Hand *Taiyin*

② The Large Intestine Channel of Hand *Yangming*, 手阳明大肠经

Miraculous Pivot: Chapter On Channels (Líng Shū:

Jīng Mài, 灵枢·经脉) states, "*The Large Intestine channel of hand yangming originates at the tip of the index finger. Running upward along the radial side of the index finger and passing through the interspace of the 1st and 2nd metacarpal bones, it dips into the depression between the tendons of m. extensor pollicis longus and brevis (the anatomical snuffbox). Following the anterior border of the forearm, it reaches the lateral side of the elbow, ascends along the lateral anterior aspect of the upper arm to the highest point of the shoulder. From there, it travels along the anterior border of the acromion, across to the 7th cervical vertebra (DU 14), and descends to the supraclavicular fossa to connect with the Lung. It passes through the diaphragm and enters the Large Intestine, its pertaining organ.*

A branch from the supraclavicular fossa ascends to the neck, passes through the neck to the cheek, and enters the gums of the lower teeth. It then curves around the upper lip and crosses the philtrum to end at the opposite side of the nose. From there, the left channel goes to the right and the right channel to the left, to both sides of the nose." (Fig. 4-6)

Zang-fu Organ Connection: Large Intestine, Lung, diaphragm.

Organs Passed Through: mouth, lower teeth, nose.

③ The Stomach Channel of Foot *Yangming*, 足阳明 胃经

Miraculous Pivot: Chapter On Channels (*Líng Shū: Jīng Mài*, 灵枢·经脉) states, "*The Stomach channel of foot yangming originates at the lateral side of the nose. It ascends to the inner canthus at the level of the root of the nose, where it meets the Bladder channel of foot taiyang. Turning downward along the lateral side of the nose, it enters the upper gum. Emerging, it curves around the lips and descends to meet the Conception vessel (Ren) at the mentolabial groove. It then runs postero-laterally across the lower portion of the cheek to ST 5. Winding along the angle of the mandible, it ascends in front of the ear and traverses GB 3 and follows the anterior hairline and reaches the forehead.*

The facial branch emerging in front of ST 5, runs downward to ST 9. From there it goes along the throat and enters the supraclavicular fossa. Descending, it passes through the diaphragm, enters the Stomach, its pertaining organ, and connects with the Spleen.

The straight portion of the channel, arising from the supraclavicular fossa, runs downward, passing through the nipple. It descends alongside the umbilicus and enters ST 30 at the inguinal region.

The branch from the pyloric orifice of the Stomach descends inside the abdomen and joins the previous portion of the channel at ST 30. Running downward, traversing ST 31, and further descending along the lateral margin of the thigh, it reaches the knee. From there, it continues downward along the anterior border of the lateral aspect of the tibia, passes through the dorsum of the foot, and reaches the lateral side of the tip of the second toe.

The tibial branch emerges from ST 36, 3 cun below the knee and ends on the lateral side of the middle toe.

The branch from the dorsum of the foot arises from ST 42 and terminates at the medial side of the tip of the great toe." (Fig. 4-7)

Zang-fu Organ Connection: Spleen, Stomach, Large Intestine, Small Intestine, and diaphragm.

Organs Passed Through: nose, eye, mouth,

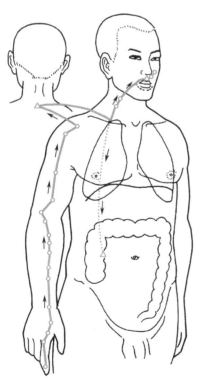

Fig. 4-6 Pathway of the Large Intestine Channel of Hand *Yangming*

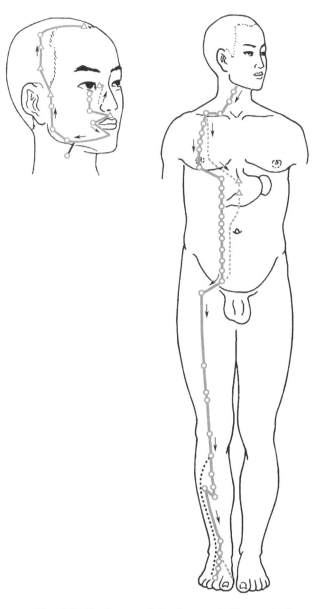

Fig. 4-7 Pathway of the Stomach Channel of Foot *Yangming*

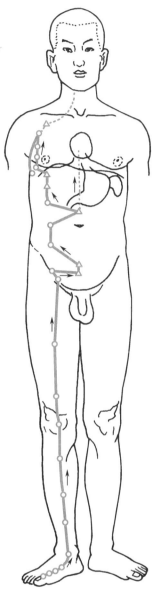

Fig. 4-8 Pathway of the Spleen Channel of Foot *Taiyin*

upper teeth, and breast.

④ The Spleen Channel of Foot *Taiyin*, 足太阴脾经

Miraculous Pivot: Chapter On Channels (Líng Shū: Jīng Mài, 灵枢·经脉) states, *"The Spleen channel of foot taiyin at the great toe. It runs along the medial aspect of the foot at the junction of the red and white skin and ascends anterior to the medial malleolus, and upward to the medial aspect of the leg. It follows the posterior aspect of the tibia, crosses and goes in front of the Liver channel of foot jueyin, passes through the anterior medial aspect*

of the knee and thigh, enters the abdomen, then the Spleen, its pertaining organ, and connects with the Stomach. From there, it ascends, passing through the diaphragm and running alongside the esophagus. When it reaches the root of the tongue, it spreads over its lower surface.

A branch from the Stomach goes upward through the diaphragm, and flows into the Heart." (Fig. 4-8)

Zang-fu Organ Connection: Spleen, Stomach, Heart, and diaphragm.

Organs Passed Through: tongue, esophagus,

and pharynx.

⑤ The Heart Channel of Hand *Shaoyin*, 手少阴心经

According to *Miraculous Pivot: Chapter On Channels* (*Líng Shū: Jīng Mài*, 灵枢·经脉), "*The Heart channel of hand shaoyin originates in the Heart. Emerging, it spreads over the "Heart system" (the tissues connecting the Heart with the other zang-fu organs). It passes through the diaphragm to connect with the Small Intestine.*

The ascending branch from the "Heart system" runs alongside the esophagus to connect with the "eye system"(the tissues connecting the eyes with the brain).

The straight branch from the "Heart system" goes upward to the Lung. It then descends and emerges from the axilla, travels along the posterior border of the medial aspect of the upper arm behind the Lung channel of hand taiyin and the Pericardium channel of hand jueyin, down to the cubital fossa. It then descends along the posterior border of the medial aspect of the forearm to the pisiform bone along the ulnar side of the palm to the tip of the little finger." (Fig. 4-9)

Zang-fu Organ Connection: Heart, Small Intestine, Lung, and diaphragm.

Organs Passed Through: Heart system, esophagus, eye system.

⑥ The Small Intestine Channel of Hand *Taiyang*, 手太阳小肠经

Miraculous Pivot: Chapter On Channels (*Líng Shū: Jīng Mài*, 灵枢·经脉) states, "*The Small Intestine channel of hand taiyang starts from the ulnar side of the tip of the little finger. Following the ulnar side of the dorsum of the hand, it reaches the wrist where it emerges from the styloid process of the ulna. From there it ascends along the posterior border of the forearm, passes between the olecranon process of the ulna and the medial epicondyle of the humerus. It continues along the posterior border of the lateral aspect of the upper arm to the shoulder joint. Circling around the scapular region, it meets Du 14 on the superior aspect of the shoulder. Then, turning downward to the supraclavicular fossa, it connects with the Heart. From there it descends along the esophagus, passing through the diaphragm, reaches the Stomach, and finally enters the Small Intestine, its pertaining organ.*

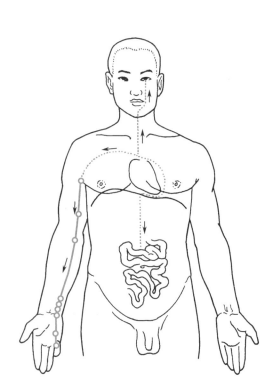

Fig. 4-9   Pathway of the Heart Channel of Hand *Shaoyin*

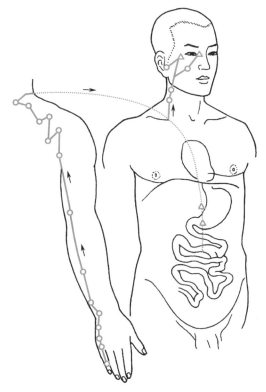

Fig. 4-10   Pathway of the Small Intestine Channel of Hand *Taiyang*

The branch from the supraclavicular fossa ascends to the neck, and on to the cheek. It enters the ear via the outer canthus.

The branch from the neck runs upward to the infraorbital region and further to the lateral side of the nose. It then reaches the inner canthus." (Fig. 4-10)

Zang-fu Organ Connection: Small Intestine, Heart, Stomach, and diaphragm.

Organs Passed Through: esophagus, eye, ear, nose.

⑦ The Bladder Channel of Foot *Taiyang*, 足太阳膀胱经

Miraculous Pivot: Chapter On Channels (Líng Shū: Jīng Mài, 灵枢·经脉) states, *"The Bladder channel of foot taiyang starts from the inner canthus of the eye. Ascending to the forehead, it joins the Governing vessel (Du) at the vertex, where a branch arises, running to the temple in the region above the ear.*

The straight portion of the channel enters and communicates with the brain from the vertex. It then emerges and bifurcates to descend along the posterior aspect of the neck. Running downward alongside the medial aspect of the scapula region and parallel to the vertebral column, it reaches the lumbar region, where it enters the body via the paravertebral muscles to connect with the Kidney and join its pertaining organ, the Bladder.

The branch of the lumbar region descends through the gluteal region and ends in the popliteal fossa.

The branch from the posterior aspect of the neck runs straight downward along the medial border of the scapula. Passing through the gluteal region downward along the lateral aspect of the thigh, it meets the preceding branch descending from the lumbar region in the popliteal fossa. From there it descends to the leg and further to the posterior aspect of the external malleolus. Then, running along the tuberosity of the 5th metatarsal bone, it reaches the lateral side of the tip of the little toe." (Fig. 4-11)

Zang-fu Organ Connection: Bladder, Kidney, brain, other *Zang-fu* organs in the cavity.

Organs Passed Through: eye, nose.

⑧ The Kidney Channel of Foot *Shaoyin*, 足少阴肾经

According to *Miraculous Pivot: Chapter On*

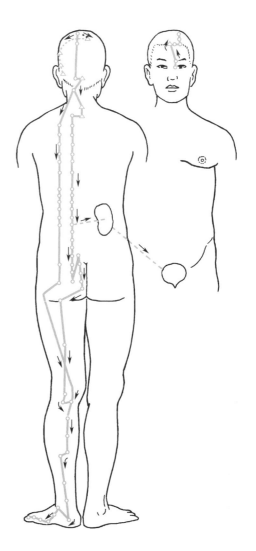

Fig. 4-11　Pathway of the Bladder Channel of Foot *Taiyang*

Channels (Líng Shū: Jīng Mài, 灵枢·经脉), "The Kidney channel of foot shaoyin starts from the interior aspect of the small toe and runs obliquely towards the sole. Emerging from the lower aspect of the tuberosity of the navicular bone, and running behind the medial malleolus, it enters the heel. Then, it ascends along the medial side of the leg to the medial side of the popliteal fossa and continues upward along the posterior border to the medial aspect of the thigh toward the spinal column, where it enters the Kidney, its pertaining organ, and connects with the Bladder.

One branch of the channel reemerges from the Kidney. Ascending and passing through the Liver and diaphragm, it enters the Lungs, runs along the throat, and terminates at the root of the tongue.

A branch springs from the Lung, joins the Heart,

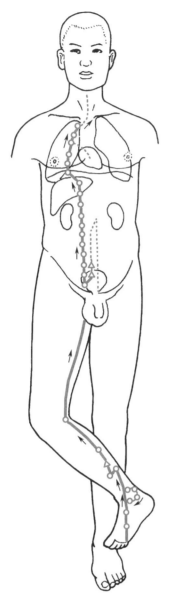

Fig. 4-12 Pathway of the Kidney Channel of Foot *Shaoyin*

it descends through the diaphragm to the abdomen, connecting successively with the upper, middle, and lower Jiao's (i.e. Sanjiao).

A branch arising from the chest runs inside the chest, emerges from the costal region at a point 3 cun below the anterior axillary crease and ascends to the axilla. Following the medial aspect of the upper arm, it runs downward between the Lung channel of hand taiyin and the Heart channel of hand shaoyin to the cubital fossa, and continues to the forearm between the tendons of m. palmaris longus and m. flexor carpi radialis, along the middle finger, ending at the tip of the middle finger.

Another branch arises from the palm at PC 8 and runs along the ring finger to its tip." (Fig. 4-13)

Zang-fu Organ Connection: Pericardium, San Jiao, diaphragm.

⑩ The *San Jiao* Channel of Hand *Shaoyang*, 手少阳三焦经

Miraculous Pivot: Chapter On Channels (Líng Shū: Jīng Mài, 灵枢·经脉) records, "The San Jiao channel of hand shaoyang starts from the tip of the ring finger, runs upward between the 4th and 5th metacarpal bones along the lateral aspect of the forearm between the radius and ulna. Passing

and runs into the chest." (Fig. 4-12)

Zang-fu Organ Connection: Kidney, Bladder, Liver, Lung, Heart, and diaphragm.

Organs Passed Through: tongue, throat, spinal column (marrow).

⑨ The Pericardium Channel of Hand *Jueyin*, 手厥阴心包经

Miraculous Pivot: Chapter On Channels (Líng Shū: Jīng Mài, 灵枢·经脉), "The Pericardium channel of hand jueyin originates from the chest. Emerging, it enters its pertaining organ, the Pericardium. Then

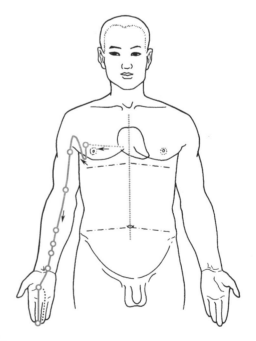

Fig. 4-13 Pathway of the Pericardium Channel of Hand *Jueyin*

through the olecranon process and along the lateral aspect of the upper arm, it reaches the shoulder region, where it goes across and passes behind the Gallbladder channel of foot shaoyang. Winding over to the supraclavicular fossa, it spreads in the chest to connect with the Pericardium. It then descends through the diaphragm to the abdomen and joins its pertaining organ, the upper, middle, and lower Jiao (San Jiao).

A branch originates from the chest. Running upward, it emerges from the supraclavicular fossa. From there, it ascends to the neck, runs along the posterior border of the ear, and on to the corner of the anterior hairline. Then, it turns downward to the cheek and terminates in the infraorbital region.

Another branch arises from behind the ear and enters the ear. Then, it emerges in front of the ear, crosses the previous branch at the cheek, and reaches the outer canthus." (Fig. 4-14)

Zang-fu Organ Connection: *San Jiao*, Pericardium, and diaphragm.

Organs Passed Through: eye, ear.

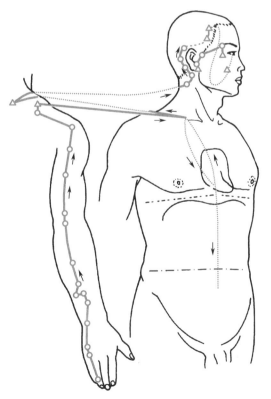

Fig. 4-14   Pathway of the *San Jiao* Channel of Hand *Shaoyang*

⑪ The Gallbladder Channel of Foot *Shaoyang*, 足少阳胆经

According to *Miraculous Pivot: Chapter On Channels* (*Líng Shū: Jīng Mài*, 灵枢·经脉), *"The Gallbladder channel of foot shaoyang originates from the outer canthus, ascends to the corner of the forehead, curves behind the ear and runs along the side of the neck in front of the San Jiao channel of hand shaoyang to the shoulder. It then returns, traverses, and passes behind the San Jiao channel of hand shaoyang, and continues down to the supraclavicular fossa.*

One branch arises from the behind the ear and enters the ear. It then emerges and passes in front of the ear to the outer canthus.

Another branch arising from the outer canthus runs downward to ST 5 and meets the San Jiao channel of hand shaoyang at the infraorbital region. Then, passing through ST 6, it descends to the neck and enters the supraclavicular fossa, where it meets the main channel. From there, it descends further into the chest and passes through the diaphragm to connect with the Liver before entering its pertaining organ, the Gallbladder. It then runs inside the hypochondriac region, and emerges from the lateral side of the lower abdomen near the femoral artery at the inguinal region. From there, it runs superficially along the margin of the pubic hair and travels transversely into the hip.

The straight branch runs downward from the supraclavicular fossa, passes in front of the axilla along the lateral aspect of the chest, and through the free ends of the floating ribs to the hip region, where it meets the previous branch. Then, it descends along the lateral aspect of the thigh to the lateral side of the knee. Going further downward along the anterior aspect of the fibula, all the way to its lower end, it reaches the anterior aspect of the external malleolus. It then follows the dorsum of the foot to the lateral side of the tip of the 4th toe.

One branch arises from the dorsum of the foot, runs between the 1st and 2nd metatarsal bones to terminate at the distal portion of the great toe." (Fig. 4-15)

Zang-fu Organ Connection: Liver, Gallbladder, and diaphragm.

Organs Passed Through: eye, ear.

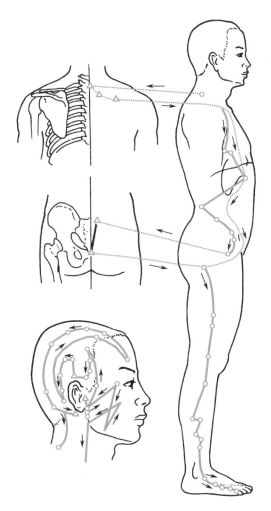

Fig. 4-15　Pathway of the Gallbladder Channel of Foot *Shaoyang*

⑫ The Liver Channel of Foot *Jueyin*, 足厥阴肝经

According to *Miraculous Pivot: Chapter On Channels* (*Líng Shū: Jīng Mài*, 灵枢·经脉), "*The Liver channel of foot jueyin originates at the lateral side of the great toe, runs along the dorsum of the foot, passes through a point 1 cun anterior to the medial malleolus, and ascends to an area 8 cun above the medial malleolus. From there, it runs across and behind the Spleen channel of foot taiyinand up to the medial aspect of the knee and along the medial aspect of the thigh to the pubic region. There, it curves around the external genitalia and continues up to the lower abdomen, runs upward and curves around the Stomach, enters the Liver, its pertaining organ, and connects with the Gallbladder. From there, it continues to ascend, passing through the diaphragm, and branching out in the costal and hypochondriac*

region. Then, it ascends along the posterior aspect of the throat to the nasopharynx and connects with the "eye system.. Running further upward, it emerges from the forehead and meets the Du vessel at the vertex.

The branch that arises from the "eye system" runs downward into the cheek and curves around the inner surface of the lips.

The branch arising from the Liver passes through the diaphragm, runs into the Lung."(Fig. 4-16)

Zang-fu Organ Connection: Liver, Gallbladder, Stomach, Lung, diaphragm.

Organs Passed Through: external genitalia, throat, nasopharynx, eye, cheek, inner surface of the lip.

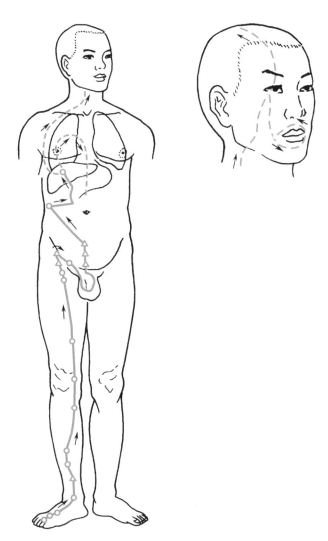

Fig. 4-16　Pathway of the Liver Channel of Foot *Jueyin*

Section 3   The Eight Extraordinary Channels

The Concept and Function of the Eight Extraordinary Channels

① The Concept of the Eight Extraordinary Channels

(1) The names of the eight extraordinary channels

The eight extraordinary channels are generic names for the *Du vessel*, *Ren vessel*, Penetrating vessel, girdling vessel, yin motility vessel, yang motility vessel, yin linking vessel, and yang linking vessel.

(2) The difference between the eight extraordinary channels and the twelve primary channels (Table 4-7)

"Extraordinary (*qí* in Chinese, 奇)" means uniquely different. The eight extraordinary channels are another category of channels that are different from the twelve primary channels.

The main difference is their distribution: compared with the twelve primary channels, none of The eight extraordinary channels are distributed on the interior, the exterior, the upper, the lower, the left and the right parts of the whole body, none of them pertains to or connects with *zang-fu* organs, and also there is no yin-yang or exterior-interior relation among them. There are eight extraordinary vessels, hence the name.

Classic of Questioning: The Twenty-seventh Question (Nàn Jīng: Èr Shí Qī Nàn, 难经·二十七难) says: *"There are The eight extraordinary channels that are not restrained by the twelve channels. What is the reason? The answer is: The eight extraordinary channels include the Yin Linking Vessel, Yang Linking Vessel, yin motility vessel, yang motility vessel, Penetrating vessel, Du vessel, Ren vessel, and Girdling vessel. The eight ones are not restrained by the twelve channels, and hence all of them are named The eight extraordinary channels."*

Table 4-7   The Difference between the eight extraordinary channels and the twelve primary channels

Distribution	Twelve Primary Channels	Eight extraordinary vessels
Distribution Regions	All over the body	Except the upper limbs
Rule of Distribution	Having regular circulating paths in the interior, the exterior, the upper, the lower, the left, and the right	Fewer rules of distribution
Pertaining to and connecting *Zang-Fu* Organs	Direct pertaining and connecting relationship with *zang-fu* organs	None
Exterior-Interior Relation	Exterior-interior relation of the yin and yang channels	None

The Genuine Meanings of Classic of Questioning (Nàn Jīng Běn Yì, 难经本义) says: *"There are regular and extraordinary vessels; the twelve primary channels are regular. The eight extraordinary channels are not restrained, and hence they are named the extraordinary vessels. Compared with the regular, the extraordinary is just like the extraordinary and regular military affairs. Doctor Yú said that the extraordinary means odd, not even. The eight extraordinary channels are different from the twelve primary channels, there is not the yin-yang or exterior-interior relation among them, and they distribute in different ways, therefore they are named the eight extraordinary channels."*

② The Function of the Eight Extraordinary Channels

(1) Strengthening the connecting of the twelve channels

The eight extraordinary channels crisscross among the twelve channels, and strengthen the connection of the twelve channels, and hence form the multi-connections among them, making closer the relationships between channels and all tissues and organs of the body.

(2) Regulating the qi and blood of the twelve channels

The channels and collaterals have the function of transporting qi and blood, the twelve channels are main pathways, and the eight extraordinary channels crisscross among the twelve channels and regulate the qi and blood of them. When the qi and blood of the twelve channels are overflowing, they will pour into the eight extraordinary channels to be stored for use; when those of the twelve channels are insufficient, the stored qi and blood of the eight extraordinary channels will brim over and supplement them in order to keep the qi and blood of the twelve channels invariable. In order to describe the function, the ancients compared primary channels to rivers and the extraordinary vessels to lakes.

Besides this, the eight extraordinary channels have a close connection with the extraordinary *fu*-organs such as the brain, marrow, uterus, and *zang* organs such as the Liver, Spleen and so on, and hence the eight extraordinary channels have certain effects on the physiological functions and pathological changes.

Classic of Questioning: The Twenty-eighth Question (Nàn Jīng: Èr Shí Bā Nàn, 难经·二十八难) says: *"The eight extraordinary channels are not restrained by the twelve channels. Where do they start and travel?...This can be compared to the sage attempting to build a canal: when the canal is overflowing, the water will pour into the deep lake, and the sage cannot restrain this situation. In the same way, when the qi and blood of the channels are overflowing, they will pour into the eight extraordinary channels, and not circulate. Hence the twelve channels cannot restrain them."*

Elucidation of Fourteen Channels: Chapter the Eight Extraordinary Channels (Shí Sì Jīng Fā Huī: Qíng Jīng Bá Mài Piān, 十四经发挥·奇经八脉篇) says: *"There are regular and extraordinary vessels: the twelve primary channels are regular; the eight extraordinary channels are not restrained, and hence they are named the extraordinary vessels. The qi and blood of the human body usually flows in the twelve channels, and when qi and blood are overflowing, they will pour into the eight extraordinary channels."*

The Distributing Course and Physiological Functions of the Eight Extraordinary Channels

① The *Du* Vessel, 督脉

(1) The distributing course

Trunk: the *Du vessel* starts from the inside of uterus, descends and emerges from RN 1 (*huì yīn*), then runs backward along the median line of the back, ascends along the interior of the spinal column to reach DU 16 (*fēng fǔ*) on the nape, enters the cranial cavity to connect with the brain, again returns to emerge from the neck and ascend along the median line of the head, passes through the forehead, nose, and upper lip, and reaches the frenulum of the upper lip [DU 28 (*yín jiāo*)]

Branch: one branch diverges from the interior of the spine and connects with the Kidney.

Branch: one branch diverges from the lower abdomen, ascends through the center of the naval, passes through the Heart, reaches the throat, and ascends to the mandible, then curves around the lip, again ascends to the center below the eyes. (Fig. 4-17)

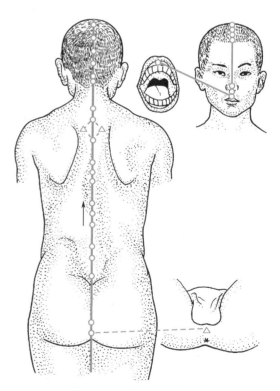

Fig. 4-17   The *Du* Vessel

(2) The physiological function

a. Regulating qi and blood of the yang channels: the *Du vessel* runs along the median line of the back, intersects the six yang channels of hand-foot at DU 14 (*dà zhuī*), and regulates the qi and blood of the yang channels. It can govern all yang channels, and hence it is named the sea of the yang channels.

b. Reflecting the functions of the brain, marrow and Kidney: the *Du vessel* ascends along the interior of the spinal column, enters the cranial cavity and connects with the brain which is the sea of marrow, and hence the *Du vessel* has a certain relationship with the brain and marrow. Usually it reflects the pathological changes of the brain and marrow. One branch also connects with the Kidney, and therefore the *Du vessel* has a certain relationship with the function of the Kidney. The Kidney governs reproduction; when there are pathological changes due to yang deficiency of the Kidney and infertility due to cold semen, the method of reinforcing the *Du vessel* can be adopted.

Classic of Questioning: The Twenty-eighth Question (Nàn Jīng: Èr Shí Bā Nàn, 难经·二十八难) says: "*The Du vessel starts from DU 1 (cháng qiáng), ascends along the interior of the spinal column, and then reaches the DU 16 (fēng fǔ) and enters the cranial cavity to connect with the brain.*"

② The *Ren* vessel, 任脉

(1) The distributing course

Trunk: the *Ren vessel* starts from the inside of the uterus, descends and emerges from RN 1 (*huì yīn*), runs forward through the pubes, and then ascends along the median line of the chest and abdomen, reaches the throat, ascends to the mandible, then curves around the lips and intersects the *Du vessel* at DU 28 (*yín jiāo*), again runs along the cheek and branches to reach the infraorbital region.

Branch: one branch emerges from the inside of the uterus, runs backward and passes through the spine, and ascends along the back. (Fig. 4-18)

(2) The physiological function

Ren means bearing or nourishing. The main functions of the *Ren vessel* are as follows:

a. Regulating qi and blood of the yin channels: the *Ren vessel* runs along the median line of the abdomen, intersects the three yin channels of the foot and the Yin Linking Vessel, and controls the interrelation of the yin channels. It has the function of regulating the qi and blood of the yin channel, and hence it is named the sea of the yin channels.

b. Related to reproduction: the *Ren* channel starts from the inside of uterus, and has the functions of regulating menstruation and nourishing embryos, and hence it is known that "the *Ren* vessel governs the embryo". Because it regulates menstruation and nourishes embryos, the Ren vessel is related to reproduction.

Classic of Questioning: The Twenty-eighth Question (Nàn Jīng: Èr Shí Bā Nàn, 难经·二十八难) says: "*The Ren vessel starts from the region below RN 3 (zhōng jí), ascends through the pubes, then runs upward along the inside of the abdomen to RN 4 (guān yuán) and hypopharynx.*"

Volume 1 in *Taiping Holy Benevolent Prescriptions (Tài Píng Shèng Huì Fāng, 太平圣惠方)* says: "*Ren means pregnancy. It is the root of production and nutrition.*"

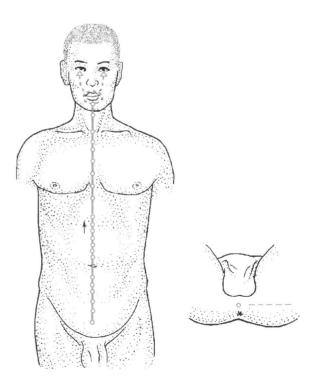

Fig. 4-18 The *Ren* Vessel

③ The Penetrating vessel, 冲脉

(1) The distributing course

Trunk: the Penetrating vessel starts from the inside of the uterus, descends and emerges from RN 1 (*huì yīn*), combines with the Kidney channel of foot *shaoyin* at the *Qi Jie*, ascends by the umbilicus and spreads in the chest, again runs upward, passes the throat, curves around the lips and reaches the infraorbital region.

Branch: one branch derives from the point of *Qì Jiē* (气街), runs along the medial side of the thigh, enters the popliteal fossa, again descends along the medial side of the tibia to the sole of the foot.

Branch: one branch derives from the region of the medial malleolus, obliquely runs forward into the dorsum of the foot and reaches the big toe.

Branch: one branch derives from the inside of the uterus, runs backward to communicate with the *Du vessel* and ascends along the interior of the spinal column. (Fig. 4-19)

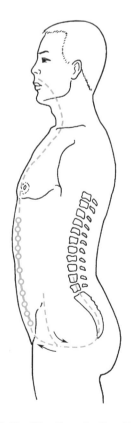

Fig. 4-19　The Penetrating Vessel

(2) The physiological function

Penetrating (*Chong* in Chinese, 冲) means the communication center. The main functions of the Penetrating vessel are as follows:

a. Regulating the qi and blood of the twelve channels: the Penetrating vessel ascends to the head, descends to the foot, runs backward to the back and forward to the abdomen. It passes through the whole body, acts as the communication center for qi and blood, and can regulate the qi and blood of the twelve channels. Therefore the penetrating channel is named the sea of the twelve channels, the sea of the five *zang* and six *fu* organs and the sea of blood.

b. Related to reproduction: the Penetrating vessel starts from the inside of the uterus, which is also the sea of blood and has the function of regulating menstruation, hence it is related to reproduction.

Miraculous Pivot: Chapter On the Four Seas (Líng Shū: Hǎi Lùn, 灵枢·海论) says: "The Penetrating vessel is the sea of the twelve channels."

Miraculous Pivot: Chapter Different Acupuncture Therapies to People of Different Fat and Lean Physiques and the Adverse and Agreeable Conditions of the Twelve Channels (Líng Shū: Nì Shùn Féi Shòu, 灵枢·逆顺肥瘦) says: "The Penetrating vessel is the sea of the five zang and six fu organs, and it can nourish these organs."

Plain Questions: Chapter Ancient Ideas on Flow to Preserve Natural Healthy Energy (Sù Wèn: Shàng Gǔ Tiān Zhēn Lùn, 素问·上古天真论) says: "For a woman...Tiangui (天癸) appears at the age of fourteen (the second seven years). At this time, the Ren vessel gets opened, and the Penetrating vessel becomes prosperous and menstruation begins to appear. As all her physiological conditions become mature, she is able to be pregnant and bear a child...After the age of forty-nine (the seventh seven years), her Ren vessel and Penetrating vessel both decline, and her menstruation stops as her Tiangui is exhausted. Her physique turns old and feeble, and by then, she can no longer conceive."

④ The Girdling Vessel, 带脉

(1) The distributing course

The Girdling vessel originates from the 11th rib,

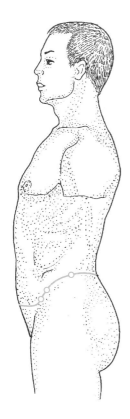

Fig. 4-20   The Girdling Vessel

runs obliquely downwards to GB 26 (*dài mài*), and circles around the waist and the abdomen. At GB 26 it again runs obliquely downward to the lateral lower abdomen along the upper border of the hipbone. (Fig. 4-20)

(2) The physiological function

Girdling (*Dai* in Chinese, 带) means a belt. The main functions of the Girdling vessel are as follows:

a. Binding all the channels: Circling around the waist like a belt, the Girdling vessel has the function of binding all the channels. The twelve channels and other seven vessels of the eight extraordinary channels distribute longitudinally, but only the Girdling vessel runs transversely like a belt, and it can bind all the longitudinal channels and regulate the channel qi.

b. Consolidating embryos and controlling leucorrhea: if the Girdling vessel is deficient, there will be problems with un-consolidation of embryos and the amount of leucorrhea will increase.

Classic of Questioning: The Twenty-eighth Question (Nàn Jīng: Èr Shí Bā Nàn, 难经 · 二十八难)

says: "*The Girdling vessel starts from the 11th rib, and Circles around the waist.*"

Volume 1 in *Taiping Holy Benevolent Prescriptions (Tai Píng Shèng Huì Fāng, 太平圣惠方)* says: "*Girdling means belting, i.e. the Girdling vessel binds all the channels and makes them harmonious and gentle.*"

Fu Qing-zhu's Obstetrics and Gynecology: Chapter Leukorrhea (Fù Qīng Zhú Nǔ Kē: Dài Xià, 傅青主 女科 · 带下) says: "*All leukorrheal diseases can be attributed to dampness syndrome, and the reason why they are called dai is that the Girdling vessel doesn't bind. The girdling vessel communicates with the Ren vessel and the Du vessel, and when there are disorders of the Ren and Du vessels, there is also a disorder of the Girdling vessel. The Girdling vessel binds the embryos. If the Girdling vessel is too weak to bind, the embryo will surely be unconsolidated. Thus if the Girdling vessel is weak, miscarriage will be easy to appear; and if the Girdling vessel is impaired, the embryo is unconsolidated.*" (Note: Leukorrhea is called *Dai* (带) in Chinese, which shares the same word with the Girdling Vessel.)

⑤ The Yin Motility Vessel and the Yang Motility Vessel, 阴跷脉, 阳跷脉

(1) The distributing course

The yin motility vessel starts from the region of the medial malleolus where KI 6 (*zhào hǎi*) of the Kidney channel of foot *shaoyin* lies, and the vessel ascends at the back of the medial malleolus and passes through the medial side of the leg and thigh, passes through the external genitalia, runs along the abdomen and chest to enter the supraclavicular fossa, then emerges from the anterior of ST 9 (*rén yíng*), passes through the lateral side of the nose and reaches the inner canthus, and joins with the channels of hand and foot *taiyang* and the yang motility vessel. (Fig. 4-21)

The yang motility vessel starts from the region of the lateral malleolus where BL 62 (*shēn mài*) of the Bladder channel of foot *taiyang* lies, and the vessel ascends at the back of the lateral malleolus and passes through the lateral side of the leg and thigh, ascends along the lateral side of the abdomen and chest, passes through the shoulder, ascends from the lateral aspect of the neck and presses close to the angle of the mouth, and then reaches the inner canthus to join with the channels of hand and foot *taiyang* and the yin motility vessel, again ascends into the hair line, then descends to the rear of the ear, and connects with GB 20 (*fēng chí*), which lies on the nape and belongs to the Gallbladder channel of the foot *shaoyang*. (Fig. 4-22)

(2) The physiological function

Motility (*Qiao* in Chinese, 跷) means light and swift. The functions of the motility vessels are as follows:

a. Controlling the motion of the lower limbs: the Yin and yang motility vessels start from the malleolus, respectively ascend along the medial or lateral side of the lower limbs to the head and face, they govern the yin-yang of the left and

right body, and make the motion of lower limbs light and swift.

b. Governing the opening and closing of the eyes: the yin motility vessel and the yang motility vessel intersect on the inner canthus, and they govern the eyelids' opening and closing.

Miraculous Pivot: Chapter Cold and Heat Syndrome (Líng Shū: Hán Rè Bìng, 灵枢·寒热病) says: "*The yin motility vessel and the yang motility vessel intersect, and then the yang motility vessel enters the Yin one, and the yin motility vessel comes out from the Yang one: they intersect at the outer canthus. When yang qi is overabundant, the eyes stay wide open; when yin qi is overabundant, the eyes stay closed.*"

Classic of Questioning: The Twenty-eighth Question (Nàn Jīng: Èr Shí Bā Nàn, 难经·二十八难) says: "*The yang motility vessel starts from the*

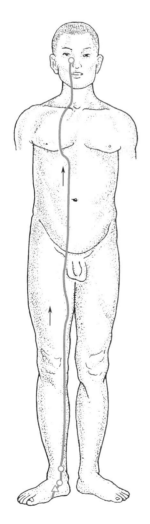

Fig. 4-21   The Yin Motility Vessel

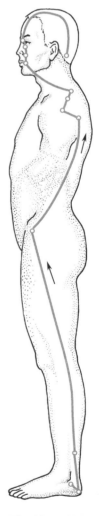

Fig. 4-22   The Yang Motility Vessel

heel, and ascends along the lateral malleolus, and then enters GB 20 (fēng chí). The yin motility vessel also starts from the heel, but it ascends along the medial malleolus to the throat, and connects with the Penetrating vessel."

Volume 1 in *Taiping Holy Benevolent Prescriptions (Tài Píng Shèng Huì Fāng,* 太平圣惠方) says: *"The motility vessels are spry and swift. It is the lynchpin of walking and the reason of motion, hence they are called the motility vessels."*

⑥ The Yin Linking Vessel and the Yang Linking Vessel, 阴维脉, 阳维脉

(1) The distributing course

The yin linking vessel starts from the medial side of the leg where the three yin channels of foot intersect, ascends along the medial side of the lower limbs to the abdomen, and then runs along with the Spleen channel of foot *taiyin*, reaches the lateral thorax to connect with the Liver Channel of foot *jueyin*, then ascends to the throat and connect with the *Ren* vessel. (Fig. 4-23)

The yang linking vessel starts from the region below the lateral malleolus, runs along with the Gallbladder channel of foot *shaoyang*, ascends along the lateral side of the lower limbs, passes through the posterior and lateral side of the trunk, runs upward to the shoulder from the rear of the armpit, passes through the neck and the rear of the ear, then runs forward to the forehead, and it is distributed on the lateral side of the head and the posterior nape to connect with the *Du* vessel. (Fig. 4-24)

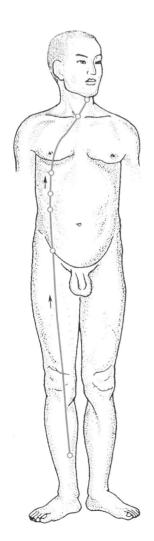

Fig. 4-23   The Yin Linking Vessel

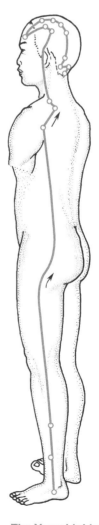

Fig. 4-24   The Yang Linking Vessel

(2) The physiological function

Linking (*Wei* in Chinese) means connecting. The function of the linking vessels is to connect all channels of the body. The yin linking vessel connects all yin channels and the yang linking vessel, all yang channels.

Classic of Questioning: The Twenty-eighth Question (*Nàn Jīng: Èr Shí Bā Nàn,* 难经 · 二十八难) says: "*The yang and yin linking vessels bind all channels of the body. Compared with the circulation of the twelve channels, they can store the overflowing qi but not circulate throughout the body. Therefore, the yang linking vessel starts from the confluence of all yang channels and the yin linking vessel from the confluence of all yin channels*".

Variorum of Classic of Questioning: The Twenty-eighth Question (*Nàn Jīng Jí Zhù: Èr Shí Bā Nàn,* 难经集注 · 二十八难) says: "*The yang linking vessel connects all yang channels, and it starts from the confluence of all yang channels; the yin linking vessel connects all yin channels, and it starts from the confluence of all yin channels.*"

Section 4 Divergent Channels, Divergent Collaterals, Sinew Channels and Cutaneous Regions

The Divergent Channels

① The Signification

The divergent channels (经别), namely the twelve divergent channels, which diverge out from the twelve channels, penetrate into the interior of the trunk and distribute through the chest, abdomen and head. They pertain to the category of the twelve channels, hence the name. (Fig. 4-25)

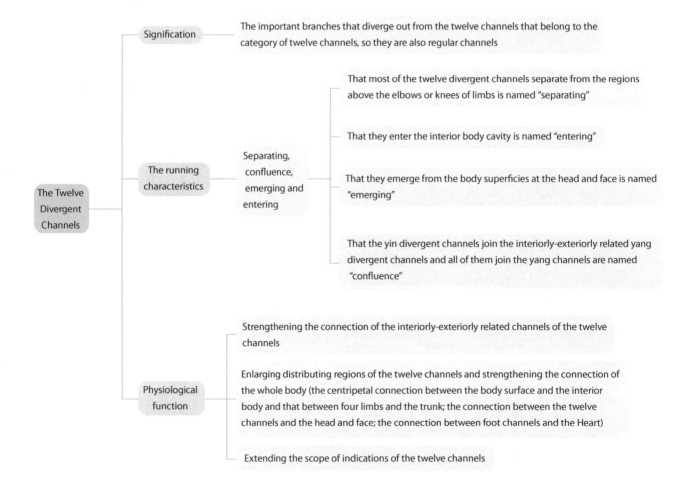

Fig. 4-25 The Twelve Divergent Channels

The twelve divergent channels are the primary ones that diverge out from the twelve channels, so their names are the same, basically, as the twelve channels. The twelve divergent channels are classified into the three yin and three yang of hand and foot, and they are named *the main channel-branch* in *Miraculous Pivot: Chapter Branches of the Twelve Channels (Líng Shū: Jīng Bié, 灵枢·经别)*. For example, the divergent channel of foot *taiyang* is named "the channel-branch of foot *taiyang*", and the others are named according to the same method.

② The Distributing Course

The distributing characteristic of the twelve divergent channels is "separating, entering, emerging and confluence". That most of the twelve divergent channels separate from the regions above the elbows or knees of limbs is called "separating"; that they enter the interior body cavity is called "entering"; that they emerge from the body superficies at the head and face is called "emerging"; that the yin divergent channels join the interiorly-exteriorly related yang divergent channels and all of them join the yang channels is called "confluence". Each pair of interiorly-exteriorly related divergent channels forms one "confluence", so the three yin and yang channels of hand and foot form 6 pairs of confluences that are named the "six confluences".

(1) The divergent channels of foot taiyang and foot shaoyin (1st confluence)

The divergent channel of foot *taiyang*: the divergent channel of foot *taiyang* diverges from the popliteal fossa of the channel of foot *taiyang*, one branch diverges from five *cun* below the sacrococcygeal region, enters the anus, pertains to the Bladder and spreads over the Kidney, then ascends along both sides of the spine, reaches the Heart and spreads into the interior of the Heart; another branch runs straight, ascends from both sides of the spine, emerges from the nape, and joins its same primary channel of foot *taiyang*.

The divergent channel of foot *taiyin*: the divergent channel of foot *taiyin* separates from

the popliteal fossa of the channel of foot *taiyin*, one branch joins the divergent channel of foot *taiyang* and runs along with the latter, ascends to the Kidney, and connects with the girdling vessel at the location of 14th vertebra; another branch ascends straight to link with the root of tongue, comes out from the nape, and joins the divergent channel of foot *taiyang*.

Miraculous Pivot: Chapter Branches of the Twelve Channels (Líng Shū: Jīng Bié, 灵枢·经别) says: "*The main channel-branch of the foot taiyang separates from the popliteal fossa of the human body, descends to reach five cun below the sacrococcygeal region, enters the anus and inside of the abdomen, pertains to the Bladder and spreads over the Kidney, then ascends along the inside of the spine and spreads into the interior of the Heart; another branch runs straight, ascends from both sides of the spine, emerges from the nape, and again joins its same primary channel of foot taiyang. The main channel-branch of the foot taiyin separates from the popliteal fossa of the channel of foot taiyin, one branch joins the divergent channel of foot taiyang and runs along with the latter, ascends to the Kidney, and connects with the girdling vessel at the location of the 14th vertebra; another branch ascends straight to link with the root of tongue, again comes out from the nape, and joins the divergent channel of foot taiyang.*"

(2) The divergent channels of foot shaoyang and foot jueyin (2nd confluence)

The divergent channel of foot *shaoyang*: The divergent channel of foot *shaoyang* separates from the lateral side of the thigh and winds along the anterior of the thigh, enters the pubes and joins the Liver channel of foot *jueyin*, ascends to enter the 11th ribs, runs along the interior of the chest and pertains to the Gallbladder, then scatters over the Liver, passes the Heart, ascends along the throat, comes out from the location between the mandible and mouth, spreads over the face, links the ocular cord and joins the channel of foot *shaoyang* at the outer canthus.

The divergent channel of foot *jueyin*: the divergent channel of foot *jueyin* separates from the dorsum of the foot, ascends to reach the pubes and joins the divergent channel of foot *shaoyang* and runs along with the latter.

Miraculous Pivot: Chapter Branches of the Twelve Channels (Líng Shū: Jīng Bié, 灵枢·经别) says: *"The main channel-branch of foot shaoyang separates and winds along the thigh, enters the pubes and joins the channel of foot jueyin. Another channel enters the 11th rib, runs along the interior of the chest and pertains to the Gallbladder, then scatters over the Liver, penetrates the Heart, ascends along the throat, comes out from the location between the mandible and mouth, spreads over the face, links the ocular cord and joins the channel of foot shaoyang at the outer canthus. The main channel-branch of foot jueyin separates from the dorsum of the foot, ascends to reach the pubes and connects with the foot shaoyang channel of Gallbladder and joins the divergent channel of foot shaoyang and runs along with the latter. This is the second confluence."*

(3) The divergent channels of foot yangming and foot taiyin (3rd confluence)

The divergent channel of foot *yangming*: the divergent channel of foot *yangming* separates from the anterior side of the thigh, enters the abdomen, pertains to the Stomach and scatters over the Spleen, then passes through the Heart, ascends along the throat, comes out from the mouth to reach the bridge of the nose and infraorbital region, encircles the ocular cord and joins the channel of foot *yangming*.

The divergent channel of foot *taiyin*: the divergent channel of foot *taiyin* separates from the medial side of the thigh, reaches the anterior side of the thigh, then joins the divergent channel of foot *yangming* and runs along with the latter, then ascends to the throat and passes through the root of the tongue.

Miraculous Pivot: Chapter Branches of the Twelve Channels (Líng Shū: Jīng Bié, 灵枢·经别) says: *"The main channel-branch of the foot yangming ascends to reach the thigh, enters the abdomen, pertains to the Stomach and scatters over the Spleen, then ascends to reach the Heart, runs along the throat, comes out from the mouth to reach the bridge of the nose and infraorbital region, encircles the ocular cord and joins the channel of foot yangming. The main channel-branch of the foot taiyin ascends to reach the thigh, joins the channel of yangming and runs along with the latter, then ascends to communicate with the*

throat and links with the root of tongue. This is the third confluence."*

(4) The divergent channels of hand taiyang and hand shaoyin (4th confluence) (inner canthus)

The divergent channel of hand *taiyang*: the divergent channels of hand *taiyang* separates from the joint behind the shoulder, enters the armpit, reaches the Heart, connects with the Small Intestine, and joins the channel of hand *taiyang*.

The divergent channel of hand *shaoyin*: the divergent channels of hand *shaoyin* separates from the region between the two sinews under the armpit, pertains to the Heart, then ascends to the throat, emerges, then reaches the face and joins the divergent channel of hand *taiyang* at the inner canthus.

Miraculous Pivot: Chapter Branches of the Twelve Channels (Líng Shū: Jīng Bié, 灵枢·经别) says: *"The main channel-branch of hand taiyang descends from the upper to the lower. It separates from the joint behind the shoulder, enters the armpit, reaches the Heart and connects with the Small Intestine. The main channel-branch of the hand shaoyin enters GB22 (yuān yè) that is between the two sinews under the armpit, pertains to the Heart, then ascends to the throat, reaches the face and joins the divergent channel of hand taiyang at the inner canthus. This is the fourth confluence."*

(5) The divergent channels of hand shaoyang and hand jueyin (5th confluence)

The divergent channel of hand *shaoyang*: the divergent channel of hand *shaoyang* separates from the head and face, enters the supraclavicular fossa downwardly, then passes through the upper burner, middle burner, lower burner, scatters over the chest, and joins the channel of hand *shaoyang*.

The divergent channel of hand *jueyin*: the divergent channels of hand *jueyin* separates three *cun* below the armpit, enters the chest, pertains to the upper burner, middle burner, and lower burner, ascends along the throat, emerges from the rear of the ear, reaches the mastoid process, and joins the divergent channel of hand *shaoyang*.

Miraculous Pivot: Chapter Branches of the Twelve Channels (Líng Shū: Jīng Bié, 灵枢·经别) says: *"The main channel-branch of hand shaoyang descends from above to below. It separates from the top of the head and enters the supraclavicular fossa, then descends again to reach the San Jiao and scatters on the chest. The main channel-branch of hand jueyin separates from three cun under GB 22 (yuān yè), enters the chest, pertains to the San Jiao, runs along the throat to reach the rear of the ear, and joins the channel of hand shaoyang below GB 12 (wán gǔ). This is the fifth confluence."*

(6) The divergent channels of hand yangming and hand taiyin (6ᵗʰ confluence)

The divergent channel of hand *yangming*: the divergent channel of hand *yangming* separates from LI 15 (*jiān yú*), enter the cervical vertebrae, descends to the Large Intestine, again ascends and pertains to the Lung, then runs along the throat, emerges from the supraclavicular fossa and joins the channel of hand *yangming*.

The divergent channel of hand *taiyin*: the divergent channel of hand *taiyin* separates from GB 22 (*yuān yè*), runs along the front of the divergence of hand *shaoyin*, enters the Lung, scatters over the Large Intestine, ascends and emerges from the supraclavicular fossa, runs along the throat and joins the divergent channel of hand *yangming*.

Miraculous Pivot: Chapter Branches of the Twelve Channels (Líng Shū: Jīng Bié, 灵枢·经别) says: *"The main channel-branch of the hand yangming separates from the hand and ascends along the location between the lateral side of the chest and the breast to reach LI 15 (jiān yú), passes the cervical vertebrae, reaches the Large Intestine, then pertains to the Lung, runs along the throat to enter the supraclavicular fossa and joins the channel of hand yangming. The main channel-branch of hand taiyin separates to reach GB 22 (yuān yè) and in front of hand shaoyin, enters the Lung, scatters over the Large Intestine, ascends to pass the supraclavicular fossa, runs along the throat and again connects to the channel of hand yangming. This is the sixth confluence."*

③ Physiological Function

The twelve divergent channels derive from the twelve channels and reach some organs and body

constituents where the twelve channels do not arrive, so they extend the distributing courses of the twelve channels, strengthen the connections between the channels and all parts of the body, and have some effect on physiology, pathology, treatment, etc.

(1) Strengthening the connection of the interiorly-exteriorly related channels of the twelve channels

After the twelve divergent channels enter the body cavity, the interiorly-exteriorly related divergent channels distribute together; when they emerge from the body superficies, the yin divergent channels join the yang divergent channels and both of them join the yang channel on the body surface, and hence the divergent channels strengthen the connection between the interiorly-exteriorly related channels.

(2) Enlarging distributing regions of the twelve channels and strengthening the connection of the whole body

In the regions where the twelve channels are not distributed, the divergent channels strengthen the connections between the channels and all parts of the trunk and *zang-fu* organs, enlarge the distributing regions and strengthen the connection of the whole body.

For example, the twelve divergent channels separate from the twelve channels of the limbs, and distribute centripetally after they enter the interior of the body. This has played an important role in extending the centripetal connection of the body surface with the interior body, limbs and trunk, and transmitting the information from the interior to the exterior.

The yang divergent channels distribute along the head and face, and the yin divergent channels also ascend to the head and face. This strengthens the connection between the twelve channels and the head and face, and offers the theoretical basis for treatments such as ear acupuncture, facial acupuncture and nasal acupuncture, etc.

The three yin and yang divergent channels of the foot ascend through the abdomen and chest, and connect with the Heart. This strengthens the connection between the channels of the foot and the Heart. Therefore, the divergent channels have the important significance of analyzing the physiological and pathological associations of the abdominal organs and the Heart.

(3) Extending the scope of indications of the twelve channels

The distribution of the twelve divergent channels make up for the distributing courses of the twelve channels, so that the twelve divergent channels extend the scope of indications of the twelve channels.

The Divergent Collaterals

① The Significance

The divergent collaterals (别络), being the largest of the collaterals, are those that separate from the twelve channels to the adjacent ones. The fifteen divergent collaterals include the 12 divergent collaterals respectively diverging from the twelve channels, the 2 collaterals of the *Du vessel* and *Ren vessel* and the major collateral of the Spleen.

The divergent collaterals are the main parts of the collateral system, and they have regular distribution and names. They are named after the names of the points from which the divergent collaterals separate from the channels. For example, the divergent collateral of hand *taiyin* separates from the LU 7 (*liè quē*), which belongs to the channel of hand *taiyin*, so it is called the divergent collateral of hand *taiyin* and the name is *liè quē*. (Fig. 4-26)

② The Distributing Course

The fifteen divergent collaterals have regular distributing courses. The twelve divergent collaterals of the twelve primary channels separate from the regions below the elbows or knees of the limbs, and the divergent collaterals of the exteriorly-interiorly related channels connect with each other; the divergent collaterals of the *Ren vessel* are distributed on the abdomen, the ones of the *Du vessel* are distributed on the back, and those of the major collateral of the Spleen are distributed on the chest and hypochondrium.

Miraculous Pivot: Chapter Branches of the Twelve Channels (Líng Shū: Jīng Bié, 灵枢·经别) says: "The divergent collateral of hand taiyin is named liè quē. It starts from the muscular layers of the wrist, runs parallel with the channel of hand taiyin and enters the center of the palm and then spreads on the thenar eminence."

"The divergent collateral of hand shaoyin is named tōng lǐ. It starts from one and a half cun behind the wrist, ascends along the channel of hand shaoyin to enter the Heart, links to the root of tongue and connects with the ocular cord."

"The divergent collateral of hand jueyin is named nèi guān. It starts from two cun above the wrist, passes in the middle of the two sinews and ascends along the channel of hand jueyin to link to the Pericardium."

"The divergent collateral of hand taiyang is named zhī zhèng. It starts from five cun above the wrist to join the channel of hand shaoyin; another branch ascends, passes the elbow and reaches LI15 (jiān yú)."

"The divergent collateral of hand yangming is named piān lì. It separates from three cun above the wrist to connectwith the channel of hand taiyin; its branch ascends to the arm, passes LI15 (jiān yú) and the curve of the jaw and the root of teeth; another channel enters the ear and converges with the general assemblage of the channels of hand taiyang, hand shaoyang, foot shaoyang and foot yangming."

"The divergent collateral of hand shaoyang is named wài guān. It starts from two cun above the wrist, ascends to bypass the medial side of the arm, enters the chest and joins the Pericardium channel."

"The divergent collateral of foot taiyang is named fēi yáng. It separates seven cun above the lateral malleolus and connects the channel of foot shaoyin."

"The divergent collateral of foot shaoyang is named guāng míng. It separates from five cun above the lateral malleolus and connects with the channel of foot jueyin and spreads on the dorsum of the foot."

"The divergent collateral of foot yangming is

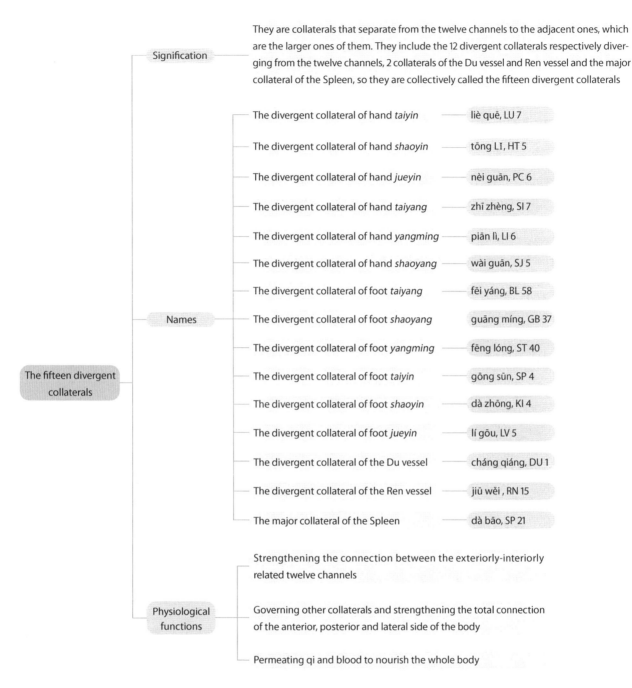

Fig. 4-26 The Fifteen Divergent Collaterals

named fēng lóng. It separates eight cun above the lateral malleolus and connects to the channel of foot taiyin; its branch ascends along the lateral border of the tibia to communicate with the head, and converges with the qi of various channels there, and then descends to reach the throat."

"The divergent collateral of foot taiyin is named gōng sūn. It separates one cun behind the basic joint of the big toe and connects to the channel of foot yangming; another branch penetrates into the abdomen and connects with the intestine and Stomach."

"The divergent collateral of foot shaoyin is named dà zhōng. It separates from the rear of the medial malleolus, winds around the heel and connects to the channel of foot taiyang; its branch runs parallel with the channel of foot shaoyang to reach the Pericardium and descends to link with the back."

"The divergent collateral of foot jueyin is named lí gōu. It separates five cun above the medial malleolus to connect to the channel of foot shaoyin; its branch ascends along the channel of foot jueyin to reach the testis and penis."

"The divergent collateral of the Ren vessel is named wěi yì. It separates from the xiphoid process and descends to spread over the abdomen."

"The divergent collateral of the Du vessel is named cháng qiáng. It ascends to press close to the spine and reaches the neck, spreads over the head, descends to the scapula and connects to the channels of shaoyin and taiyang, and then penetrates along the side of the spinal column."

"The major collateral of the Spleen is named dà bāo. It starts from three cun under GB 22 (yuān yè) and spreads over the chest and hypochondrium."

③ The Physiological Function

(1) Strengthening the connection between the exteriorly-interiorly related twelve channels

The divergent collaterals of the yin channels distribute to the yang channels and the divergent collaterals of the yang channels runs to the yin channels, and hence the connection is realized.

(2) Governing other collaterals and strengthening the total connection of the anterior, posterior and lateral sides of the body

The divergent collateral of the *Ren vessel* spreads over the abdomen, the divergent collateral of the *Du vessel* spreads over the back, and the divergent collateral of the Spleen spreads over the chest and hypochondrium, hence the divergent collaterals strengthen the total connection of the anterior, posterior and lateral side of the body and govern other collaterals.

(3) Permeating qi and blood to nourish the whole body

The superficial collaterals and minute collaterals separate from the divergent collaterals. The divergent collaterals are largest, the superficial collaterals are smaller and finer, and the minute collaterals are the smallest and finest. They spread like nets to the whole body. Hence the divergent collaterals are permeated with the qi and blood of the channels in the linear course, then extends in regional dispersion, and nourishes the whole body.

The Sinew Channels

① The Significance

The sinew channels (经筋) are the system, in which the qi of the twelve channels joins, knots, disperses and connects to the sinews, muscles and joints. They are the connecting regions of the twelve channels, and hence they are named the twelve sinew channels.

The names of the sinew channels are the same as the names of the twelve channels; they are classified into the three yin and three yang of hand and foot, and are called *the sinew channel* in Chapter *The Tendons Distributed Along the Channels (Jīng Jīn)* in *Miraculous Pivot (Líng Shū)*. For example, the sinew channel of the channel of foot *taiyang* is called the sinew channel of foot *taiyang*.

② The Distributing Course

The twelve sinew channels are the system where the twelve channels connect with the sinews and muscles. The sinew channels of the three yang channels of the hand and foot are distributed on the lateral side of the limbs; the sinew channels of the three yin channels of the hand and foot are distributed on the medial side of the limbs. The twelve sinew channels are distributed over the sinews and muscles of the body, and most of them knot, join, disperse and connect around the bones and joints; some enter the chest and abdomen, but they do not pertain to or connect with the *zang-fu* organs. The twelve sinew channels start from the terminal ends of the limbs and distribute centripetally to the head and trunk.

③ The Physiological Function

The sinew channels are attached to the bones and joints, and have the function of controlling the motion of the joints.

Plain Questions: Chapter Discussion on Flaccidity (Sù Wèn: Wěi Lùn, 素问·痿论) says: *"The sinew channels control the bones and muscles and smooth the joints."*

The Cutaneous Regions

① The Significance

The cutaneous regions (皮部) are certain areas of the body surface on which the twelve channels reflect their functions. The entire area of the body is divided into twelve parts that pertain to the twelve channels, so they are called the twelve cutaneous regions.

② The Distribution

The twelve cutaneous regions are the division of the twelve channels and their subordinate collaterals, so the body surface distribution of the twelve cutaneous regions is the same as that of the twelve channels. The cutaneous regions, being the body surface division of the twelve channels, are different from the channels and collaterals: the channels are distributed linearly, and the collaterals are distributed like a net, and the cutaneous regions are distributed in more of a flat shape, and wider than the distribution of channels and collaterals.

③ Physiological Function

The cutaneous regions depend on the qi and blood's nutrition in the twelve channels. They are the most superficial part of the body exposed to the outside, which contacts the environment directly, they have inducing and regulating functions in response to environmental changes, and along with defensive qi they defend the body against exterior evil.

Furthermore, in diagnosis, inspecting changes in complexion and appearance for the different cutaneous regions will contribute to diagnosing disorders of some *zang-fu* organs, channels and collaterals. In treatment, plastering therapy, moxa-wool moxibustion, hot compress therapy and plum blossom needle therapy applied on the skin can cure disorders of the internal organs.

Plain Questions: Chapter Discussion on Skin Divisions (Sù Wèn: Pí Bù Lùn, 素问 · 皮部论*) says:*

"When one wants to determine to which channel the part of skin belongs, it should be based upon the locations where the channel reaches and passes...The conditions of all the twelve channels are the same. The yang collaterals of the yangming Channel (the cutaneous region of the channel of yangming)...are mostly greenish, it shows there is pain; if they are mostly blackish, it shows there is Bi (the disease of blocking of extremities, channels and viscera by evils); if they are mostly yellowish and reddish, it shows there is heat; if they are mostly whitish, it shows there is cold; if all the five colors are existing it shows there is a disease with alternating heat and cold. The skin is the region where the collaterals spread."

Section 5   The Functions of the Channels and Collaterals

The channel-collateral system crisscrosses and spread throughout the whole body, and has the functions of communicating between the interior, exterior, upper and lower, connecting the *zang-fu* organs, transporting qi and blood, inducing and transmitting, regulating functions and so on. (Fig. 4-27)

The Function of Communicating and Connecting

The channels and collaterals are components of body structure. They crisscross and network the whole body, and have the functions of communicating between the interior, exterior, upper and lower parts, and connecting the *zang-fu* organs. The human body is composed of tissues and organs, such as the five *zang* and six *fu* organs, the five sense organs and nine orifices, and the limbs and bones. Although the functions of these tissues and organs are different, they cooperate with each other to assist the organic and unitary activities to keep coordination and harmony between the interior, exterior, upper and lower parts of the body. Their mutual connection and organic cooperation mainly depends on the

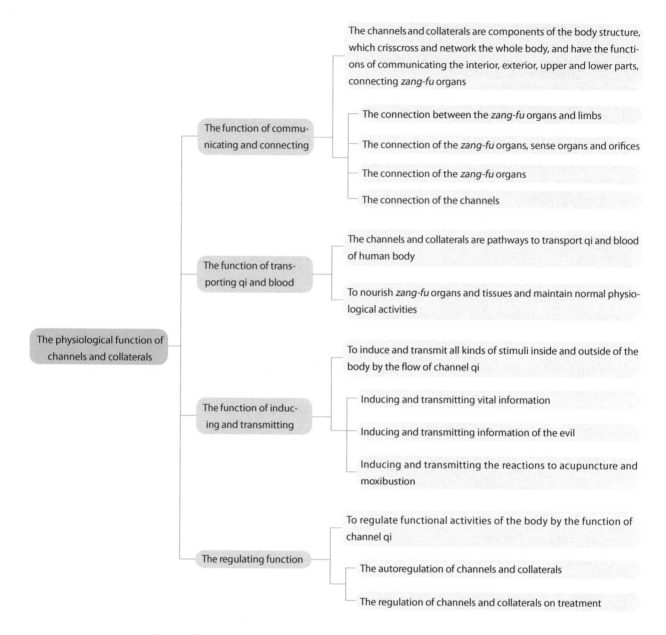

Fig. 4-27　The Physiological function of channels and collaterals

communication and connection of the channel-collateral system. The main connections are as follows:

(1) The Connection between the *Zang-fu* Organs and the Limbs

The *zang-fu* organs and the limbs are connected mainly through the communication and connection of the twelve channels. The three yin channels of the hand and foot distribute along the medial sides of the upper and lower limbs, and the three yang channels of the hand and foot along the lateral sides. The twelve channels pertain to or connect with the internal organs; and through the twelve sinew channels and twelve cutaneous regions, they connect with external tissues such as the sinews, muscles, joints and skin. Thus, the *zang-fu* organs and limbs are mutually communicated with by the internal pertaining function and the external connecting function of the twelve channels.

Miraculous Pivot: Chapter On the Four Seas (*Líng Shū: Hǎi Lùn*, 灵枢·海论) says: "*The twelve channels pertain to zang-fu organs inside, and connect with the limbs and joints outside.*"

② The Connection of the *Zang-fu* Organs, Apertures and Orifices (Table 4-8)

The twelve channels pertain to the *zang-fu* organs inside, and they also distribute through the sense organs and orifices such as the eyes, tongue, mouth, nose, ears, external genitalia and anus. In this way, the *zang-fu* organs, the sense organs and orifices are connected through communication of the channels.

The channels connect with the eyes: the Heart channel of hand *shaoyin* links to the ocular cord; the Small Intestine channel of hand *taiyang* reaches the outer and inner canthus; the Bladder channel of foot *taiyang* starts from the inner canthus; the *San Jiao* channel of hand *shaoyang* reaches the outer canthus; the Gallbladder channel of foot *shaoyang* starts from the outer canthus; and the Liver channel of foot *jueyin* connects with the ocular cord.

The channels connect with the tongue: the Spleen channel of foot *taiyin* connects with the root of the tongue and spreads under the tongue; the Kidney channel of foot *taiyin* links to the root of the tongue.

The channels connect with the mouth: the Large Intestine channel of hand *yangming* runs along the mouth, the Stomach channel of foot *yangming* runs along the mouth and encircles the lips, and the Liver channel of foot *jueyin* encircles the lips.

The channels connect with the nose: the Large Intestine channel of hand *yangming* runs along the nostril, the Stomach channel of foot *yangming* starts from the nose, and the Small Intestine

Table 4-8　The Connection of the twelve channels and major organs

Name of channels	Connected organs
Lung Channel of hand *taiyin*	Reaches the throat
Large Intestine Channel of hand *yangming*	Reaches the lower teeth，runs along the mouth and reaches both sides of the nose
Stomach Channel of foot *taiyang*	Starts from the nose, enters the upper teeth, Runs along the mouth, encircles the lips, ascends to reach the front of the ear and runs along the throat
Spleen Channel of foot *taiyin*	Runs along the throat, connects with the root of the tongue and spreads under the tongue
Heart Channel of hand *shaoyin*	Runs along the throat, links to the ocular cord
Small Intestine Channel of foot *taiyang*	Runs along the throat, reaches the outer canthus, enters the interior of the ear, reaches the nose, and reaches the inner canthus
Bladder Channel of foot *taiyang*	Starts from the inner canthus, reaches the upper part of the ear，enters and connects with the brain
Kidney Channel of foot *shaoyin*	Runs along the throat, and runs along the root of the tongue
Pericardium Channel of hand *jueyin*	
San Jiao Channel of hand *shaoyang*	Links the rear of the ear, reaches the upper part of the ear, enters the interior of the ear, emerges and reaches the front of the ear, and reaches the outer canthus
Gallbladder Channel of foot *shaoyang*	Starts from the outer canthus, descends along the rear of the ear, enters the interior of the ear, emerges and reaches the front of the ear, and reaches the back region of the outer canthus
Liver Channel of foot *jueyin*	Encircles the external genitalia, runs along the throat, links the ocular cord, and encircles the inside of the lips

channel of hand *taiyang* reaches the nose.

The channels connect with the ears: the Small Intestine channel of hand *taiyang* enters the interior of the ear; the *San Jiao* channel of hand *shaoyang* enters the interior of the ear from the rear of the ear, emerges and reaches the front of the ear; the Gallbladder channel of foot *shaoyang* enters the interior of the ear from the rear of the ear, emerges and reaches the front of the ear; the Bladder channel of foot *taiyang* reaches the upper part of the ear.

The channels connect with the external genitalia and anus: the Gallbladder channel of foot *shaoyang* bypasses the pubes; the Liver channel of foot *jueyin* reaches the pubes and encircles the external genitalia; and the *Du* vessel,

Ren vessel and penetrating vessel all descend and emerge from RN 1 (*huì yīn*).

The five sense organs, nine orifices and internal organs are connected through the communication of the channels.

Miraculous Pivot: Chapter *The Visceral Diseases Caused by Evil Qi* (*Líng Shū: Xié Qì Zàng Fǔ Bìng Xíng*, 灵枢·邪气脏腑病形) says: "*The circulation of qi and blood in the twelve channels and the three hundred and sixty five collaterals circulate upwardly to the head and face infusing into the various sense organs.*"

③ The Connection of the *Zang-fu* Organs (Table 4-9)

On the one hand, there is the pertaining-connecting relation between the twelve channels

Table 4-9   Connections of the twelve channels and *zang-fu* organs

Name of Channels	Pertaining-and-connecting *zang-fu* organs	Other connected *zang-fu* organs
Lung Channel	Pertains to the Lung, and connects with the Large Intestine	Returns to pass orifice of Stomach
Large Intestine Channel	Pertains to the Large Intestine, and connects with the Lung	
Stomach Channel	Pertains to the Stomach, and connects with the Spleen	
Spleen Channel	Pertains to the Spleen, and connects with the Stomach	Reaches the Heart
Heart Channel	Pertains to the Heart, and connects with the Small Intestine	Ascends to the Lung
Small Intestine Channel	Pertains to the Small Intestine, and connects with the Heart	Reaches the Stomach
Bladder Channel	Pertains to the Bladder, and connects with the Kidney	
Kidney Channel	Pertains to the Kidney, and connects with the Bladder	Ascends to pass the Liver, enters the Lung, and connects with the Heart
Pericardium Channel	Pertains to the Pericardium, and connects with the *San Jiao*	
San Jiao Channel	Pertains to the *San Jiao*, and connects with the Pericardium	
Gallbladder Channel	Pertains to the Gallbladder, and connects with the Liver	
Liver Channel	Pertains to the Liver, and connects with the Gallbladder	Presses close to the Stomach, and ascends to reach the Lung

and the *zang-fu* organs. That is to say, each channel pertains to or connects with one *zang* or *fu* organ, and this theory is the structural basis of the interconnection between *zang-fu* organs.

On the other hand, there are connections between channels and other *zang-fu* organs in their distributing courses. Besides given pertaining-connecting relation between channels and *zang-fu* organs, some channels can still connect with many other *zang-fu* organs. For example, the channel of foot *shaoyin* pertains to the Kidney and connects with the Bladder, and it also penetrates into the Liver, enters the Lung, connects with the Heart, and infuses into the chest. The channel of foot *jueyin* pertains to the Liver and connects with the Gallbladder, and it also runs along the Stomach and infuses into the Lung. Some organs are connected with many channels. For example, the channels which connect with the Lung are as follows: the channel of hand *taiyin* pertains to the Lung, the channel of hand *yangming* connects with the Lung, the channel of foot *jueyin* joins the Lung, the channel of foot *shaoyin* enters the Lung, the channel of hand *shaoyin* passes the Lung, etc. Furthermore, the divergent channels make up for any deficiency of the primary channels. For example, the divergent channel of foot *yangming* ascends to communicate with the Heart; the divergent channel of foot *shaoyang* passes through the Heart, etc. This forms a multi-connection among *zang-fu* organs.

④ The Connection of the Channels

Through the communication and connection of channels and collaterals, there are close relationships among each part of the channel-collateral system. For example, there is a given sequence of joining and circulating for the interiorly-exteriorly related channels. The trunks and branches of the channels intersect in their distributing courses. The twelve divergent channels and divergent collaterals strengthen the connection between exteriorly-interiorly related channels. The eight extraordinary channels crisscross among the twelve channels and strengthen the connections among the channels. Further, the collaterals network the whole body

and reach everywhere, so the channel-collateral system forms the complete and reticular connecting system.

The communicating and connecting function of the channels and collaterals is the structural basis of their other functions.

The Function of Transporting Qi and Blood

This function indicates that the channels and collaterals are pathways to transport the qi and blood of human body, possessing the function of transporting both of them. Qi and blood are the main substances of the vital activities of human body. Only when all tissues and organs are nourished by qi and blood can they maintain their normal physiological functions. Through the circulating function of the channels and collaterals, qi and blood reach all over the body, irrigate internal *zang-fu* organs, moisten external striae and interstitial spaces, and nourish organs and tissues to maintain their normal physiological functions.

Miraculous Pivot: Chapter The Various Conditions of Internal Organs Relating Different Diseases (Líng Shū: Běn Zàng, 灵枢·本脏) says: *"The functions of the channels of a man are to circulate blood and qi, operate yin and yang, moisten the sinews and bones and smooth the joints."*

Miraculous Pivot: Chapter The Length of Channels (Líng Shū: Mài Dù, 灵枢·脉度) says: *"Just like the flowing of water and constant movement of the sun and the moon, the flow of the channel qi cannot cease. The yin channel qi nourishes the five zang organs and the yang channel qi nourishes the six fu organs; they pour into each other like a ring, going round and round. As to the channel qi that is overflowing, it permeates the zang-fu organs inside, and moistens the muscles and skin outside."*

The Function of Inducing and Transmitting

The function of inducing and transmitting means that the channel-collateral system induces and transmits all kinds of stimuli. The channel-collateral system is the pathway through which qi and blood circulates, and through the flow of the channel qi the reactions to the stimuli can be transmitted.

① Inducing and Transmitting Vital Information

Vital activity is a very complex process, and large quantities of information vital to life are constantly emitted. The channel-collateral system is the information net that can exchange and propagate information. When the body surface, sense organs and orifices are stimulated, the information will be internally transmitted to the correlated *zang-fu* organs along the channels; when the functions of the *zang-fu* organs vary, the information also can be transmitted to the body surface, sense organs and orifices, and eventually all parts of the body can be harmonized and balanced.

② Inducing and Transmitting Information about Evil Qi

When the normal functions of the *zang-fu* organs and tissues are damaged, disorders can be induced and transmitted by the channels and collaterals, and then the body will show different symptoms and syndromes. For example, when the superficies are attacked by exterior evil, the information will be internally transmitted to the *zang-fu* organs; when there are disorders of the *zang-fu* organs, the syndromes are reflected in the superficies by the transmission.

Plain Questions: *Chapter Discussion on Skin Divisions (Sù Wèn: Pí Bù Lùn, 素问·皮部论)* says: "*When evil qi invades the skin, the striae and interstitial spaces will be open; when the striae and interstitial spaces are open, the evil qi will invade into the collaterals; when the collateral is fully filled with evil qi, it will be poured into the channel; when the channel is fully filled, it will go further and retain in the zang-fu organs.*"

③ Inducing and Transmitting the Reactions to Acupuncture and Moxibustion

The channels and collaterals can sensitively induce and transmit reactions to stimuli such as acupuncture, hot medicinal compresses and *tui na*. For example, the methods of obtaining qi, promoting qi and causing qi to arrive at the location of a disease show that the channels and collaterals can induce and transmit reactions to acupuncture and moxibustion.

The Regulating Function

The channel-collateral system can communicate, connect, and transport qi and blood as well as induce and transmit. On this basis, the channel-collateral system can regulate functions of *zang-fu* organs, body constituents, sense organs and orifices as well as maintain the balance of internal and external environments through the action of the channels' qi.

① The Auto-regulation of Channels and Collaterals

When the internal and external environment of the body vary, or the body is invaded by evil qi, some functional disorders will appear, and the channel qi will move to the location of disease, the channel qi will expel the pathogen or regulate the body's functions, and the body can keep a balanced state of yin and yang without any treatment. This is the autoregulation of the channel qi (right qi).

② The Regulation of Channels and Collaterals on Treatment

When there are some pathological changes of the human body, therapies such as acupuncture can activate channel qi, make qi arrive at the location of disease, regulate the functions of *zang-fu* organs and tissues and make them recover physiological balance. Therefore, simulating therapy such as acupuncture can activate the regulating and harmonizing functions of the channel qi to cure diseases.

Miraculous Pivot: *Chapter On Channels (Líng Shū: Jīng Mài, 灵枢·经脉)* says: "*One can determine the survival or death of the patient, can treat various diseases and find out whether the disease is excess or deficient according to the condition of the channel, and one must master it.*"

Miraculous Pivot: *Chapter The Beginning and End of the Channel (Líng Shū: Gēn Jié, 灵枢·根结)* says: "*The essential effect of acupuncture is to regulate yin and yang. When yin and yang are adjusted, the essence qi of the patient will be abundant, physique and function will be combined, and the spirit will be able to be stored inside."*

Miraculous Pivot: Chapter the Nine Kinds of Needles and the Twelve Source Points (*Líng Shū: Jiǔ Zhēn Shí Èr Yuán,* 灵枢·九针十二原) *says: "The most important thing in acupuncture is to get acupuncture feeling: when it appears, the curative effect will appear in the wake of it."*

Section 6 The Applications of the Channel–collateral Doctrine

The channel-collateral doctrine is a component of the theoretical system of Chinese medicine. It is widely applied in Chinese medicine to illuminate physiological functions, explain pathological changes, guide diagnosis and treatment, and so on. (Fig. 4-28)

Explaining Pathological Changes

In normal physiological conditions, the channels and collaterals have the function of transporting qi and blood and inducing transmission. In pathological changes, the channels and collaterals may serve as the pathways of transmitting evil qi and reflecting disorders.

(1) The Channels and Collaterals are the Pathways through which Exogenous Evil Enters the Body From the Exterior to the Interior

The channels and collaterals interiorly pertain to the *zang-fu* organs and exteriorly connect with the extremities and joints, so when evil qi attacks the body surface, it may be transmitted to the internal organs from the exterior to the interior and from the superficial to the deep. For example, exterior evil attacks the body surface, symptoms of chills,

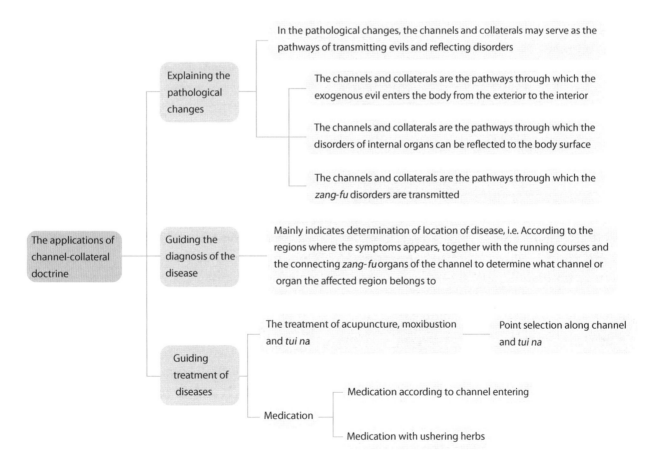

Fig. 4-28 The applications of channel-collateral doctrine

fever, headache and so on will appear first, then cough, chest pain and so on appear. This is because the exterior evil transmits interiorly to the Lung through the channels and collaterals.

(2) The Channels and Collaterals are the Pathways through which Disorders of the Internal Organs can be Reflected to the Body Surface

The channels and collaterals closely connect the internal organs, external body constituents, sense organs, and orifices, and so disorders of zang-fu organs can be reflected in the exterior by the channels and collaterals, manifesting some symptoms and syndromes of the body constituents, sense organs, and orifices.

For example, the Liver channel of foot jueyin encircles the external genitalia, reaches the lower abdomen, branches out in the chest and lateral thorax and goes up to the ocular cord, and hence the syndrome of stagnation of Liver qi includes the symptoms of eczema, itch, etc. As another example, the Stomach channel of foot yangming enters the upper teeth and the Large Intestine channel of hand yangming into the lower teeth, so the syndrome of accumulated heat of Stomach and intestines includes the symptoms of swelling and pain of the gums; the divergent Heart collateral of hand shaoyin goes up to the tongue, so the syndrome of flaring up of Heart fire includes the symptoms of redness and pain in the tongue or oral aphthae.

(3) The Channels and Collaterals are the Pathways through which the Zang-fu Disorders are Transmitted

The zang-fu organs communicate and connect with one another through the channels and collaterals, so disorders of the zang-fu organs can be transmitted to each other through the channels and collaterals. For example, the Liver channel of foot jueyin curves around the Stomach and runs into the Lung, and hence Liver disease may invade the Stomach and Liver fire may invade the Lung; The Kidney channel of foot shaoyin enters the Lung and connects with the Heart, so water overflowing due to Kidney deficiency may attack the Heart and reach the Lung. The Heart channel of hand shaoyin and the

Small Intestine of hand taiyang have pertaining-connecting relationship, so Heart fire may move downward to the Small Intestine and result in the symptoms of urgent micturition, odynuria and dark urine (a syndrome of excessive heat of the Small Intestine).

Plain Questions: Chapter Discussion on Contralateral Needling Therapy (Sù Wèn: Miù Cì Lùn, 素问·缪刺论) says: "*When evil qi invades the body, it will start with the skin and soft hair; if it is retained there and does not leave, it will enter the collateral; if it retains again, it will enter the channel to join the five zang organs and then disperse to the intestines and Stomach. In the way, the yin and yang will become even more overabundant alternately and the five zang organs will be impaired. This is the sequence of evil-qi transmission from the skin and soft hair to the five zang organs.*"

Miraculous Pivot: Chapter the Nine Kinds of Needles and the Twelve Source Points (Líng Shū: Jiǔ Zhēn Shí Èr Yuán, 灵枢·九针十二原) says: "*When the five zang organs have a disease, it will reflect on the twelve source points, and each of the source points belongs to a certain zang organ. When one understands the attribute of the source point and perceives its response, the disease condition of the five zang organs can be known.*"

Guiding the Diagnosis of the Disease

As each channel has its certain distributing courses and pertaining-connecting zang-fu organ, it may reflect the disorders of the regions it passes and the zang-fu organs they pertain to. Thus in clinical application, according to the regions where the symptoms appear, together with the distributing courses and the pertaining-connecting zang-fu organs of the channel, the channel and organ to which the disorder belongs can be determined to provide basis for treatment.

For example, headaches can be analyzed according to location of the pain: a headache on the forehead is most related to the yangming channel; on both sides of the head, it is most related to the shaoyang channel; on the occiput and neck, it is mostly related to the taiyang channel; on the vertex, it is most related to the *jueyin* channel or the *Du vessel*. As for toothaches: pain of the superior teeth is most related with the Stomach channel of foot *yangming*; pain of the lower teeth is most related with the Large Intestine channel of hand *yangming*. Hypochondriac pain is most related with Liver and Gallbladder diseases; the pain in the supraclaveicular fossa is most related with the lungs.

The syndrome differentiation of six channels theory recorded in the book *Treatise on Cold Pathogenic Diseases* (*Shāng Hán Lùn*, 伤寒论) is also a syndrome differentiation system, which developed on the basis of the channel-collateral doctrine.

In clinical practice, the special changes of channels and back-*Shu* points can assist in diagnosing diseases. Some obvious tenderness or reactive changes such as tubercles or cord-like things may occur along distributing courses or on some points where the channel qi gathers, and changes of complexion, appearance and temperature of the local skin can also help diagnose diseases. For example, tubercles may be found on BL 13 (*fèi shū*) or tenderness on LU 1 (*zhōng fǔ*) in Lung diseases; tenderness may be found on the *lán wěi* point in acute appendicitis; some abnormal changes may be found on BL 20 (*pí shù*) in chronic Spleen-Stomach diseases.

Miraculous Pivot: Chapter The Various Conditions of Internal Organs Relating Different Diseases (*Líng Shū: Běn Zàng*, 灵枢·本脏) says: "When one examines the corresponding conditions outside, one will be able to estimate the changes of the internal organs, and thereby, the disease will be diagnosed."

Miraculous Pivot: Chapter Each According to His Ability (*Líng Shū: Guān Néng*, 灵枢·官能) says: "When one examines the pain of the patient's five zang and six fu organs, and integrates with the colors displayed on the left, right, upper and lower sides of the face, he will be able to know the cold or heat nature of the disease and the involved channel. In treatment, examining the cold, warm, slippery or choppy conditions of the skin of the anterolateral side of the forearm, one can determine the patient's

disease."

Guiding the Treatment of Diseases

(1) The Treatment of Acupuncture, Moxibustion and *Tui na*

According to pathological changes of channels and *zang-fu* organs, acupuncture, moxa-wool moxibustion and *tui na* (推拿) treatment are therapies where physical stimulations such as needling, fuming with moxa, and massaging certain regions of the body surface are used to activate the induced transmission of channel qi and regulate the balance of the function, and then to achieve the therapeutic purpose. Acupuncture, moxibustion and *tui na* treatment must abide by the principles of point selection in accordance with the channel. Point selection in accordance with the channel means to determine which channel the disease pertains to according to the syndrome differentiation of channel-collateral doctrine, and then select points to treat the disease according to the distributing course and the connecting range of the channel. In clinical practice, the methods of point selection such as nearby and distant point selection in accordance with the channel, lower point selection in treating upper diseases, upper point selection in treating lower diseases, left-right point combination, and superior-inferior point combination are applications of the principle of point selection in accordance with the channel.

(2) Medication

Medication is also transmitted through the pathways of channels and collaterals. Through the function of channel-collateral transmission, the medicine reaches the location of the disease and plays its therapeutic role. Ancient doctors based the theory of channel tropism on long-term clinical practice. The theory of channel tropism is a method to analyze and categorize medicines by the application of the channel-collateral doctrine. That is to say those medicines have actions special to the *zang-fu* organs, channels and collaterals, and they are attributed to the each channel and can be made systematic in nature.

The main value of the theory of channel tropism is to guide the clinical medication in accordance with different channels. That is to say that when doctors treat disease, they grasp the properties of the medicine, and select the medicines attributed to the channel to which the disease is attributed. For example, *chái hú* (Radix Bupleuri, 柴胡), *xiāng fù* (Rhizoma Cyperi, 香附), and *qīng pí* (Pericarpium Citri Reticulatae Viride, 青皮) have the function of dispersing stagnated Liver qi, and hence they are attributed to the Liver channel of foot *jueyin*, and they are called medicines attributed to Liver channel and selected to cure the syndrome of stagnation of Liver qi.

Ancient doctors also founded the theory of channel-ushering according to the theory of channel tropism. A channel-ushering herb can guide the medical force to the location of the disease, and it is usually called a medicinal usher. For example, if a headache is attributed to the channel of *yangming*, *bái zhǐ* (Angelicae Dahuricae, 白芷) can be selected for treatment; if the headache is attributed to the channel of *shaoyang*, *chái hú* (Radix Bupleuri) can be selected, and if the headache is attributed to the channel of *taiyang*, *qiāng huó* (Rhizomza Seu Radix Notopterygii, 羌活) can be selected. Not only *bai zhǐ*, *chái hú* and *qiāng huó* respectively are attributed to the channels of hand and foot *yangming*, *shaoyang* and *taiyang*, but also they can act as channel-ushering herbs for other herbs and usher other medicines to the corresponding channels for treatment.

Besides this, in clinical practice ear acupuncture, electro-acupuncture, point injection therapy and point-ligating therapies are also guided by the channel-collateral doctrine.

Chapter 5
Body Constitution

The theory of body constitution is the study of the concept, formation, characteristics, and types of the human body and the correlating relationship with the occurrence, development, variation, diagnosis, prevention and treatment of disease, first discussed in *The Yellow Emperor's Internal Classic* (*Huáng Dì Nèi Jīng*, 黄帝内经). Focusing on the study of constitution is helpful for analyzing the regularity of the occurrence, development and variation of disease, and contributes to the improvement of their prevention, diagnosis and treatment.

Section 1   Basic Concept of Body Constitution

Concept of Body Constitution

The term "body constitution, 体质", or diathesis, refers to the relatively stable characteristics of an individual either genetically inherited or acquired during development that manifest in various aspects of morphology and structure, physiological function and psychological activity. (Fig. 5-1) An individual's constitution is determined by factors both genetically inherited and acquired during development. It is a relatively constant attribute formed over the long-term growth, development and aging process in response to natural and social environmental factors and manifests in the form of variations in morphology, physiology and psychology.

Miraculous Pivot: Chapter *On the Relation between Firmness and Softness of Body and One's Life-span* (*Líng Shū: Shòu Yāo Gāng Róu*, 灵枢·寿夭刚柔) states: "*People are born of different diathesis, firm or soft, weak or strong, tall or short, yin or yang.*"

Formation of Body Constitution

Normal everyday activities are a harmonized unity of physique and spirit, one of the basic characteristics of the presence of life and good health. The two aspects of spirit and physique are mutually dependent upon each other and exert a reciprocal influence, with certain physical structures resulting in corresponding physiological functions and psychological characteristics. Healthy physiological functions and psychological character are the result of sound physical structure, and are reflected in the intrinsic characteristics of the individual's constitution. It is thus evident that the body constitution consists of variation in physical structure, physiological function and psychological character.

1 Variation in Physical Structure

Variation in physical structure, including internal and external structures, is an important component of an individual's constitutional character. External

221

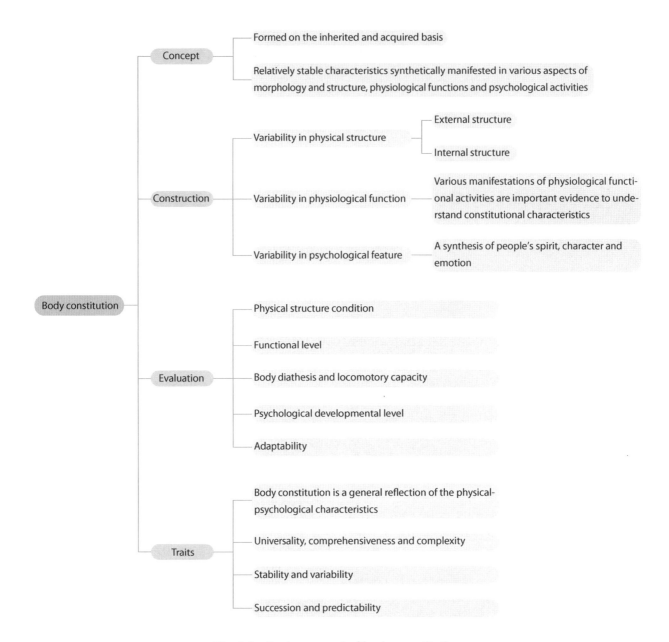

Fig. 5-1 Basic concept of body constitution

structure points to external appearance, while internal structure is the internal foundation of body constitution. Together, the two aspects form an organic whole that is represented through external variation in such aspects as appearance, physique and figure.

External appearance includes a person's physique, figure, body weight, character, gestures, complexion, and hair. As a whole, they can reflect their level of growth and development, nutritional state and physical fitness. These factors are intimately related to the occurrence and treatment of disease. For instance, overweight people are prone to develop damp syndromes, and thin people fire syndromes.

② Variation in Physiological Function

Variation in physiological function is another important factor in an individual's constitutional character. It is a reflection of the integrity and cooperation of internal physical structures, and a reflection of the functional activity of the viscera and channels, qi, blood and body fluids. The various manifestations of physiological activities are important evidence for understanding constitutional character.

③ Variation in Psychological Character

The psychological element of an individual is a synthesis of spirit, character and emotion, the major aspects in which the variations of a person's psychological nature are embodied.

The psychological element is a reflection of physical structure and physiological function. It manifests in different forms based upon the functional status of the viscera, qi and blood in ways such as short temper, depression, courage or bashfulness. Physical structure and physiological function are the material basis for psychological character, mutually affecting each other in a manner that leads to various psychological or behavioral characteristics.

Psychological character is also closely related to an individual's life experience and socio-cultural environment. Therefore, an individual may present different psychological states under different circumstances.

Evaluation of Body Constitution

Evaluation of body constitution should be an integrated consideration of physical structure, physiological function and psychological character.

① Criteria for Evaluating Body Constitution

(1) *Physical structure and condition*, including external appearance, physique, figure, and internal integrity and coordination.
(2) *Functional level*, including the functions of all organs and systems, especially cardiovascular and respiratory.
(3) *Body diathesis and motor capacity*, including speed, strength, endurance, sensitivity, coordination, and basic activities of walking, jumping, running, throwing and climbing, etc.
(4) *Level of psychological development*, including intelligence, emotions, behavior, sensibility, consciousness, personality, temperament, and volition.
(5) *Adaptability*, including the capability to adapt to various changes in natural and social environments, as well as resistance to illness and the ability to recover from it.

② Criteria for an Ideal Healthy Constitution

An ideal body constitution refers to a state of harmonized unity between physique and spirit, beginning with ample development of genetic potential and proper nurturing and care for the body that results in harmony of the physical structure, physiological functions, psychological character and a strong adaptability to environment. A healthy constitution includes both physical and psychological health. The identification of ideal constitution should be based on the following:

a. Sound physical development, strong physique, balanced figure, proper body weight.

b. Moist and slightly ruddy complexion, clear eyesight, lustrous beard and hair, fine skin and muscular elasticity.

c. Loud, clear voice, solid teeth, proper hearing, adequately rested, normal urine and stool, peaceful pulse manifestation.

d. Agile movements, with sound motor activity.

e. Optimistic and energetic, with tactile awareness and motivation.

f. A positive attitude, calm and with clear objectives, rational and creative.

g. Strong ability to adapt, comfortable in various environments, able to manage stress and resist negative stimuli and disease.

Characteristics of Body Constitution

① Body Constitution is a Summary of an Individual's Unique Physical-psychological Character

Body constitution is a reflection of the unique characteristics of physical structure, physiological function and psychological activity, and represents an outline of an individual's physical and psychological qualities.

② Universality, Comprehensiveness and Complexity

Body constitution exists universally within each individual. An individual's physical and psychological characteristics are fully expressed in the body's structure, function, and emotional state. The constitution of each individual is inherently unique and complex.

③ Stability and Variability

Body constitution is both inherited genetically and acquired during development. Genetic endowment determines the inherent stability and unique features of an individual's body constitution, traits that remain relatively stable for a given period of one's life. Body constitution also exhibits a certain degree of variability, or, evolution, based on a variety of environmental factors such as diet and nutrition, psychological factors, age, and illness or injury.

④ Continuity and Predictability

The continuity of body constitution refers the existence of different individuals and the continuous nature of variation. The characteristics of body constitution accompany an individual from the beginning to the end of the life process. People exhibit individual developmental and evolutionary patterns associated with their body constitution, therefore making future change predictable to a certain degree. This predictability provides clues for the practice of "preventing future illness before it occurs".

Section 2   Formation of Body Constitution

The formation of body constitution is the sum of various complicated factors both internal and external, which can be divided into the two main categories of congenital and acquired factors.

Congenital Factors

Congenital factors, or genetic endowment, refer to all characteristics inherited from the parents prior to birth and include genetic inheritance as determined by the parents' sex cells at conception, blood relationship between parents, their age, as well as any factors that may have influenced proper development or health of the fetus during pregnancy.

Genetic endowment is the material foundation for determining body constitution and represents the preset conditions that will affect its strength or weakness.Important influential factors include (Fig. 5-2):

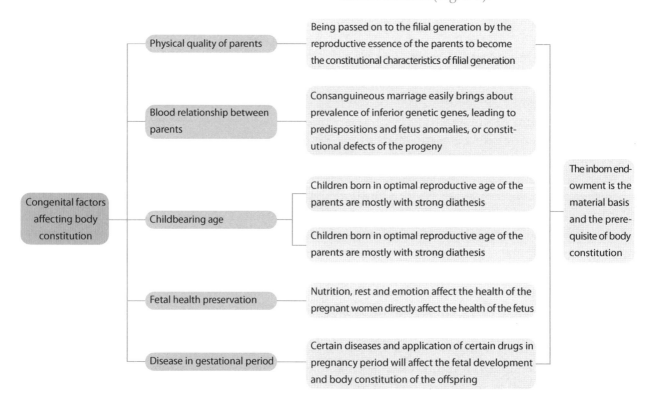

Fig. 5-2   Influential congenital factors on the formation of body constitution

① Physical Quality of the Parents

The life of the filial generation originates from the reproductive essence of the parents. Their physical quality and diathetic features are passed on to the filial generation and become the constitutional characteristics of the filial generation. Parental characteristics such as strong or weak, fat or thin, hard or soft, tall or short, skin color, disposition, temperament, and inherited defects and hereditary disorders (pigeon chest, humpback, epilepsy, asthma), are all related to genetic factors. Thus, parents with good diathesis and abundant kidney essence produce strong filial offspring, while those with weak diathesis and deficient kidney essence produce weak filial offspring.

Miraculous Pivot: The Dredge of Qi (Líng Shū: Jué Qì, 灵枢·决气*)* states: *"The two essences converge and a new life is formed."*

Miraculous Pivot: The Natural Span of Life (Líng Shū: Tiān Nián, 灵枢·天年*)* states: *"The beginning of human life...takes the mother as foundation and father as the frame."*

Induction on Pediatrics: Fetal diseases (Yòu Kē Fā Huī: Tāi Jí, 幼科发挥·胎疾*)* states: *"The filial generation is the branch of the parents."*

② Blood Relationship between Parents

Modern biomedicine holds that consanguineous marriage often leads to the prevalence of genetic defects, fetal abnormalities, constitutional defects such as physical weakness or mental retardation, also mentioned in early ancient classics.

The Twenty Third Year of Duke Xi, Zuo's Commentary (Zuǒ Zhuàn, Xī Gōng Èr Shí Sān Nián, 左传·僖公二十三年*): "Couples of the same surname do not proliferate."*

③ Age of the Parents

Childbearing age has a direct influence on the constitution of the offspring. Children with strong diathesis are mostly born to parents of optimal reproductive age, with strong vital energy and kidney essence. Children born to parents either too old or too young are susceptible to inherit a weak constitutional foundation.

Effective Prescription for Women (Fù Rén Liáng Fāng, 妇人良方*)* states: *"People should be married at the appropriate age. Though men sexually mature at sixteen, they should marry at thirty; though a woman's kidney essence begins to function at fourteen, she should wed at twenty. With both yin and yang in their prime, the couple unites and the woman conceives, giving birth to a strong and robust baby."*

④ Nurturing the Fetus

A pregnant woman should take special care in maintaining a healthy diet, daily lifestyle, physical and psychological state in order to guarantee the normal development of the fetus. Nutrition, rest and emotions all affect the health of a pregnant woman and directly affect the health of the fetus, and consequently, the baby following birth. Proper attention to health during pregnancy is therefore very important. A pregnant woman should avoid inappropriate air temperature or diet, maintain a regular daily rhythm and a pleasant mood, and abstain from sexual activity.

⑤ Disease during Pregnancy

Certain diseases during pregnancy will affect fetal development and the body constitution of the child. Certain herbs and pharmaceuticals may also adversely affect the fetus. Pregnant women should take care to avoid disease and illness.

Acquired Factors

In comparison to congenital factors which form the material foundation for body constitution, acquired factors affect the variation and evolution of an individual's constitution. A favorable living environment and peaceful emotions may promote physical and mental health and allow the full potential of an individual's constitution to be expressed; poor living conditions and emotional instability lead to weakened body constitution, and eventually, disease. (Fig. 5-3)

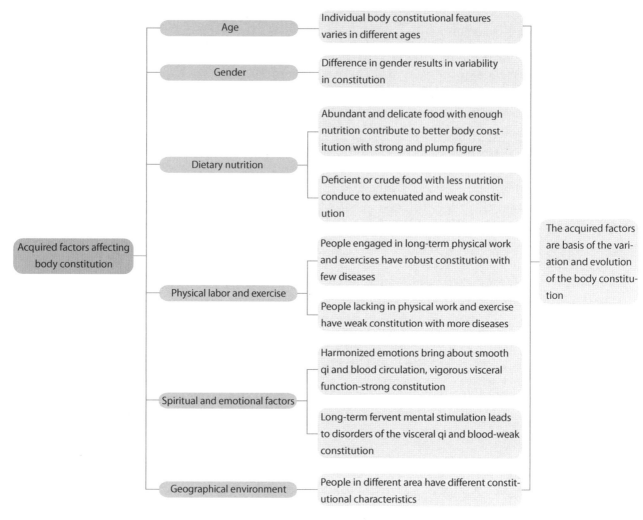

Fig. 5-3　Acquired Factors Affecting Body Constitution

① Age

The variation in individual body constitution at different ages originates from the changes in the physiological functions of the viscera, channels, qi, blood, essence and bodily fluids. Therefore, different stages in life result in correlative differences in constitution.

Childhood is the earliest stage of development of the human body. It grows vivaciously, however, the viscera are still very delicate and the qi and blood still immature, a state characterized as "infantile yin and yang". When afflicted by illness, children easily become excess or deficient, hot or cold. Because the body's vitality is strong yet unstable, children easily become ill and quickly recover.

Adolescence, or puberty, is a period during which the human body gradually matures, physical form continues to grow, and the body's physiological functions become complete. In the end of this stage, the body's diathesis is mostly fixed.

Young adulthood is the period during which the human body is at its peak, robust in visceral functions and rich in qi and blood. An individual reaches both physiological and psychological maturity and the body constitution is in its healthiest state with plenty of vigor and few illnesses. Even if disease does occur, it usually presents as an excessive syndrome that is easily cured.

In the elderly stages of life, visceral functions decline, qi and blood wane, and consequently, the body constitution is weakened. It manifests in the appearance of senility and the decline of mental faculties. Aged people become more susceptible to illness and it becomes more difficult for them to make a complete recovery.

The influence of age on body constitution is most important during puberty and young adulthood. Puberty is the first transitional stage of life when sexual maturity is reached. It is also a period when physical structure, physiological functions and metabolism all undergo dramatic changes and is a time when individuals should take care to exercise and nurture the body properly in order to strengthen the constitution. It is the turning point from adulthood to old age, and represents the second transitional stage toward gradual decline of the life systems and organs, both structurally and functionally. Cultivation of good health should be emphasized in order to preserve the remaining constitutional strength and extend life expectancy.

Miraculous Pivot: The Natural Span of Life (*Líng Shū: Tiān Nián*, 灵枢·天年) states: "*At the age of ten, the five zang organs begin to be settle, circulation of qi and blood is complete; qi flourishes in the lower half of the body, making children very active. At the age of twenty, qi and blood begin to flourish; the muscles grow strong, making people apt to move quickly. At the age of thirty, the viscera are completely settled, the muscles are solid, and the blood becomes full, making people prefer to walk. At forty, all the viscera and channels are fully developed and stable, the striae starts to loosen, the luster of the complexion begins to fade and hair grays, people prefer to sit. At fifty, the liver qi begins to decline and the gall fluid becomes thin, vision begins to blur. At sixty, the heart qi starts to decline, circulation of qi and blood becomes sluggish, people often suffer from sorrow and grief, and tend to lie down. At seventy, the spleen qi becomes deficient and the skin withers. At eighty, the lung qi starts to fade and the vigor departs, people are prone to senility and mistakes in speech. At ninety, the kidney qi is consumed causing the other four viscera and the channels to become vacant. At the age of one hundred, the five viscera are deficient and both spirit and qi perish, leaving the human body alone until life concludes.*"

Plain Questions: Major Discussion on the Theory of Yin and Yang and the Corresponding Relationships Among All the Things in Nature (*Yīn Yáng Yìng Xiàng Dà Lùn*, 素问·阴阳应象大论) states: "*At the age of forty, half the yin essence is lost, and people begin to grow weak in daily life. At fifty, the body feels heavy, the eyes and ears begin to decline. At sixty, sexual function in males is reduced, qi greatly declines, the orifices no longer function appropriately and yang qi becomes deficient in the lower body and excessive in the upper body, secretions of the nose and eyes appear.*"

② Gender

The most basic type of human constitutional division is that of male and female. Due to the differences in genetic character, body configuration, visceral structure, physiological function and psychological character between them, the body constitutions differ accordingly.

Generally speaking, the male is virile, staunch and strong, with a robust physique, powerful visceral functions and physical work capacity, with an open and extroverted character; the female is feminine, gentle and amicable, with a soft and slim figure, relatively weak physically, with a reserved and introverted character. Diseases in males are mostly those that injure the essence and qi, such as nocturnal and spontaneous emissions; female diseases mostly centered on the blood with illnesses relating to the menstrual cycle, vaginal secretion, pregnancy and child birth.

Miraculous Pivot: The Five Tones and Five Tastes (*Líng Shū: Wǔ Yīn Wǔ Wèi*, 灵枢·五音五味) states: "*Women are born with an excess of qi and a deficiency of blood, due to the unavoidable loss of blood throughout life.*"

③ Diets and Nutrition

Nutrition from food and drink is an important factor in determining the strength of body diathesis. Following birth, it is the source of all nourishment for the human body. Different living condition and dietary habits, different quantity and quality of food intake together gradually lead to constitutional discrepancy.

Generally speaking, the nutritional intake of those with an abundant and well-rounded diet is sufficient and contributes to a better constitution with a strong, full figure; an insufficient or overly-simple diet poor in nutrition leads to a weak constitution with a thin, underdeveloped figure. However, overeating or addiction to greasy, rich foods may cause obesity, qi deficiency and excessive phlegm. Simple, whole foods enough to alley hunger are good for smooth circulation of qi and blood and prevent the generation of phlegm, resulting in a favorable constitution.

The human body needs various nutritive substances, so a proper diet is a diverse one. Addiction to a certain type of food leads to a deficiency of certain nutrients and an excess of others, which in turn can lead to yin-yang deficiency or excess of the *zang* organs, qi and blood, over time, a partial diathesis, and even disease. For instance, addiction to sweet, greasy, rich foods may aid the generation of damp, forming a damp phlegm constitution; addiction to pungent and spicy foods leads to generation of fire, burning bodily fluids, forming a yin-deficient constitution with hyperactive fire; over consumption of salty foods damages the heart, forming constitution with weak heart qi; overeating raw and cold foods injures the spleen and stomach, forming a constitution with deficient spleen and stomach qi; addiction to alcohol results in the generation of damp heat, which tends to impair the liver and spleen.

Proper dietary habits with appropriate nutritional intake are therefore of utmost significance for an ideal body constitution.

Plain Questions: Discussion on Special Disease (Sù Wèn: Qí Bìng Lùn, 素问·奇病论) states: *"Fatty foods lead to internal heat and sweet foods cause abdominal distension."*

Plain Questions: Discussion on Interrelationship Between Life and Nature (Sù Wèn: Shēng Qì Tōng Tiān Lùn, 素问·生气通天论) states: *"Addiction to sour foods leads to excessive liver qi that over restricts the spleen qi; addiction to salty foods causes damage to the skeleton, short muscles, and depresses heart qi; addiction to sweet foods leads to obstruction of the heart qi, a dark complexion, and imbalance of kidney*

qi; addiction to bitter foods leads to loss of the spleen qi and thickness of the stomach qi; addiction to pungent foods leads to slackening of the tendons and a wearied spirit."

④ Physical Labor and Exercise

Proper labor and exercise may loosen one's muscles, tendons and bones, relax the joints, promote the circulation of qi and blood, enhance visceral activity, and facilitate the digestion and absorption of food. People engaged in long-term physical work have strong muscles, tendons and bones, prosperous visceral function, a robust constitution with few illnesses. On the contrary, being lazy, living a comfortable and luxurious life leads to sluggish qi and blood circulation, muscles, tendons and bones are slack, visceral function declines, and a weak constitution is formed, even causing illness. Physical labor and exercise should be done in proper amount. Over exertion leads to injuries of the tendons and bones, consumption of qi and blood, declined visceral functions, and finally formation of a weak constitution.

Plain Questions; Discussion on Pain (Sù Wèn: Jǔ Tòng Lùn, 素问·举痛论) states: *"Over exertion consumes qi."*

Plain Questions: Discussion on the Elucidation of Five-Qi (Sù Wèn: Xuān Míng Wǔ Qì Piān, 素问·宣明五气篇) states: *"Excessive observation hurts the blood, excessive bed rest impairs qi, prolonged sitting injures the muscles, extended standing injures the bones, and constant walking injures the tendons. These are known as the five impairments of over exertion."*

⑤ Psychological and Emotional Factors

Psychological and emotional activities take the visceral qi and blood as their material basis. Emotional changes are accompanied by changes in qi and blood of the viscera and affect the body constitution. Positive emotions bring about smooth qi and blood circulation, vigorous visceral functions, and a strong constitution, whereas long-term fervent mental stimulation or persistent emotional strain will exceed the range of physiologic adjustment, leading to deficiency or disorders of the visceral qi and blood (discussed in detail in Chapter 7), harm the body constitution, and even cause disease. People who unpredictably fluctuate between rage and depression are of the "wood-fire constitution", and are prone to dizziness and apoplexy; those who fall into long-term melancholy and sadness have a "stagnant liver constitution", which may be related to the development of cancer. The maintenance of a favorable mental state is beneficial to the preservation of good health and boosts the constitution.

⑥ Geographical Environment

The differences in topography, properties of water and earth, natural resources, climatic characteristics, dietary habits, living conditions, life style, and social customs, etc., among different geographic regions, contribute to variation in physical structure, physiological function and psychological behavior among various peoples of different regions.

In general, a rough geographical environment rears individuals with a strong, muscular physique and forceful temperament; a more mild geographical environment produces a delicate physique and gentle temperament. As far as the geography and climate of China are concerned, the south is damp and hot, the north is dry and cold; the eastern coastal area has an oceanic climate, the western hinterlands has an interior, continental climate. As a result, the people of northwestern China are strong in physique with closed striae, tough temperament, and have a sound resistance to disease, whereas those in south eastern China have a relatively weak physique with loose striae, gentle temperament, and inferior resistance to illness.

Moreover, the economic conditions, living standards, marital and child rearing customs, treatment of disease and difference between city and countryside are also important factors that affect the body constitution.

Treatise on the Headstream of Medicine: Discussion on Diversified Treatments of People of Different Places (Yī Xué Yuán Liú Lùn: Wǔ Fāng Yì Zhì Lùn, 医学源流论 · 五方异治论) states: *"Humans are born with the endowment of heaven and earth, so the body constitution varies according to different places."*

Section 3 Categorization of Body Constitution

Categorization Method of Body Constitution

The theoretical system of Chinese medicine takes the concept of holism as its guiding concept, with the theory of yin and yang and the five phases as its conceptual framework, and the doctrines of visceral organs, qi, blood and bodily fluids as its theoretical basis for determining the various body constitutions of different individuals within a given population. For instance, the yin-yang grouping method places special emphasis on the yin or yang; the visceral grouping method uses visceral structure and function; the qi, blood, bodily fluids grouping method emphasizes the shortage of these substances and their metabolic abnormalities; the physical appearance grouping method considers the external appearance of the body: and the personality grouping method places importance on personality traits such as rough or gentle, brave or timid, etc. The yin-yang grouping method will be discussed in further detail in the section below.

Miraculous Pivot: Connecting with the Heavens (Líng Shū: Tōng Tiān, 灵枢 · 通天) states: *"There are the five kinds of individuals: Taiyin, Shaoyin, Taiyang, Shaoyang and Balanced Yin-Yang, whose body constitutions are different due to the diversity of tissue, bone, qi and blood."*

Commonly Used Constitutional Categories and Their Characteristics

An ideal, healthy constitution is one of balanced yin and yang. However, yin and yang are in the constant process of waxing and waning change, leading to yin-superior or yang-superior states of the normal constitution. As a result, the normal constitutions include the balanced yin-yang constitution, yang-superior constitution and yin-superior constitution. (Fig. 5-4)

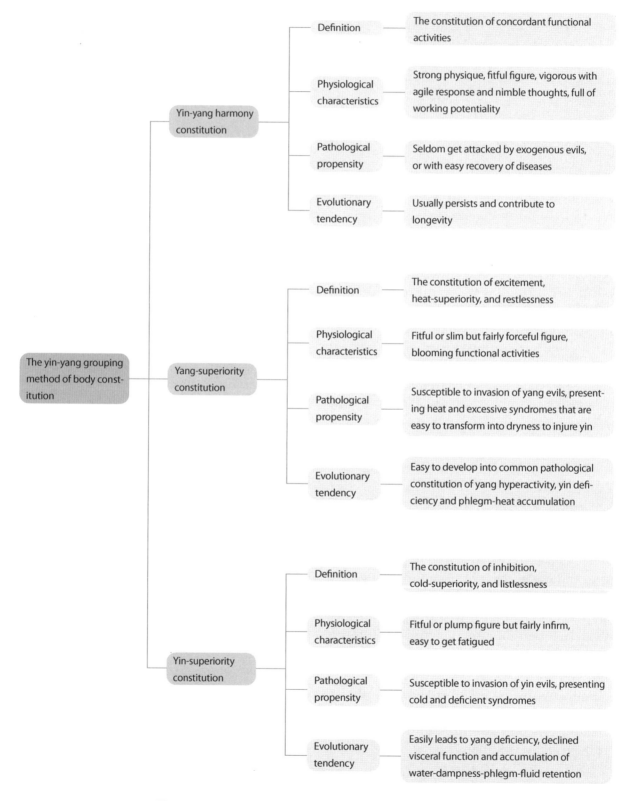

Fig. 5-4   Yin-yang grouping method of body constitution

Plain Questions: Discussion on the Regulation of Channels (*Sù Wèn: Tiáo Jīng Lùn*, 素问·调经论) states: "People with balanced yin and yang... are named healthy or normal people."

Plain Questions: Discussion on Interrelationship Between Life and Nature (*Sù Wèn: Shēng Qì Tōng Tiān Lùn*, 素问·生气通天论) states: "With yin and yang in relative equilibrium, the life activities are maintained."

① Balanced Yin-Yang Constitution

(1) Definition

This refers to a constitution of well-coordinated body functions.

(2) Physiological characteristics

Physiological characteristics appear as a strong, fit physique, or slightly plump but not obese, or thin, but energetic; a lustrous and bright facial complexion and skin color, with the possibility of a slight tendency toward any of the five colors; open and agreeable personality; proper diet, normal urine and stool; peaceful sleep at night with sound recuperation; vigorous with agile responses and focused thoughts, full of working potential; red and moist tongue with peaceful and forceful pulse.

(3) Pathological predisposition

People of this constitution are rarely afflicted by exogenous evils owing to their strong self-regulatory ability and adaptability to external environment and seldom fall ill. When struck with illness, they mostly suffer from external and excessive syndromes with a quick recovery, often without the need for medicine.

(4) Evolutionary tendency

Provided that external injury and chronic disease are avoided, the constitution of balanced yin and yang, assisted by proper nurturing and living habits, will continue and contribute to longevity.

Miraculous Pivot: Connecting with the Heavens (*Líng Shū: Tōng Tiān*, 灵枢·通天) states: "Those having a constitution of balanced yin and yang, living in quiet and non-interference, who do not easily become frightened or delighted, who do not contend for power but conform to the changing environment, being modest and courteous to others. This is of utmost importance to the physical and psychological balance."

Miraculous Pivot: The Natural Span of Life (*Líng Shū: Tiān Nián*, 灵枢·天年) states: "With strong zang viscera, well regulated qi and blood circulation, properly functioning muscles, and compacted striae, with evenly flowing nutritive and defensive qi, normal respiration, the six fu viscera working well in transforming food and water, bodily fluids evenly distributed, things are as they should be. People in possession of these traits will enjoy long life and good health."

② Yang-Superior Constitution

(1) Definition

This refers to a constitution of excitability, dominant heat, and restlessness.

(2) Physiological characteristics

The physiological characteristics of a yang-superior constitution manifest as a slightly thin, but solid figure; reddish or darkish complexion with oily skin; outgoing character, fidgety or irritable, with weak self-control; healthy appetite with good digestion and absorption; prone to constipation and dark and scanty urinations; preference for cold drinks with an aversion to heat, or relatively high body temperature, with heavy sweating and thirst; very energetic with agile motions, and strong libido; reddish tongue and lips with thin, yellow coating, with a yang-natured pulse.

(3) Pathological predisposition

People of this constitution are susceptible to invasion of yang evils such as wind, heat and summer-heat, and suffer from hot and excessive syndromes, with a tendency to transform into dryness and injure yin. Skin lesions and ulcers often appear. Various internal diseases result in syndromes of excessive fire, hyperactive yang and deficient yin. Symptoms include dizziness, headache, palpitations, insomnia and various types of bleeding.

(4) Evolutionary tendency

The long term hyperactivity of yang in people of this constitution, with excessive motion and insufficient rest, eventually consumes yin. Unbalanced life style, excessive strain, excessive contemplation and worry, excessive sexual activity, improper diet (especially of spicy foods) or excessive smoking or drinking results in metabolic hyperactivity that damages yin, with tendencies toward excessive yang, yin deficiency, and fire-phlegm pathological development.

③ Yin-Superior Constitution

(1) Definition

This refers to a constitution of inhibition, dominant cold, and listlessness.

(2) Physiological characteristics

The physiological characteristics of a yin-superior constitution manifest as a fit, or slightly overweight, but soft physique, easily fatigued; dull, pale complexion; introverted character, timid and easily frightened with little movement and a preference for quiet; limited appetite with normal digestion and absorption; preference for heat and aversion to cold, or relatively low body temperature; lethargic with sluggish motions, dull reactions, and a weak libido; pale tongue and lips, with a yin-natured pulse.

(3) Pathological predisposition

People of this constitution are susceptible to the invasion of yin evils such as cold and damp, and suffer from cold and deficient syndromes, easy transmitted internally leading to visceral damage. Frostbite is commonly observed. Various internal diseases result in syndromes of dominant yin, together with yang deficiency. Damp accumulation, edema, phlegmatic fluid retention and blood stasis may also appear.

(4) Evolutionary tendency

The long-term dominance of yin in people of this constitution eventually damages yang, leading to yang deficiency, declined visceral function and accumulation of water-damp, phlegmatic fluid retention, and blood stasis.

It should be pointed out that the terms of yin deficiency, yang deficiency, yin dominant, yang dominant, qi deficiency, blood deficiency, phlegmatic fluid, blood stasis, etc., are conceptually different from those cognominal syndrome names in the theoretical system of syndrome differentiation and treatment determination. Constitutional groups reflect the characteristics of an individual's health that are present during times when the individual is free from illness, such as a yin deficient constitution or qi deficient constitution. A syndrome is an analysis of the pathological nature of a given stage in a disease course, such as yin deficiency and qi deficiency. However, constitution is the basis for disease. The type of an individual's constitution exerts a strong influence on the type of syndrome that ensues, especially with chronic disease. When illness occurs, the syndrome type often coincides with the constitutional type, proving the intimate relationship between the two.

Section 4　Application of the Doctrine of Body Constitution

Variation in body constitution originates from the rise and decline of the viscera and the channels and the wax and wane of qi, blood and body fluids, which are reflections of the rise and decline of the right qi of the body. This contributes to the difference in susceptibility to disease, its development and the individual's response to therapy among various constitutional types. Therefore body constitution is closely related to etiology, onset of disease, pathomechanics, syndrome differentiation, determination of treatment, health maintenance and disease prevention. It represents an important factor in "suiting treatment to fit the individual", an important guideline in clinical practice. (Fig. 5-5)

Body Constitution and Etiology

Body constitution determines the individual's susceptibility to certain pathogens. The yin or yang inclination of body diathesis reflects different functional states and selectivity to external stimulation, hence the susceptibility to different pathogens. Generally speaking, an individual of yang superior constitution is

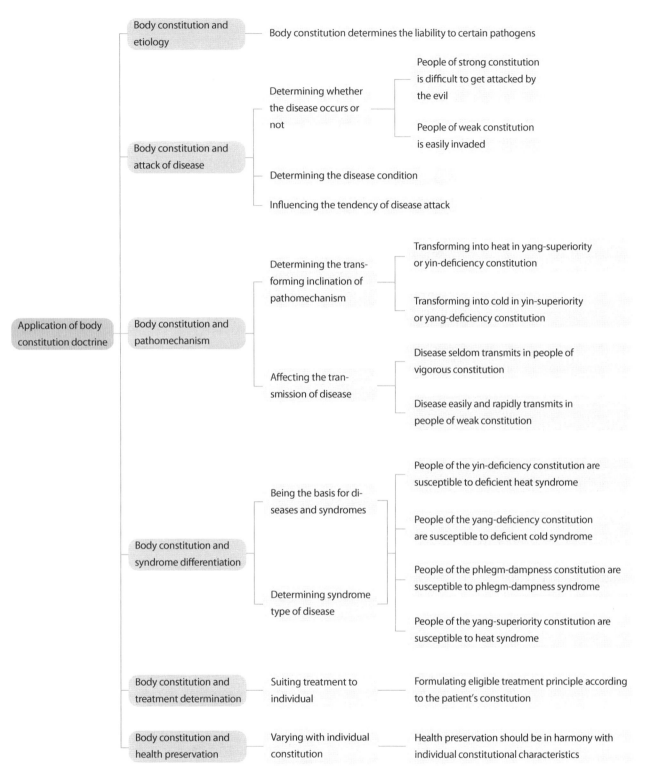

Fig. 5-5   Application of the doctrine of body constitution

susceptible to heat or summer-heat pathogens but resistant to cold; and a yin superior constitution is liable to cold and damp evils but resistant to heat.

Body Constitution and Onset of Disease

Body constitution determines whether or not

disease occurs. The Chinese medical theory of pathogenesis holds that, the pathogen invasion is an important condition and the deficiency of right qi is the internal foundation for the onset of disease, and that the result of the struggle between vital and evil qi is the key determining factor. Consequently, the rise and decline of right qi is closely related to the strength or weakness of the constitution. A strong constitution with vigorous vial qi and efficient resistance to disease is difficult for pathogens to attack, whereas a weak constitution with feeble right qi and inferior resistance to disease is easily invaded.

The body constitution determines the conditions of disease. After initial invasion, the conditions of disease vary according to different types of body constitution, making the onset of disease sudden, latent, or recurrent.

Constitution also influences the tendencies of the onset of disease. Usually children, with delicate viscera and a tender constitution are prone to coughing, diarrhea, food stagnation; aged people, with depressed visceral function and a weak constitution are liable to phlegmatic fluid retention, coughing, dyspnea, palpitations, and diabetes; obese people or people with profuse internal damp phlegm are susceptible to apoplexy and dizziness; thin or yin deficient people commonly suffer from pulmonary tuberculosis and coughing.

Miraculous Pivot: The Five Kinds of Affections (*Líng Shū: Wǔ Biàn*, 灵枢·五变): *"People with flabby muscles and loosened striae are easily attacked by the wind...those with weak zang viscera are prone to diabetes(xiao dan, 消瘅) ...those with a small and fragile physique are liable to suffer from chills and fever.. .those with flaccid muscles and rough skin are susceptible to joint inflammation."*

Body Constitution and Pathomechanics

Body constitution determines the patterns of transformation of pathomechanics. After invasion by a pathogen, the pathological nature of the disease often changes according to the type of constitution. The general law is,

the pathological nature of the disease usually transforms into heat in yang superior or yin-deficient constitutions with relatively excited metabolic activity, and into cold in yin-superior or yang-deficient constitutions with relatively inhibited metabolic activity; transforms into dryness in blood-fluid deficient constitution and into damp in a constitution of qi-deficiency with profuse dampness. Due to the inherent nature of the body, there arise the transformations of heat, cold, dryness, and damp.

Constitution also affects the transmission of disease. Disease transmission is related to the strength of the evil and whether it is properly treated, but more importantly it is determined by constitutional factors, that is, the strength of the right qi. An individual of vigorous constitution is full of right qi, the resistance is strong and so disease is seldom transmitted; an individual of weak constitution is lacking in right qi, resistance is feeble and disease is transmitted easily and rapidly, resulting in a worsened or even life threatening condition.

Body Constitution and Syndrome Differentiation

Body constitution is the foundation for the development of disease and their syndrome diagnoses. Many syndromes are derived from their correlating type of constitution. As an example, an individual with a yin deficient constitution is susceptible to syndromes of yin deficiency; the same holds true for a damp phlegm constitution.

Body constitution determines the type of syndrome. One possibility is when the same pathogen attacks people of different constitutional types and leads to different syndrome types, i.e. the same disease with different syndromes. For instance, if a cold pathogen arises, the right qi of people with a strong constitution can resist the evil at the body's surface, manifest as exterior wind-cold syndrome with chills, fever, lack of sweating, general aching; people of a weak constitution deficient in right qi and will be unable to resist the pathogen, allowing the evil to invade internally and cause interior cold syndrome of spleen yang deficiency, with aversion to cold, cold limbs, lack of appetite, cold pain in the abdomen and diarrhea. Another example is the common cold may manifest as an exterior wind-cold syndrome, exterior wind-heat syndrome, or exterior wind-damp syndrome, due to different types of body constitution.

On the other hand, when attacked by various different pathogens, people of the same or similar body constitutions may present similar or even identical syndromes, i.e. different diseases with the same syndrome. For example, an individual with a yang-heat constitution displays a heat syndrome when attacked both by wind-cold evil or summer-heat evil. Both chronic diarrhea and edema may be present in syndromes of yang deficiency of the spleen or kidney when occurring in people of the same body constitution.

Body Constitution and Treatment Determination

The relationship between body constitution and treatment determination is summarized as "suiting treatment to fit the individual", meaning to formulate proper treatment principles according to the patient's constitution, age, and gender. Age and gender also affect body constitution, therefore making body constitution the central factor in "suiting treatment to fit the individual".

There are constitution types of weak and strong, yin and yang, cold and hot. In addition to differentiating syndromes, individual variation in constitution should be paid close attention when deciding upon treatment methods. Generally speaking, people of strong constitution are prone to excessive syndromes, purging methods are to beused; weak constitution easily leads to deficiency or mixed deficiency and excess syndromes, tonification or simultaneous purging-tonifying therapy is to be utilized accordingly. When treating patients of yang superior constitution (dominant yang or deficient yin), the

use of warm and hot herbs should be restricted to avoid generation of excessive fire; when treating patients of yin superior constitution (yin dominant or yang deficient), the use of cool and cold herbs should be restricted in order to prevent further hyperactivity of yin and damage to yang. For example, a person with a yang deficient constitution is attacked by a cold pathogen, it is prone to transform through yin into cold. Hot, pungent herbs should be applied to warm yang and dispel cold. In an individual with a yin deficient constitution, internal fire is easily aroused, and similar to the above example, transforms through yang into heat. Cooling, moistening treatment methods should be used.

Body constitution also affects the selection of herbs of different natures and flavors. The four natures of cold, cool, warm and hot, and the five flavors of pungent, sweat, sour, bitter and salty should be selected with consideration for body constitution in addition to the nature of the syndrome. In most cases, patients of a yin deficient constitution are to be treated with sweet-cold, sour-cold, salty-cold, clear and moistening drugs, while herbs of pungent-heat and dispersing nature or bitter-cold descending nature should be avoided; patients of a yang deficient constitution should be treated with methods of warming and tonifying, while bitter-cold drugs should be avoided; patients of a qi deficient constitution should be treated by replenishing the primordial qi with sweet-warm herbs, while the use of purging and dissipating through bitter-cold herbs is prohibited; patients of a damp phlegm constitution should be treated by invigorating the spleen with aromatic herbs, and resolving the damp phlegm through warming, tonifying with sour and sweet herbs is prohibited.

The unique nature of an individual's constitution also effects the amount of herbs to be administered. Different constitutions react differently to different herbs and dosage should therefore be determined with consideration to body constitution. In general, people of strong constitutions are more tolerant to herbs, dosage may be relatively larger, and the nature of the herbs may be relatively intense. People of weak constitution are less tolerant to herbs; dosage should be relatively small and the nature of the herbs relatively mild and peaceful.

People with allergies should avoid administration of sensitive drugs.

Body Constitution and Health Maintenance

Health maintenance refers to the cultivation of one's physique and temperament, to boost body constitution, prevent disease and improve longevity. It should be in harmony with an individual's constitutional characteristics.

For example, in considering proper dietary health, people of heat dominant constitutions should eat foods with a cool nature and avoid heat; those of cold dominant constitutions should eat foods of warm nature and avoid cold. People with yin deficient constitutions should take in sweet and moistening foods, avoiding greasy and rich, or pungent and spicy foods; those with yang deficient constitutions should consume warm, tonifying, but not raw or cold foods. Obese people of damp phlegm constitutions should have clear and light foods and avoid sweet and oily foods.

In the respect to the cultivation of mental health, introverted people, being prone to depression, unhappiness and frustration, should find outlets for their emotions, participate in more group activities, or converse with other people in order to alleviate the negative internal stasis. For irritable people who are easily agitated, patience and tolerance should be cultivated.

Chapter 6
Etiology

Concept of Pathogen

The term 'pathogen' refers to the cause of a disease, and is also called "etiological factor", "evil", "pathogenic factor", etc.. Various factors, such as the six exogenous pathogens, pestilential pathogens, seven emotions, inappropriate diet, irregular work and rest, trauma, etc., can function as pathogens and lead to disease.

During the disease process, certain pathological byproducts are retained within the body, sometimes leading to new illnesses, thus becoming pathogenic factors themselves. Pathological byproducts such as phlegm, blood stasis, and calculus, etc. originate from pathogenic factors, and are also termed secondary pathogens.

Etiology is an important part of the CM theoretical model that focuses on the formation, nature and characteristics of various pathogenic factors.

As stated in *The Origin and Development of Medicine: Various Pathogens of Same Disease* (*Yī Xué Yuán Liú Lùn: Bìng Tóng Yīn Bié Lùn*, 医学源流论·病同因别论), "*What people suffer from is called disease, and what causes disease are called pathogens.*"

Categorization of Pathogens

Medical scholars of past dynasties maintained different methods of classification for pathogens.

The Yellow Emperor's Classic of Internal Medicine (*Huáng Dì Néi Jīng,* 黄帝内经) holds that the pathogens can be categorized according to the two basic aspects of Yin and Yang. It is raised in *Plain Questions: Regulating the Channels* (*Sù Wèn: Tiáo Jīng Lùn,* 素问·调经论) , "*The evil emerges from either yin or yang. The wind, rain, coldness and summer heat usually generate yang evils, while inappropriate dietary and living habits, as well as uncontrolled emotions, may result in yin evils.*" That is, in other words, evils invading the body surface by exogenous ways such as climatic anomaly, are called "yang evils", and those affecting the internal organs of the body by endogenous ways, like improper dietary, living, sexual or emotional habits, are called "yin evils". Therefore, diseases are accordingly divided into two aspects of exogenous and endogenous.

Zhang Zhong-jing (张仲景) of the *Han* dynasty created a theory of dividing pathogens into 3 classes，as discussed in *Golden Chamber of Miscellaneous Diseases: Syndromes and Pulse Manifestations of Various Viscera and Channels* (*Jīn Kuì Yào Luè: Zàng Fǔ Jīng Luò Xiān Hòu Bìng Mài Zhèng,* 金匮要略·脏腑经络先后病脉证), "*The diversity of pathogens may be reduced to no more than three classes. Firstly, the evil that invades the viscera through the channels and collaterals, is endogenous; secondly, the evil that causes stagnation of the blood vessels of the extremities and orifices, is exogenous;*

and finally, improper sexual activities, metal blades, and animal and insect bites make up the third class, thus completing the categorization of the various causes of disease."

In the *Jin* Dynasty, Ge Hong (葛洪) proposed the principle of three types of pathogenic factors as *"endogenous, exogenous and invasive"* in his *Handbook of Prescriptions for Emergency: Three Kinds of Pathogens (Zhǒu Hòu Bèi Jí Fāng: Sān Yīn Lùn,*肘后备急方·三因论*)*.

Chen Wu-ze (陈无择) in *Song* dynasty established his theory of three pathogens in *Treatise on Three Categories of Pathogens: Volume 2 (Sānyīn Jí Yī Bìngzhèng Fāng Lùn: Juàn Èr,*三因极一病证方论·卷二*)* on the basis of *Golden Chamber of Miscellaneous Diseases (Jīn KuìYào Luè,* 金匮要略*)* and wrote, *"...there are three causes (of disease): the endogenous, exogenous and neither endogenous nor exogenous 'other' factors. The endogenous includes the seven emotional factors, the exogenous the six climatic pathogens, and the neither endogenous nor exogenous refers to those factors that cannot be included in the former two."* The content of this doctrine represents a great contribution to

the theoretical system of etiology and served as the foundation for following classification methods of etiology.

Modern classification systems usually divide the pathogens into four groups: exogenous, endogenous, secondary, and other pathogens, according to their different natures and the invading pathways (Fig. 6-1).

The Treatise on Three Categories of Pathogens: Volume 2, Essence of Five Subjects (Sān Yīn Jí Yī Bìng Zhèng Fāng Lùn: Juàn Èr, Wǔ Kē Fán Yào, 三因极一病证方论·卷二·五科凡要*)* states: *"The cause of a disease must be identified before treatment is decided. If the pathogen has not been properly identified, the etiology of the disease will remain unclear. The pathogens may be summed up into three groups: the endogenous, the exogenous and the neither endogenous nor exogenous... The six climatic pathogens: cold, summer-heat, the dryness, damp, wind, and heat... The seven emotional endopathogens include the excessive joy, anger, melancholy, anxiety, grief, fear, and terror. ......The former are normal climatic factors that invade the body's surface through the channels*

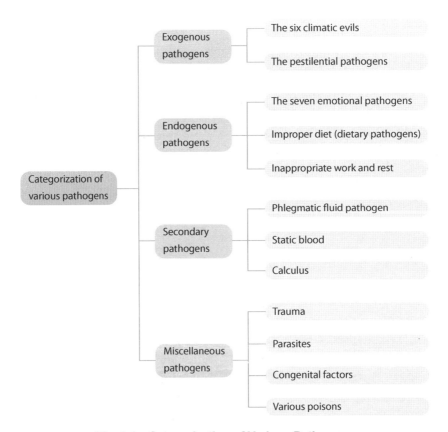

Fig. 6-1 Categorization of Various Pathogens

and collaterals and reside within the viscera, hence the name of exogenous pathogens. The latter are common human emotions, that when stirred, emerge forth from the correlated viscera when in excess and take form in the extremeties, and thus referred to as the endogenous pathogens. Others like improper diet, excessive use of the voice and breath, unconstrained mental, physical and sexual activities, animal and insect bites, metal blades, and chronic infectious disease coherence, etc., which go counter to the conventions of the nature, are categorized as the neither endogenous nor exogenous pathogens."

Methods for Understanding the Cause of Disease

The first method is interrogation, i.e. to understand the objective conditions that may have contributed to the onset of illness through detailed questioning of the disease process and other relevant factors. This is to confirm or to deduce the pathogen. Certain pathogens like emotional factors and external trauma can often be recognized through interrogation.

Syndrome differentiation can also be applied to understanding pathogens, analyzing the symptoms and signs of the disease to deduce its etiology, also known as "identification of etiology according to the differentiation of symptoms and signs". Onset of any disease is the result of pathogens acting on the human body. Symptoms and signs vary with the nature and pathogenic features of different pathogens. The etiology may therefore be identified by analysis of clinical manifestations.

In some cases there may be a discrepancy in the "cause" obtained from the "identification of etiology according to differentiation of symptoms and signs" and the "cause" obtained from the interrogation procedure. This is because the former is based on the disease's clinical manifestations, which appear only after the pathogen's attack on the human body. The cause obtained from inquiry into the patient's medical history usually matches the actual cause, or, primary pathogen, while the one surmised from syndrome differentiation often coincides with the synthesis of the pathogen and the organism's reaction to it. As a result, it may also be categorized as a pathomechanical factor. (Fig. 6-2, Fig. 6-3)

The syndrome differentiation method is the

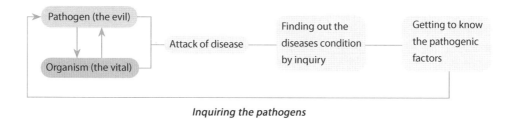

Inquiring the pathogens

Fig. 6-2　Etiological inquiry

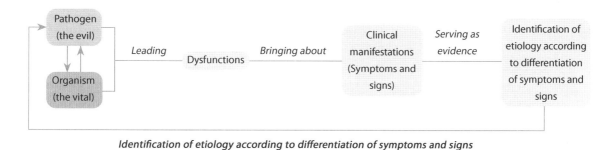

Identification of etiology according to differentiation of symptoms and signs

Fig. 6-3　Identification of etiology according to syndrome differentiation

primary method of understanding etiology. It is also one of the unique characteristics of Chinese medical etiology. Principles for treatment are also determined on the basis of this procedure, termed "determining treatment following identification of etiology".

Section 1　Exogenous Pathogens

Exogenous pathogens, or externally contracted pathogens, are those that invade the body from the external environment, through the body's surface, or by the orifices of the mouth or nose, and in turn lead to exogenous disease. In their early stages, externally contracted diseases have the characteristics of acute onset, chills, fever, and general aching pain throughout the body etc.

Exogenous pathogens include the six climatic pathogens and pestilential pathogens.

The Six Climatic Pathogens

① Basic Concepts of the Six Climatic Pathogens

The "six climatic pathogens", or "six climatic evils", is a general term for the cold, summer-heat, dryness, damp, wind, and heat (fire) evils. Under normal conditions they are called the "six climatic factors" and represent natural climatic changes.

The formation of externally contracted pathogens is closely related to abnormal climatic change. The six climatic factors may become pathogenic when they emerge in excess or deficiency, occur untimely or change abruptly. When the abnormalities of climatic change supersede the capability of the human body to adapt, or when the body's right qi is too weak to acclimatize and develops illness, the climatic abnormalities become climatic pathogens, known as the "six climatic evils". Here, the term "pathogen" has the meaning of "excessive" or "overactive", and represents deviation from natural equilibrium.

What is defined as "abnormal" climatic change is relative, and whether or not the six climatic pathogens lead to the onset of disease depends upon both the climatic anomaly and the condition of the body's right qi. Thus, although they may lead to diseases at any time, the six climatic pathogens tend to cause disease more often during periods of severe abnormality in climate change.

The six climatic pathogens are considered as externally contracted disease causing agents, or, exogenous evil, and are different from the "five evils produced by the five *zang* organs" that belong to the category of pathogenesis. To distinguish from the six climatic pathogens, i.e. cold, summer-heat, dryness, damp, wind, the heat (fire) evils, the five pathogens produced by five *zang*-organs are respectively referred to as endogenous wind, endogenous cold, the endogenous damp, endogenous dryness, and endogenous heat (fire), which are covered in detail in the chapter on pathomechanics.

② General Illness-Causing Characteristics of the Six Climatic Pathogens

The six climatic pathogens share the following common features:

A. External contraction

The six climatic pathogens attack mainly by way of the surface of the body or by the mouth and nose, and reside within the exterior. In the early stage of externally contracted illness, symptoms like chills, fever, sweating or lack of sweat, thin tongue coating, and floating pulse are commonly seen, and are collectively referred to as the exterior symptoms. Diseases caused by the exogenous pathogenic factors are also called externally contracted disease.

B. Seasonal nature

Seasonal nature is a prominent characteristic of the six climatic pathogens. They cause disease in correlation with the seasons. Wind attacks in spring, summer-heat in summer, dryness in autumn, and cold in winter. Due to this seasonal nature, externally contracted diseases are also called "seasonal diseases".

C. Regional nature

Diseases caused by the six climatic pathogens

often vary with region and environment. For instance, people living in humid areas are easily affected by damp, while those working in high temperature environments are prone to attack from heat and dryness.

D. Coexistence

Any of the six climatic pathogens may attack the human body alone or together in collusion with one or more others. Illnesses like wind-cold type common cold, damp-heat type diarrhea, and wind-cold-damp arthritis, are examples of the coexistence of multiple evils within the body.

From the point of view of modern science, aside from climatic factors, some biological, physical and chemical agents also play an important role in the pathology of the human body and the occurrence of exogenous diseases.

③ The Nature and Illness-Causing Characteristics of the Six Climatic Pathogens

The nature and characteristics of the six climatic pathogens of wind, cold, summer-heat, damp, dryness and heat (fire) evils are classified and organized according to the method of "metaphorical comparison". The symptoms and signs that manifest in the course of a disease are compared metaphorically to climatic features and material phenomena of the natural world, combined with their tendencies and inductive theory to create the nature and characteristics of corresponding illnesses of the six climatic pathogens. For example, migrant and protean clinical symptoms are comparable to the constantly moving, elusive nature of wind, so that the nature of the wind pathogen is defined as moving and constantly changing, and the illnesses it causes are characterize by migrant and protean symptoms; symptoms such lethargy in the extremities, edema of the lower limbs, thick and impure secretions coincide with the heavy, turbid, and viscous property of static water, hence the tendency of the damp pathogen to attack the lower body, resulting in sensations of weight and turbidity, viscosity and impurity of secretions in illnesses caused by damp pathogens.

The characteristics of illness vary according to the nature of each of the six climatic pathogens respectively.

(1) Wind, 风

Wind is the primary climatic feature of spring. When wind overpowers the right qi and attacks the human body, it becomes the wind pathogen or wind evil. Although wind is present in all four seasons, it is most prevalent in spring. Illnesses caused by the wind pathogen occur throughout the year, yet are most commonly seen in spring.

The Nature and Illness-Causing Characteristics of the Wind Pathogen (Table 6-1):

A. Wind is categorized as a yang pathogen

It is light and upward moving, opening and dispersing in nature. When the wind pathogen attacks, it tends to invade the yang portions of

Table 6-1　The nature and illness-causing characteristics of the wind pathogen

Nature	Illness-Causing Characteristics	Principle Symptoms and Signs
Yang evil, light and upward moving, opening and dispersing	Tends to invade the upper half of the body	Headache, nasal obstruction, itchy throat
	Tends to invade the surface of the body	Aversion to wind, fever, sweating
Migrates and changes frequently	Has no fixed position of illness Symptoms change constantly without a constant state	Migratory joint pain Itchy weals of hives, emerge at no regular interval, no fixed position
Characterized by motion	Unstable movements of the limbs	Convulsion of limbs and opisthotonos
Titled the chief pathogen of all diseases	Combines with other evils to invade the body; the most commonly seen pathogen	Combines to form wind-cold, wind-damp, wind-dry, wind-heat, wind-cold-damp

the body, namely the upper half of the body and its surface. It tends to open up the skin and striae and disperse. Once wind has entered the body, symptoms include headache, runny nose, itchy throat, aversion to wind, fever, and sweating, etc.

B. Wind pathogen migrates and changes frequently
Wind tends to move without fixed position, and changes constantly without constant form. First, there is no fixed position of illness in afflictions of the wind pathogen. A common example is the roving joint pain caused by excessive wind, also named "wind inflammation of the joints" or "migratory joint inflammation". Second, observable symptoms are constantly changing, such as the itchy weals of urticaria caused by wind pathogens that disappear, and reemerge with no discernable pattern or location.

C. The wind pathogen is characterized by motion
Unstable movements of the limbs often accompany the diseases caused by wind evil. In patients afflicted by wind, there are convulsions in the limbs and opisthotonos, facial palsy, facial muscle twitches and a loss of voluntary muscle control of the mouth and eyes. All are related to externally contracted wind.

D. Wind is the primary pathogenic agent of all diseases
"Primary" means the most important. What the wind evil as the primary pathogen of all disease stems from its tendency to combine with other evils to invade the body. It is also the most commonly observed pathogen. Cold, damp, dryness and heat pathogens often adhere to the wind evil to attack the body and cause diseases of wind-cold, wind-damp, wind-dryness, wind-heat, wind-cold-damp, etc.

Plain Questions: Chapter Discussion on Taiyin and Yangming (Sù Wèn · Tài yīn Yáng Míng Lùn, 素问·太阴阳明论*): "The wind pathogen attacks the upper body…The yang part of the body suffers from the wind evil first."*

Plain Questions: Wind (Sù Wèn: Fēng Lùn, 素问·风论*): "The wind is migrant and changes easily."*

Plain Questions: Chapter Major Discussion on the Theory of Yin and Yang and the Corresponding Relationships Among All the Things in Nature (Sù Wèn: Yīn Yáng Yìng Xiàng Dà Lùn, 素问·阴阳应象大论*): "when the wind becomes excessive it moves."*

Plain Questions: Discussion on Febrile Diseases (Sù Wèn: Píng Rè Bìng Lùn, 素问·评热病论*): "symptoms of sweating and fever indicate an attack of wind."*

Plain Questions: Hollow Bones (Sù Wèn: Gǔ Kōng Lùn, 素问·骨空论*): "The wind evil bears the title of chief pathogen of numerous diseases."*

Guide to Clinical Practice with Medical Records: Wind (Lín Zhèng Zhǐ Nán Yī Àn, 临证指南医案·风*): "Among the six climatic evils, only the wind evil can amalgamate with all other five. Together with cold it becomes wind-cold, with damp wind-damp, with dryness wind-dryness, with fire wind-fire. It is most likely because wind can invigorate the other five evils and injure the human body that it has earned the title of chief pathogen of numerous diseases. The other five don' t have this characteristic. Cold can not coexist with heat, summer-heat evil does not unite with cold, nor damp with dryness, or fire with cold. From this point of view, the wind evil has a leading role in sharing the causes of various diseases."*

(2) Cold, 寒

Cold is the primary climatic factor of winter. Excessive cold becomes the exogenous cold pathogen or cold evil, is mainly seen in winter, cold syndromes occur most commonly in winter. However, it may lead to disease in any season, whenever the temperature drops suddenly, or if exposed to wind while sweating, it is easy for cold to invade the body.

The Nature and Illness-Causing Characteristics of the Cold Pathogen (Table 6-2):

A. Cold is characterized as a yin pathogen
Cold has the characteristics of low temperature and frigidity, and is therefore a yin pathogen. Cold syndromes with damage to yang qi always accompany the diseases caused by cold. When cold invades the body surface it depresses the action of defensive yang qi. Symptoms of external contraction such as chills, fever, lack of sweat may appear. If the cold pathogen directly attacks the interior, it injures the yang of the Spleen and Stomach, resulting in symptoms like cold abdominal pain, vomiting, diarrhea, fear of cold with cold body and limbs (interior cold syndrome with deficiency of Spleen and Stomach

Table 6-2 The nature and illness-causing characteristics of the cold pathogen

Nature	Illness-Causing Characteristics	Principle Symptoms and Signs
Cold in nature; yin evils	Leads to cold syndromes and damage to yang qi	Exterior cold symptoms of chills, fever, lack of sweat when it invades the body's surface and depresses the activity of defensive yang qi; leads to the interior cold symptoms of cold abdominal pain, vomiting, diarrhea, fear of cold with cold body and limbs when it directly attacks the internal organs
Characterized by coagulation	Restricts qi and blood circulation, even resulting in blockage; leads to pain	Causes headaches and general pains when attacking the body's exterior; leads to cold abdominal pain when attacking the internal organs; results in joint pains which are aggravate by cold weather when residing in joints, channels and collaterals
Characterized by contraction	Restricts the qi-flow and closes the cutaneous striae	Chills, fever, lack of sweating when it invades the body's exterior and depresses the activity of defensive yang qi
	Contracting the tendons and vessels	Cramping of the limbs with course movements or numbness when it attacks the channels and joints

yang); if the Heart and Kidney yang is weak, the cold pathogen may directly attack the lesser yin channels, and the patient may display aversion to cold, desire to lie with limbs curled up, watery diarrhea with undigested food in the stool, polyuria, depression, faint and thready pulse, etc. (interior cold syndrome with deficiency of Heart and Kidney yang).

There are two different ways that cold invades the human body, "cold damage" and "cold attack". When the cold assaults the body surface and depresses the action of defensive yang qi, resulting in exterior cold symptoms, it is called "cold damage"; when the cold pathogen directly attacks the internal organs and damages the visceral yang, leading to symptoms of interior cold, it is called "cold attack".

B. The cold pathogen has the effect of coagulation
Cold leads to coagulation and obstruction. When it causes disease, it can restrict qi and blood circulation, even blocking it, and leading to pain. For instance, it may cause headache and dull pains when attacking the body's surface, lead to cold abdominal pain when attacking the interior organs, result in joint pain known as "cold inflammation of the joints" or "painful joint inflammation" when residing in the joints, channels and collaterals and is often aggravated by cold temperatures. Causing pains is an

important characteristic feature of cold illnesses.
C. The cold pathogen is characterized by contraction
Cold is a yin pathogen and has the property of frigidity, which leads to contraction. When attacking the body's exterior, it reduces qi-flow and closes the striae, which depresses the activity of defensive qi and results in chills, fever, lack of sweat; when attacking the channels and joints, it contracts the tendons and vessels thus resulting in cramped limbs with course movements or numbness.

Plain Questions: Chapter Major Discussion on the Theory of Yin and Yang and the Corresponding Relationships Among All the Things in Nature (Sù Wèn: Yīn Yáng Yìng Xiàng Dà Lùn, 素问·阴阳应象大论): "An overabundance of yin leads to cold", "An overabundance of yin damages yang."

Miraculous Pivot: Chapter The Treating Therapy from Oral Inquiry (Líng Shū: Kǒu Wèn, 灵枢·口问): "When cold resides in the skin, yin becomes excessive and the yang deficient, thus causing chills."

Plain Questions: Chapter Discussion on Bi-Syndrome (Sù Wèn: Bì Lùn, 素问·痹论): "pain originates from cold; cold leads to pain."

Miraculous Pivot: Era (Ling Shū: Suì Lù, 灵枢·岁露): "once attacked by the cold the cutaneous striae close."

Plain Questions: Pain (Sù Wèn: Jǔ Tong Lùn, 素问·举痛论): "cold pathogen obstructs qi. ... cold closes the cutaneous striae, blocks the flow of qi, then obstructs qi. . .the vessels get frigid when the cold evil resides within them, and leads to cramping of the limbs, then the collaterals contract and develop pain. When warmed, the pain gets is relieved."

(3) Summer-heat, 暑

Summer-heat is the predominant climatic factor of summer. It originates from the heat of summer. When it becomes overwhelming, it injures the human body and is called the summer-heat pathogen or summer-heat evil. It has an obvious seasonal relationship and is seen only during the period between summer solstice and the beginning of autumn.

Like cold evil, there are two different ways the summer-heat pathogen invades the human body, "summer-heat damage" and "summer-heat attack". Summer-heat illnesses with slow onset and light symptoms are called "summer-heat damage", while those with acute onset and severe symptoms are defined as "summer-heat attacks".

In addition, the ancient classics make division between "yin shu" and "yang shu" (*shu* here representing the illnesses of midsummer). "Yin shu" refers to illness resulting from an invasion of cold while the body is at rest (for example, while sleeping on an unusually cool night) and manifests as a cold syndrome; on the contrary, to

be attacked by excessive heat in summer while active is termed "Yang Shu" and manifests as a heat syndrome.

Plain Questions: Chapter Heat (Sù Wèn: Rè Lùn, 素问·热论): "Febrile illnesses caused by cold damage before the summer solstices are warm diseases, while those after the summer solstice are defined as summer-heat diseases."

Jing-yue's Complete Works: Summer-Heat Diseases, discussion on syndrome (Jǐng Yuè Quán Shū: Shǔ Zhèng, Lùn Zhèng, 景岳全书·暑证·论证): "The syndrome of 'Yin Shu' is caused by the attack of cold during summer. It commonly afflicts those who loathe heat and prefer the cool, chill of large buildings or shady, breezy places, or who do not take care to dress appropriately for sudden changes in temperature. The body surface is invaded by cold evil and leads to fever, headache, lack of sweating, chills, cramped limbs and aching. This describes the attack of cold evil in summer, or 'Yin Shu', and is similar to cold damage... 'Yang Shu' indicates an attack of heat in summer. It commonly afflicts those who on days of intense summer heat undertake long trips or intense physical labor, and results in headache, restlessness, high fever, extreme thirst, profuse sweating, floating pulse, shortness of breath, depletion of qi, etc. This is an attack of heat in summer, hence the name 'Yang Shu'."

The Nature and Illness-Causing Characteristics of the Summer-Heat Pathogen (Table 6-3):

Table 6-3 The nature and illness-causing characteristics of the summer-heat evil

Nature	Illness-Causing Characteristics	Principle Symptoms and Signs
Scorching	Yang and heat syndromes	High fever, thirst, flushed cheeks, bloodshot eyes, surging, large pulse
Rising and dispersing	Affects the head and eyes	Dizziness and reddish complexion
	Disturbs the Heart spirit	Sudden loss of consciousness, unresponsive to external stimuli
	Opens and disperses the cutaneous striae	Heavy sweat
	Consumes the fluid and weakens the qi of the body	Thirst with great desire to drink, dry, red tongue with, dark colored urine with reduced volume, shortness of breath, fatigue
Combines with damp evil	Causes summer-heat damp syndrome	Low fever, unrelenting thirst, fatigued limbs, thoracic discomfort, vomiting, loose stool, yellow and greasy tongue coating

A. The summer-heat pathogen is scorching in nature

The summer-heat evil originates from the heat of the season, making it a yang pathogen with a scorching nature. Symptoms of illness caused by summer-heat evil always tend to be yang and hot in nature, such as high fever, thirst, flushed cheeks, red eyes, large pulse, etc.

B. Summer-heat evil rises and disperses

The summer-heat evil is a yang pathogen and has the characteristics of rising and dispersing. When it attacks, it may affect the head and eyes, leading to symptoms like dizziness and reddish complexion. It may also disturb the shen of the Heart, resulting in sudden loss of consciousness, lack of response to external stimuli. Summer-heat also opens and the cutaneous striae causing sweating, thus injuring bodily fluids with its dispersive tendency. Qi is dispersed together with sweat, so the summer-heat evil consumes not only fluid but also qi, leading to symptoms of injury of both qi and fluids like thirst with great desire to drink, dry, red tongue, dark colored urine with reduced quantity and fatigue with shortness of breath.

C. Summer-heat pathogen carries damp evil with it as it invades the body

Summer weather is scorching hot and abundant in rain. When the rain is evaporated by the heat, the air is filled with a mixture of heat and damp. Therefore the summer-heat evil usually invades the body together with the damp, thus leads a complicated syndrome of summer-heat and damp. Symptoms include low fever, polydipsia, fatigued limbs, thoracic discomfort, vomiting, loose stool, with a yellow and greasy tongue coating.

Plain Questions: Chapter Discussion on the Interrelationship between Life and Nature (Sù Wèn: Shēng Qì Tōng Tiān Lùn, 素问·生气通天论): "Those attacked by the summer-heat evil sweat, when restless, are thirsty and short of breath, when at rest, talk a lot. The body burns like smoldering charcoal and is alleviated through perspiration."

Plain Questions: Major Discussion on the Progress of the Six Climatic Changes(Sù Wèn: Liù Yuán Zhèng Jì Dà Lùn, 素问·六元正纪大论): "The

weather turns scorching hot and the mountains and water blaze, ushering in the great summer-heat. ... so people suffer from qi deficiency...with bloodshot eyes and heat in the Heart, in extreme cases become anxious with sensations of stifling heat in the chest, and are prone to sudden death."

Miraculous Pivot: Era (Ling Shū: Suì Lù, 灵枢·岁露): "Confronted with the summer-heat, the skin becomes loose and the striae are opened."

Plain Questions: Pain (Sù Wèn: Jǔ Tong Lùn, 素问·举痛论): "When heated, the cutaneous striae is opened, nutrients and the defensive flow, sweat is dispersed and qi follows."

Plain Questions: Needling (Sù Wèn: Ci Zhi Lùn, 素问·刺志论): "Qi deficiency and fever indicates an attack of summer-heat."

Feng's Brocaded Secret Records (Féng Shì Jǐn Náng Mì Lù, 冯氏锦囊秘录):"During the hot and wet long summer, the damp earth dominates the climate, so the summer-heat evil always combines with damp."

(4) Damp, 湿

Damp is the dominating climatic factor of long summer, the sixth month of the lunar calendar, the dividing point between summer and autumn. It is the dampest season of the year, with yang heat still plentiful and rain water abundant, the humidity flourishes. When the dampness becomes overpowering and injures the body, it is damp evil. Damp evil may attack at any time throughout the year but is most prevalent in long summer. Those who have live in an area with cloudy and rainy weather, get caught out in the rain, work around water, or who favor cold and uncooked foods are all susceptible to damp illnesses.

The Nature and Illness-Causing Characteristics of the Damp Evil (Table 6-4):

A. Damp is classified as a yin pathogen

The damp pathogen is that of water, and water is classified as yin. Like water, damp is a tangible pathogen, and has the property of being heavy, turbid and viscid. It usually stagnates in the viscera and channels of the human body and blocks the flow of qi, leading to abnormalities in the rising and falling of qi. It results in thoracic discomfort and a feeling of suffocation when it hinders the qi flow of the upper *Jiao*; may cause

Table 6-4   The nature and illness-causing characteristics of the damp evil

Nature	Illness-Causing Characteristics	Principle Symptoms and Signs
Yin pathogen	Blocks the flow of qi; impairs the yang qi of the body	Causes thoracic discomfort and a feeling of suffocation when it hinders the qi flow of the upper *Jiao*; leads to a loss of appetite and proper gastric movement as well as abdominal distension when it blocks the qi flow of the Spleen and Stomach in the middle *Jiao*; causes lower abdominal distension and uncomfortable urination when affecting the qi flow of the Kidneys and Bladder in the lower *Jiao*
Heavy and turbid	Causes a wrapped and heavy feeling of the head and body, sore and ponderous limbs	Causes a feeling of heaviness in the head as if it were wrapped with cloth; general weariness; lingers in the channels and joints and causes joint inflammation and sore and laden limbs
Heavy and turbid	Thick and murky secretions and excretions	Dirty complexion and eye secretion, watery stool and diarrhea with puss and/or blood，cloudy urine
Viscid and stagnant	Sticky and viscid symptoms	Symptoms include sticky stool of dysentery, uncomfortable urination and strangury, sticky feeling or sweat taste in the mouth, thick and greasy tongue coating
Viscid and stagnant	Long, persistent course of illness	Eczema and damp inflammation of the joints with slow onset, long course, recurrent attacks, and difficulty in complete recovery
Tends to attack the lower part of the body	Attack the lower part of the body	Cloudy and uncomfortable urination, vaginal discharge, diarrhea, dysentery, edema and ulcers of the lower limbs

loss of appetite and proper gastric movement, ulcers, as well as abdominal distension, watery stool and irregular bowel movements when it obstructs the qi-flow of the Spleen and Stomach in the middle *Jiao*; may lead to lower abdominal distension and urinary irregularities when it hinders the qi flow of the Kidneys and the Bladder in the lower *Jiao*. Being a yin pathogen, damp may damage the yang qi of the body when it attacks. For instance, externally contracted damp evil usually injures the Spleen, specifically the yang qi of the Spleen. The Spleen then fails to transport and transform, thus generates water-dampness internally, leading to watery stool, reduced urination and edema, etc.

B. The damp evil is heavy and turbid in nature
Damp pathogen has the property of being heavy. Symptoms of an illness caused by damp pathogen are characterized as a wrapped and heavy feeling of the head and body, sore and laden limbs. If attacked by the damp evil, a patient may feel a weighted sensation in the head as if wrapped with a wet cloth, general lethargy,

etc. If the damp evil remains in the channels and joints, there may appear symptoms like joint inflammation, and sore and laden limbs, termed "damp inflammation of the joints" or "fixed joint inflammation".

Another characteristic of the damp evil is turbidity. There are sticky, greasy and stagnant manifestations. Symptoms include thick, murky secretions and excretions. When it attacks the upper part of the body, it leads to a dirty complexion and eye secretions; causes watery stool and diarrhea sometimes with puss or blood when residing in the Large Intestine; brings on cloudy urination and vaginal discharge in women when residing in the lower *Jiao*. It may also affect the skin causing eczema and sores that secrete puss.

C. The damp pathogen is viscid and stagnant
The damp evil has the traits of being viscid and stagnant. This refers to the sticky and viscid characteristics of damp related symptoms as well as the lingering, persistent nature of the illnesses caused by damp pathogens. The former manifests in uncomfortable bowel movements or dysentery,

filled with puss and phlegm, uncomfortable urinary discharges or strangury, a sticky, sweet taste in the mouth, a thick and greasy tongue coating, etc. The latter is reflected in the slow onset, long course, reoccurrence, and difficulty in treating damp illnesses.

D. Damp pathogen attacks the lower part of the body

Like water, the damp evil tends to go downward and tends to attack the lower part of the body, e.g. cloudy and uncomfortable urination, vaginal discharge, diarrhea or dysentery, edema and ulcers of the lower limbs, etc.

Plain Question: Major Discussion on the Progress of the Six Climatic Changes(Sù Wèn: Liù Yuán Zhèng Jì Dà Lùn, 素问·六元正纪大论): *"When damp becomes overpowering, it leads to watery excretion, extreme damp leads to edema."*

Warm-heat Diseases: Exogenous Warm-heat Diseases (Wēn Rè Lùn: Wài Gǎn Wēn Rè Piān 温热论·外感温热篇): *"As damp becomes overpowering, yang qi becomes weak."*

Plain Questions: Chapter Discussion on the Interrelationship between Life and Nature (Sù Wèn: Shēng Qì Tōng Tiān Lùn, 素问·生气通天论) : *"When injured by damp, the head feels as if it has been wrapped."*

Plain Questions: Chapter Discussion on Bi-Syndrome (Sù Wèn: Bì Lùn, 素问·痹论): *"Wind, cold, damp, when these three pathogens combine and invade the body, they lead to arthralgia. If wind is the primary pathogen, it leads to roaming arthralgia; if cold is the primary pathogen, then it leads to painful joint inflammation; if damp is the primary pathogen then there is severe joint pain."*

Guide to Clinical Practice with Medical Records: Dampness (Lín Zhèng Zhǐ Nán Yī Àn: Shī, 临证指南医案·湿): *"Damp is heavy and turbid, a pathogen with form."*

Systematic Differentiation of Damp-Heat Disorders: Chapter Shan Jiao (Wēn Rè Tiáo Biàn: Shàng Jiāo Piān, 温热条辨·上焦篇): *"Damp is thick, viscid and greasy. It is not like cold that can be alleviated through simple perspiration or warm/heat that retreats when cooled. Therefore it is difficult to heal quickly."*

Plain Questions: Chapter Discussion on Taiyin

and Yangming (Sù Wèn: Tài Yīn Yáng Míng Lùn, 素问·太阴阳明论): *"Injury from damp is first strikes the lower half of the body."*

Miraculous Pivot: Chapter *The Visceral Diseases Caused by Evil Qi (Líng Shū: Xié Qì Zàng Fǔ Bìng Xíng, 灵枢·邪气脏腑病形)*: *"Lesions in the lower half of the body result from the dampness evil attack."*: "The lower half of the body is where damp tends to strike."

(5) Dryness, 燥

Dryness is the primary climatic feature of autumn. The weather is usually clear and fine with little rain. This lack of moisture causes the dryness to dominate. When it becomes overpowering and injures the human body, it becomes the dryness pathogen or dryness evil. The dryness evil may cause disease in any season where there is a lack of rain, but mainly in autumn.

There are two kinds of dryness, i.e. warm and cool. In early autumn, the remaining summer-heat combines with the dryness of autumn. Together they invade the body and cause warm-dryness syndromes; and in late autumn, as winter draws near the air grows cool. The cool air accompanies dryness evil and invades the body, causing cool-dryness syndromes.

The warm-dryness and the cool-dryness share some common characteristics, but there is also some differences in their nature and the characteristics of illnesses they cause. The former causes warm-dryness syndrome, i.e. the symptoms are dry and tend to be hot to some degree, while the latter causes cool-dryness syndrome, with dry symptoms tend to be somewhat cold. (Table 6-5)

The Nature and Illness-Causing Characteristics of the Dryness Evil (Table 6-6):

The dryness evil has the characteristics of drying and withering: The dryness evil is arid, rough and non-lubricating. Illnesses it causes have the following features:

A. Dryness injures bodily fluids, leading to various dry symptoms

When externally contracted, it leads to dry mouth and lips, dry nose, dry throat, dry, scaly skin, short urination, and dry and hard stools.

B. The dryness pathogen injures the yin of the Lungs

Table 6-5　The differences between warm-dryness and cool-dryness pathogens

	Warm-dryness	**Cool-dryness**
Prevalent season	Early autumn	Late autumn
Climate	The dryness combines with the remaining heat of summer	The dryness combines with the approaching cold of the coming winter
Syndrome	Warm-dryness syndrome(dry and tending to be hot)	Cool-dryness syndrome(dry and tending to be cold)

Table 6-6　The nature and illness-causing characteristics of the dryness evil

Nature	Illness-Causing Characteristics	Principle Symptoms and Signs
Drying and withering in nature	Impairs the bodily fluids, leading to various dry symptoms	Dry mouth and lips, dry nose, dry throat, dry and scaly skin, short urinations, dry and hard stools
	Injures the yin of the Lungs	Dry cough with little sputum, or sticky sputum that is difficult to cough up, or blood stained sputum, extreme then gasping with chest pain

Fragile and delicate, the Lungs prefer moisture and fear dryness. They govern qi and control respiration. The Lungs open through the nose and match externally with the skin and fine hair, thus communing with the outside world directly. The dryness invades the Lungs through the skin and fine hair, the nose, and injures the fluids of the Lungs, leading to loss of the ability of the Lungs to disperse and descend, causing symptoms like dry cough with little sputum, or thick sputum difficult to cough up, or blood stained sputum, even gasping with chest pain, etc.

Plain Questions: Major Discussion on the Theory of Yin and Yang and the Corresponding Relationships Among All the Things in Nature (Sù Wè: Yīn Yáng Yīng Xiàng Dà Lùn, 素问·阴阳应象大论): *"Excessive dryness leads to dehydration."*

Mysterious Truth of Etiology of Plain Questions · Dryness (Sù Wèn Xuán Jī Yuán Bìng Shì: Zào Lèi, 素问玄机原病式·燥类): *"All the symptoms of withered, arid, sear, and chapped, desquamative, are results of dryness evil attack."*

(6) Fire (Heat), 火 (热)

Fire (heat) thrives in summer. The fire (heat) pathogen results when fire (heat) overpowers and injures the human body. The fire (heat) pathogen has no distinct seasonal nature like that of the summer-heat pathogen and leads to fire (heat)

syndromes throughout the whole year.

There is one more pathogen in the group of febrile diseases, the warm pathogen, which shares a similar yang and heat nature with the heat and the fire pathogens. They are collectively called "warm-heat pathogens" or "warm-fire pathogens", and categorized together with the externally contracted pathogens. The warm pathogen can change into heat, and the heat can change into fire; they can be understand as three different degrees of the "warm-heat pathogens" or "warm-fire pathogens", generally speaking, the warm pathogen is the lower grade of heat, and the fire is the extreme.

The Nature and Illness-Causing Characteristics of the Fire (Heat) Pathogen (Table 6-7):

The fire (heat) pathogen is a yang pathogen with a flaring, rising nature: The fire (heat) pathogen is burning hot and is categorized as a yang pathogen, flaming, even scorching. The characteristics of the illnesses it causes are:

A. The fire (heat) pathogen leads to excessive heat syndromes, particularly noticeable in the upper half of the body

The fire (heat) pathogen has a flaring nature and classified as a yang pathogen. Overabundance of yang generates heat, thus the fire (heat) pathogen leads to syndromes of excessive heat,

Table 6-7 The nature and illness-causing characteristics of the fire (heat) pathogen

Nature	Illness-Causing Characteristics	Major Symptoms and Signs
Classified as a yang pathogen with a flaring, rising nature	Manifests as excessive heat syndromes with heat symptoms mainly in the upper half of the body	High fever, aversion to heat, disruption of the Heart-spirit, thirst, sweating, dark colored urine, surging rapid pulse; red complexion, bloodshot eyes, painful, swollen red throat, sores and ulcers of the mouth cavity and tongue
	Tends to disturb the Heart-spirit	High fever, coma, delirium, or even mania
	Injures the bodily fluids and damages qi	Thirst with desire to drink, dry throat and lips, crimson tongue, dark colored and reduced urine, constipation, tiredness and lethargy, shortness of breath and unwillingness to speak
	Generates wind and disturbs the flow of blood	"generates wind": high fever, convulsions of the limbs, locked jaw, eyes rolled upward, arched trunk and limbs; "disturbs the blood flow": internal bleeding, nosebleeds, vomiting blood, bloody stool, bloody urine, and skin ulcers
	Causes skin ulcers	carbuncles, furuncles, swellings, and other cutaneous sores; localized swelling, reddening, burning sensations, aching and puss secretions

with symptoms like high fever, aversion to heat, disruption of the Heart-spirit, thirst, sweating, dark colored urine, surging rapid pulse, etc. The fire (heat) pathogen flares with the yang heat syndrome manifesting in the upper half of the body, e.g. red complexion, bloodshot eyes, painful, red swelling in the throat, sores and ulcers of the mouth cavity and tongue, etc. are all manifestations of an attack of the fire (heat) pathogen.

B. The fire (heat) pathogen disturbs the Heart-spirit

Once the fire (heat) pathogen invades the nutritious blood phase it easily disturbs the Heart-spirit, causing light symptoms like restlessness, insomnia, and severe symptoms such as high fever, coma, delirium, or even mania.

C. The fire (heat) pathogen easily injures the bodily fluids and damages qi

The fire (heat) pathogen not only burns and scorches but also forcefully disperses the bodily fluids. Therefore bodily fluids are easily injured by the fire (heat) evil. Clinically it manifests as symptoms of yin injury. Aside from obvious heat symptoms, there may also be thirst with a desire to drink, dry throat and lips, crimson tongue, dark

colored and reduced urine, and constipation. The over-activity of the fire (heat) evil can consume the right qi of the body, resulting in general depression of bodily functions. Deficiency of bodily fluids may lead to a failure to transform into qi and lead to qi deficiency. Patients may display symptoms of tiredness and lethargy, shortness of breath and unwillingness to speak, etc. with syndromes of great heat and damage to the bodily fluids.

D. The fire (heat) pathogen generates wind and disturbs the flow of blood

Excessive fire (heat) rouses the internal wind of the Liver and causes abnormal blood circulation. To "generate wind" means that the fire (heat) pathogen scorches the Liver channel and consumes fluids, bringing on failure of nourishment to the tendons and vessels that in turn leads to internal wind of the Liver. Symptoms include high fever, convulsions of the limbs, locked jaw, eyes rolled upwards, arched trunk and limbs, etc. The Liver wind caused by extreme heat is named "extreme heat causes wind syndrome".

"Disturbing the flow of blood" refers to the invasion of the fire (heat) pathogen into the blood vessels, which causes accelerated blood flow or even scorched vessels and internal bleeding in severe cases. Other symptoms include various types of bleeding: bleeding from the nose, bloody stool, vomiting blood, bloody urine, etc.

E. The fire (heat) pathogen tends to cause sores and ulcers

The fire (heat) pathogen invades the blood phase and lingers locally, corroding the blood and flesh that lead to carbuncles, furuncles, swellings, and other cutaneous diseases. Clinical manifestations include localized swelling, redness, burning sensations, aching and secretion of puss.

Plain Questions: Major Discussion on the Theory of Yin and Yang and the Corresponding Relationships Among All the Things in Nature (Sù Wèn: Yīn Yáng Yīng Xiàng Dà Lùn, 素问·阴阳应象大论): "Excessive pungent and sweet flavor medicine results in heat syndrome." "Excessive pungent and sweet flavor medicine with diaphoretic affect leads to disorder of yin." "Sthenic fire (pure yang) consumes genuine qi." "Heat (caused by qi stagnation) leads to swellings."

Plain Questions: Discussion on the Most Important and Abstruse Theory (Sù Wèn: Zhì Zhēn Yào Dà Lùn, 素问·至真要大论): *"Syndromes characterized by restlessness and mania are related to fire." "Syndromes characterized by fever, fainting and convulsion are related to fire." "Syndromes characterized by upward flow of qi are related to fire."*

Miraculous Pivot: Chapter On Carbuncle and Deep-rooted Carbuncle (Líng Shū: Yōng Jū, 灵枢·痈疽): "Excessive heat leads to corruption of the muscles, turning into pus, hence the formation of Yong (carbuncle)."

The Pestilent Pathogens

① Basic Concept of the Pestilential Pathogens

The pestilent pathogens refers to a group of externally contracted pathogens with a highly infectious nature, referred to as "pestilence", "epidemic pathogenic factor", "unusual pathogen", "perverse pathogen", "plague" in the ancient classics (Fig. 6-4).

The pestilent pathogens can attack the body through various pathways of aerial infection, oral or nasal infection, or through ingestion, insect

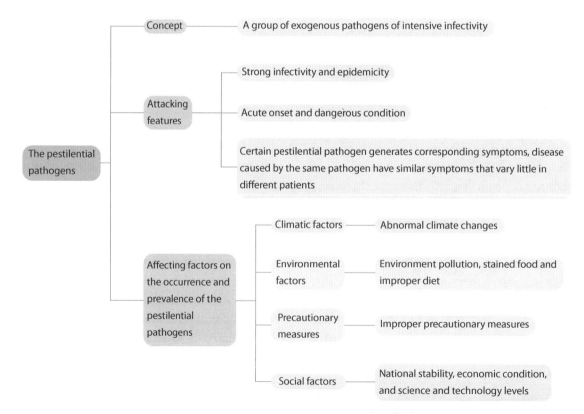

Fig. 6-4 Summary of factors that influence the occurrence and outbreak of pestilent disease

and animal bites, and skin contact.

The diseases caused by the pestilent evils are called "epidemics", "plagues", "epidemic diseases". For instance, diseases like "*da tou wen* (epidemic disease characterized by swelling and redness of face, 大头瘟)", "*ha ma wen* (frog plague, 蛤蟆瘟)", "*yi li* (ekiri, 疫痢)", "*lan hou dan sha* (skin rash with rotten throat, 烂喉丹痧)", "*bai hou* (diphtheria, 白喉)", "*tian hua* (smallpox, 天花)", "*huo luan* (cholera, 霍乱)", "*shu yi* (anthrax, 鼠疫)", etc., actually include many contagious and violent diseases of modern medicine.

Though the pestilential evils and the six climatic evils both belong to the externally contracted pathogens, the former one are stronger in toxicity, virulence, and infectious nature, and cause more severe and life-threatening damage than the latter one.

Treatise on Plague Diseases: Original Preface (Wēn Yì Lùn: Yuán Xù, 温疫论·原序): "Pestilential evils attack the human body, unlike any of the six climatic evils of wind, cold, summer-heat or dampness, in a peculiar pattern that is different from any other known pathogen."

Treatise on Plague Diseases: Original Diseases (Wēn Yì Lùn: Yuán Bìng, 温疫论·原病): "Cold-attack and summer-heat-stroke are terms of affection of common climatic factors; while plague refers to attack of the pestilent evils between heaven and earth."

② Illness-Causing Characteristics of the Pestilent Pathogens

(1) The pestilent pathogens are highly contagious and epidemic in nature

The pestilential evils are highly contagious and have a strong epidemic nature. They can be communicated in many ways including airborne infection and ingestion of contaminated food. In an area struck by infectious disease, people are infected without regard to age, gender or constitution. Pestilent diseases may occur locally throughout a large contiguous area.

(2) Pestilent pathogens have acute onset with life-threatening symptoms

Most of the pestilential pathogens are of the toxic heat category. They act quickly and usually combine with turbid and foul pathogens like smog and miasma when invading the body, so the onset is more urgent, intense and dynamic than that of the six climatic evils. Thus the patient's condition is more dangerous. Symptoms of fever, psychological disturbance, rapid blood circulation, internal wind, violent vomiting and diarrhea, etc., may appear during the course of illness.

(3) Certain pestilent pathogens generate corresponding symptoms and diseases caused by the same pathogen have similar symptoms that vary little in different patients

The pestilential pathogens are a group of various pathogens that are different in nature and selectivity. They give rise to different diseases and syndromes in different parts of the human body. Different pestilent pathogens cause different diseases, i.e. certain pestilent pathogens generate corresponding symptoms. Each pathogen has its own unique characteristics and follows a unique pattern of progression and transmission with similar clinical manifestations. Therefore, it was noted that diseases caused by the same pathogen have similar symptoms varying little in different patients. For instance, the virus that leads to parotitis acts mainly on the parotid gland. All infected patients have the same symptom of swelling and pain of the parotid gland. The ekiri pathogen attacks the intestines and causes abdominal pain, tenesmus, dysentery with blood and white puss-stained stool.

Treatise on Plague Diseases: Original Diseases (Wēn Yì Lùn: Yuán Bìng, 温疫论·原病): "When pestilent evil...comes, the aged and the young, the strong and the weak, whosoever, once gets in touch with it, will unexceptionally get sick."

Plain Questions: Major Discussion on the Progress of the Six Climatic Changes (Sù Wèn: Liù Yuán Zhèng Jì Dà Lùn, 素问·六元正纪大论): "When pestilent evils come tempestuously, people are liable to sudden death."

Plain Questions: Discussion on Acupuncture Methods (Sù Wèn: Cì Fǎ Lùn, 素问·刺法论): "When the five pestilences arise, people are easily infected contagiously, no matter young or old, the symptoms are alike."

③ Factors that Influence the Occurrence and Outbreak of Pestilent Disease

A. Climatic factors

Abnormal climate changes like long drought,

extreme heat, flooding, wet fog and smog, contribute to the generation of various pestilent pathogens (pathogenic microorganisms) and ensuing harm to the human body. In other words, the attack of pestilent pathogens is facilitated by abnormal climatic phenomena.

B. Environmental factors

Poor environmental sanitation, such as the compiling or storage of corrupt and contaminated objects, propagation of mosquitoes and flies, or polluted water sources and air can all breed pestilent pathogens and contribute to the spread the etiological agents. Contaminated food and water or improper dietary habits may also bring about the occurrence of epidemic disease.

C. Precautionary measures

Pestilent pathogens are highly contagious and infect anyone exposed to them. Poor or improper precautionary measures will lead to the spread of disease.

D. Social factors

Social factors including national stability, economic conditions, and levels of science and technology may influence the occurrence and prevalence of the pestilent diseases.

Section 2   Endogenous Pathogens

The endogenous pathogens refer to a class of pathogens that lead to disease through internal damage. In comparison with the exogenous diseases, the diseases they cause occur internally, hence the label of internal injury. The term 'endogenous disease' refers to a group of diseases caused by dysfunction and imbalance of qi and blood, yin and yang due to internal visceral damage for various reasons, and are thus referred to as the 'various internal diseases'. In contrast to illnesses caused by externally contracted pathogens, the endogenous diseases are not usually accompanied with an external syndrome.

The endogenous pathogens are divided into three groups of internal injury caused by excesses of the seven emotions, improper diet, and inappropriate work and rest.

The Seven Emotional Pathogens

① Basic Concept of the Seven Emotional Pathogens

A. The Significance of the seven emotions

The seven emotions refer to the seven emotional states of joy, anger, sadness, contemplation, melancholy, fear and fright, which are emotional response to the various external stimuli, both environmental and social. They are normal physical and psychological reactions that usually do not lead to disease. When abnormal emotional activity or imbalance leads to disease, then they are referred to as 'the seven emotional pathogens'.

B. Pathology of the seven emotional pathogens

When external psychological stimuli attack suddenly and intensely beyond the threshold for adaptation, persist for an extended period of time, or when the individual's ability to cope and adapt are compromised and fails to properly manage external stimuli, dysfunction of the qi and blood and of the five zang-fu viscera ensues and the internal balance of yin and yang is lost.

Treatise on Three Categories of Pathogenic Factors: Volume 2, Discussion on Three Categories of Pathogens (Sān Yīn Jí Yī Bìng Zhèng Fāng Lùn: Juàn Zhī Èr, Sān Yīn Lùn, 三因极一病证方论·卷之二·三因论): *"Seven emotions refer to joy(happiness), anger(rage), melancholy (worry), pensiveness (anxiety), sorrow (grief), terror (fear) and fright."*

② Relationship between the Seven Emotional Factors, *Zang-Fu* Organs and Qi and Blood

An individual's emotional and psychological activities are closely related with the qi and blood of the *zang-fu* organs. The former are products of the physical activities of the latter, i.e. the qi and blood of the organs serve as the material basis for emotional activity, or, in other words, human emotional and mental activities are the external manifestations of the qi and blood of the *zang-fu* organs. *The Internal Classic (Nèi Jīng,* 内经) outlined the idea of matching the emotional activities with the five *zang* viscera respectively, i.e. fright and joy are the emotions of the Heart, anger the emotion of the Liver, contemplation the emotion of the Spleen, sadness and melancholy the emotions of the Lung, and fear the emotion of the Kidney. Therefore, dysfunction of the viscera and bowels or disorder of qi and blood may result in emotional imbalance.

On the other hand, emotional imbalance may in turn affect the functions of the *zang-fu* organs and the flow of qi and blood, leading to the following pathological circles: excessive fright or joy damages the Heart, excessive anger damages the Liver, excessive contemplation damages the Spleen, excessive sadness sorrow and melancholy damages the Lungs, while excessive fear damages the Kidneys.

Plain Questions: *Chapter Major Discussion on the Law of Motions and Changes in Nature (Sù Wèn: Tiān Yuán Jì Dà Lùn, 素问·天元纪大论)*: *"Five Zang-viscera produce five qi in the body, to generate emotions of joy(happiness), anger(rage), pensiveness (anxiety), sorrow (grief), and terror (fear)."*

Miraculous Pivot: *Chapter The Issue of Distribution and Operation of The Defensive Qi and Nutritive Qi (Líng Shū: Yíng Wèi Shēng Huì, 灵枢·营卫生会)*: *"Blood is the miraculous qi." (Following the sentence "Nutritive and defensive are the essential qi (营卫者, 精气也)", compared with the nutritive and defensive, Blood is transformed from the essence of water and food, the process is miraculous, so it is said that blood is the miraculous qi.)*

Plain Questions: Chapter Major Discussion on the Theory of Yin and Yang and the Corresponding Relationships Among All the Things in Nature (Sù Wèn: Yīn Yáng Yìng Xiàng Dà Lùn, 素问·阴阳应象大论): *"Anger (rage) is the emotion of the Liver"*, and *"over anger (rage) injures the Liver"*; *"joy (happiness) is the emotions of the Heart"*, and *"joy (happiness) impairs the Heart"*; *"pensiveness (anxiety) is the emotion of the Spleen"*, and *"over pensiveness (anxiety) harms the Spleen"*; *"sorrow (grief) is the emotions of the Lung"*, and *"sorrow (grief) damages the Lung"*; *"terror (fear) is the emotion of the Kidney"*, and *"over terror (fear) disservices the Kidney"*.

Miraculous Pivot: Chapter The Diseases Caused by Spiritual Activities (Líng Shū: Běn Shén, 灵枢·本神): *"Deficient Liver qi leads to terror, and excessive Liver qi results in anger…deficiency of the Heart qi leads to sorrow, and excessive Heart qi results in ceaseless laughter."*

③ General Illness-Causing Characteristics of the Seven Emotional Pathogens (Fig. 6-5)

A. The pathology of the seven emotional pathogens is related to psychological stimuli, with most diseases manifesting as mental disorders

The occurrence of a diseases caused by the seven emotional pathogens is related to psychological stimuli and the manifest most often as emotional imbalance, such as depression, psychosis, and mania. These are termed mental disorders or mental diseases.

B. The seven emotional pathogens directly damage the viscera and bowels

Mental and emotional activities take the essence and qi of the viscera as their material foundation. When emotions become excessive, the viscera may therefore be injured directly. The seven emotional pathogens exhibit a selective quality when damaging the organs, specifically, excessive fright or joy damages the Heart, excessive anger damages the Liver, excessive contemplation damages the Spleen, excessive sadness sorrow and melancholy damages the Lungs, while excessive fear damages the Kidneys. The Heart is the commanding viscus of the five *zang-fu* organs and the primary agent of all mental activity. All injuries caused by the seven emotional pathogens eventually relate back to the Heart. Clinically, the Heart, the Liver and the Spleen are the three viscera most commonly injured by emotional factors.

C. The seven emotional pathogens affect the flow of qi of the five *zang* viscera

The seven emotional pathogens primarily affect the five *zang* viscera by disturbing the flow of qi within them, leading to disorders of qi and blood circulation. Different emotional pathogens affect the qi flow of the corresponding viscus in a specific manner. Excessive anger drives the qi upward, excessive joy slackens the qi, excessive fright throws qi into disorder, excessive contemplation causes qi to stagnate, excessive sadness consumes qi, excessive melancholy depresses qi, and excessive fear forces the qi downward.

D. Emotional changes influence the condition of a patient's illness

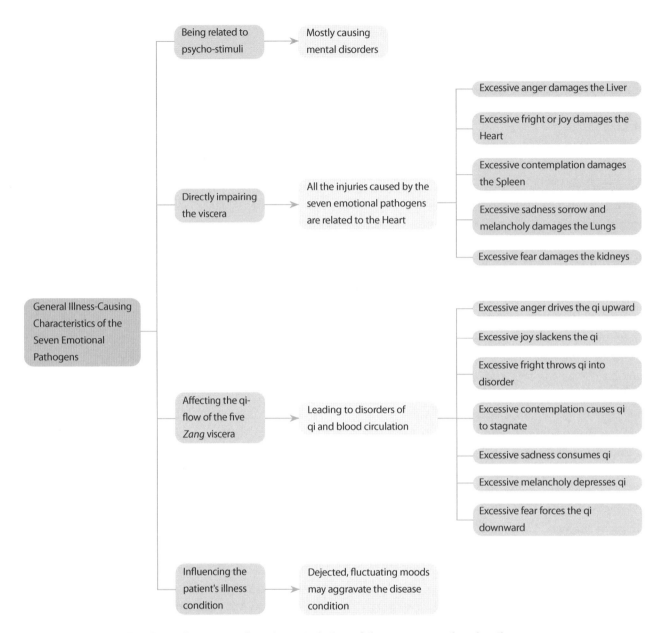

Fig. 6-5 Illness-causing characteristics of the seven emotional pathogens

Emotional changes may strongly affect the condition of a patient's illness in two main ways. First, a positive, optimistic or euphoric mood may help smooth the qi flow, thus contribute to the healing process; In contrast, depression or intense mood swings may further disrupt the flow of qi of the organs and aggravate the condition.

Miraculous Pivot: The Initiation of Various Diseases (Líng Shū: Bǎi Bìng Shǐ Shēng, 灵枢·百病始生): *"Intemperance of emotions hurts the viscera."*

Plain Questions: Chapter Major Discussion on the Theory of Yin and Yang and the Corresponding

Relationships Among All the Things in Nature (Sù Wèn: Yīn Yáng Yìng Xiàng Dà Lùn, 素问·阴阳应象大论): *"Over fright or joy (happiness) impairs the Heart"*, *"Over anger (rage) injures the Liver"*, *"Over pensiveness (anxiety) harms the Spleen"*, *"Over sorrow (grief) or melancholy (worry) damages the Lung"*, and *"Over terror (fear) disserves the Kidney"*.

Treatise on Three Categories of Pathogenic Factors: Volume 2, Discussion on Three Categories of Pathogens (Sān Yīn Jí Yī Bìng Zhèng Fāng Lùn: Juàn Zhī Èr, Sān Yīn Lùn, 三因极一病证方论·卷之二·三因论): *"The seven emotions are normal mental activities of human.*

Once stirred, they accumulate and grow excessive internally in the corresponding viscera and then get represented externally in the corresponding parts, thus turn into endogenous pathogens."

Plain Questions: Pain (Sù Wèn: Jǔ Tong Lùn, 素问·举痛论): "All diseases result from qi disorders, over anger (rage) drives qi upward, over joy(happiness)slackens qi, excessive sorrow (grief) consumes qi, over fear (terror) collapses qi...over fright disorders qi...over pensiveness (anxiety) causes qi stagnation."

Miraculous Pivot: Chapter The Diseases Caused by Spiritual Activities (Líng Shū: Běn Shén, 灵枢·本神): "Qi flow in those who are in deep melancholy and sorrow is always stagnant."

④ Respective Characteristics of the Seven Emotional Pathogens

The emotions of joy, anger, melancholy, contemplation, sadness, terror and fright injure different organs respectively, generate corresponding pathogenesis and lead to different syndromes accordingly. Thus, they have certain individual illness-causing features of their own.

A. Excessive fright or joy damages the Heart; excessive joy slackens qi; excessive fright throws qi into disorder (Table 6-8)

Joy, or happiness, is a positive mental state. Proper

Table 6-8   Illness-Causing Characteristics of Excessive Joy and Fright

Emotional Pathogen	Illness-Causing Characteristics		Major Symptoms and Signs(examples)
Excessive joy	Damages the Heart and slackens qi	Disordered Heart qi in mild cases	Palpitations, insomnia and inability to concentrate
		Upset Heart-spirit in severe cases	Constant laughter, crazed speech and actions
Sudden fright	Damages the Heart and throws qi into disorder	Disordered circulation of the Heart qi; separation of the Heart-spirit	Anxiety and paranoia, palpitations and insomnia in mild cases; panic, incoherent speech and psychological disorder in extreme cases

joy or happiness may help qi and blood circulate smoothly and brings comfort to the body, which is beneficial to health. Joy is the Heart's emotion; as a result, excessive joy damages the Heart and leads to disruption of the Heart qi, and may upset the calm of the Heart-spirit. In mild cases symptoms such as palpitations, insomnia and inability to concentrate may appear, while in severe cases constant laughter, crazed speech and actions may be seen.

Fright, or panic, represents a sudden, strenuous emotional reaction. Fright is one of the Heart's emotional activities; therefore, excessive fright damages the Heart and throws the circulation of qi into disorder, in extreme cases leading to complete separation of the Heart-spirit. Symptoms such as anxiety or paranoia, palpitations and insomnia may be seen in mild cases, while panic, incoherent speech and psychological disorder indicate severe damage to the Heart.

Plain Questions: Chapter Major Discussion on the Theory of Yin and Yang and the Corresponding Relationships Among All the Things in Nature (Sù Wèn: Yīn Yáng Yìng Xiàng Dà Lùn, 素问·阴阳应象大论): "Over joy (happiness) impairs the Heart."

Plain Questions: Pain (Sù Wèn: Jǔ Tong Lùn, 素问·举痛论): "Over joy(happiness)slackens qi...joy makes people feel full of satisfaction, with the nutritive and defensive circulating smoothly and qi flows slowly." "Over fright disorders qi...fright makes people feel having nothing to mentally depend on, and nowhere to shield the spirit, and the thoughts go astray thus forming a state of disorders of qi."

Miraculous Pivot: Chapter The Diseases Caused by Spiritual Activities (Líng Shū: Běn Shén, 灵枢·本神): "Over joy makes the spirit exhausted and it leaves the viscera."

B. Excessive anger injures the liver, and drives qi upward (Table 6-9)

Anger, rage, or wrath, is a furious and agitated emotional state that corresponds to the Liver. Thus, excessive anger injures the Liver, driving qi upward, carrying the blood upward with it, with possible side-effects of the Spleen and Stomach. Upward driven Liver qi manifests as irritability and sudden outbursts, headache and distention of the head, flushed cheeks and bloodshot eyes; if the upward-moving qi stirs the blood and causes and adverse rising of both qi and blood, it may cause vomiting or spitting up blood, or even fainting. If the Liver fails to govern free coursing and influences the Spleen and Stomach, it may cause belching, vomiting, abdominal distension, diarrhea, loss of appetite, etc.

Table 6-9   Illness-causing characteristics of excessive anger

Emotional Pathogen	Illness-Causing Characteristics		Major Symptoms and Signs
Excessive anger	Damages the Liver, driving qi upward	Adverse rising of Liver qi	Irritability and sudden outbursts, headache and distention of head, flushed cheeks and bloodshot eyes
		Upward driven qi stirs the blood	Vomiting or spitting blood, even fainting
		Affects the Spleen and Stomach	Belching, vomiting, abdominal distension, diarrhea, and loss of appetite

Plain Questions: Chapter Major Discussion on the Theory of Yin and Yang and the Corresponding Relationships Among All the Things in Nature (Sù Wèn: Yīn Yáng Yìng Xiàng Dà Lùn, 素问·阴阳应象大论): "Over anger (rage) injures the Liver."

Plain Questions: Pain (Sù Wèn: Jǔ Tong Lùn, 素问·举痛论): "Over anger (rage) drives qi upward…anger leads to abnormal rising of qi, even causes hematemesis and stagnant-food-diarrhea, thus driving qi upward."

Plain Questions: Chapter Discussion on the Interrelationship between Life and Nature (Sù Wèn: Shēng Qì Tōng Tiān Lùn, 素问·生气通天论): "Excessive anger leads to segregation of qi from the configuration, and blood stasis in the upper part of the body, causing raged syncope (or emotional syncope, furious syncope, a serious condition due to qi and blood rushing up to the head, obstruction of viscera and channels)."

Jǐng-yue's Complete Works: Vomiting (Jǐng Yuè Quán Shū: Ǒu Tù, 景岳全书·呕吐): "Vomiting due to abnormal rising of qi is mainly caused by depression and rage, which stir up the Liver qi and affect the Stomach, then result in vomiting."

C. Excessive contemplation harms the spleen and causes qi to stagnate (Table 6-10)

Contemplation, or anxiety, is an emotional activity of concentrated thinking and deliberation,

Table 6-10   Illness-causing characteristics of excessive contemplation

Emotional Pathogen	Illness-Causing Characteristics		Major Symptoms and Signs(examples)
Excessive Contemplation	Harms the Spleen and causes stagnation of the Spleen qi	Stagnation of the Spleen qi	Anorexia, abdominal distension, diarrhea
		Disrupts the calms of the Heart-spirit	Palpitations, insomnia, excessive dreaming, even dementia
		Affects the Liver and Kidney	Premature ejaculation in males, and irregular menstruation and vaginal discharge in females

the emotion of the Spleen. Thus excessive contemplation harms the Spleen, and causes stagnation of the Spleen qi, in turn affecting the Liver and Kidneys as well as disrupting the calm of the Heart-spirit. Stagnant Spleen qi may result in a loss of transportation and transformation that manifests as a loss of appetite, abdominal distension, and diarrhea. The Heart may also be affected by long-term excessive pensiveness, disturbing the calm of the Heart-spirit, and resulting in palpitations, insomnia, excessive dreaming, even dementia. When constant anxiety affects the Liver and the Kidney, it can cause impotence, nocturnal emissions and premature ejaculation in males, and irregular menstruation and vaginal discharge in females.

Plain Questions: Chapter Major Discussion on the Theory of Yin and Yang and the Corresponding Relationships Among All the Things in Nature (Sù Wèn: Yīn Yáng Yìng Xiàng Dà Lùn, 素问·阴阳应象大论): "Over-pensiveness (anxiety) harms the Spleen."

Plain Questions: Pain (Sù Wèn: Jǔ Tong Lùn, 素问·举痛论): "Over pensiveness (anxiety) causes qi stagnation…pensiveness causes concentration of the mind, and qi remains instead of being dispersed, forming qi Stagnation."

D. Excessive sadness and melancholy damage the Lungs; excessive sorrow consumes qi while excessive melancholy depresses qi (Table 6-11)

Sadness, or sorrow, is a depressed, painful emotional state and is the emotion of the Lungs. Thus, excessive sadness injures the Lungs and consumes the Lung qi, leading to low voice, weakness and shortness of breath, listlessness, depression, and low spirits.

Table 6-11 Illness-causing characteristics of excessive melancholy (worry)

Emotional Pathogen	Illness-Causing Characteristics		Major Symptoms and Signs
Excessive sadness	Injures the Lungs and consumes qi	Causes consumption of the Lung qi	Low voice, weakness and shortness of breath, listlessness, depression, low spirits
Long-term melancholy	Damages the Lungs and depresses qi	Causes depression and stasis of the Lung qi	low and pessimistic spirits, thoracic discomfort and feeling of suffocation, shortness of breath

Melancholy, or worry, is a distressed and gloomy emotional state, also belonging to the Lungs. Long-term melancholy may damage the Lungs and cause depression of the Lung qi, and lead to low and pessimistic spirits, thoracic discomfort and feeling of suffocation, shortness of breath, etc.

Plain Questions: Chapter Major Discussion on the Theory of Yin and Yang and the Corresponding Relationships Among All the Things in Nature (Sù Wèn: Yīn Yáng Yìng Xiàng Dà Lùn, 素问·阴阳应象大论): "Over sorrow (grief) or melancholy (worry) damages the Lung".

Plain Questions: Pain (Sù Wèn: Jǔ Tong Lùn, 素问·举痛论): "Excessive sorrow (grief) consumes qi…… sorrow leads to stiffness of the Heart channels and distension of the Lung, the upper-Jiao is obstructed and nutrient and defensive qi disordered,

transforming into heat and consumes qi."

Miraculous Pivot: Chapter The Diseases Caused by Spiritual Activities (Líng Shū: Běn Shén, 灵枢·本神): "Sorrow leads to obstruction of qi."

E. Excessive fear damages the Kidney and forces the qi downwards (Table 6-12)

Fear, horror, or terror is a scared emotional state and is associated with the Kidneys. As a result, excessive fear damages the Kidneys, making the Kidney qi scatter and consuming the blood and essence. The qi and blood tend to move downward which manifests as urinary and fecal incontinence, premature ejaculation, spermatorrhoea, nocturnal emissions, a pale, white complexion, dizziness and fainting.

Plain Questions: Chapter Major Discussion on the Theory of Yin and Yang and the Corresponding Relationships Among All the Things in Nature (Sù

Table 6-12　Illness-causing characteristics of excessive fear

Emotional Pathogen	Illness-Causing Characteristics		Major Symptoms and Signs
Excessive Fear	Damages the Kidneys, and forces qi downward	Qi and blood tend to flow downward	Pale, white complexion, dizziness and fainting
		Scatters the Kidney qi and consumes the blood and essence	Urinary and fecal incontinence, premature ejaculation, spermatorrhoea, withered bones

Wèn: Yīn Yáng Yìng Xiàng Dà Lùn, 素问·阴阳应象大论): *"Over terror (fear) disserves the Kidney."*

Plain Questions: Pain (Sù Wèn: Jǔ Tong Lùn, 素问·举痛论): *"Over-fear (terror) collapses qi."*

Miraculous Pivot: Chapter The Diseases Caused by Spiritual Activities (Líng Shū: Běn Shén, 灵枢·本神): *"Unchecked fear tends to damage the essence, leading to bone aching and flaccid syndrome with cold limbs, and emission due to unconsolidated Kidney qi."*

In addition, fright and fear often attack together. However, there is a definite difference between the two. The term "fright" emphasizes the suddenness and lack of expectation of the shock received; while "fear" points to the psychological uneasiness that is accompanied by a certain degree of self-awareness. Fright arises suddenly and without warning while fear tends to accumulate gradually, making the former easy to recover from and the latter very difficult. (Table 6-13)

Table 6-13　Differences between fright and fear

	Emotional Presentation	Known or Unknown	Timing	Difficulty of Recovery
Fright	Surprise, sudden tension	Absence of self-awareness of the fright received; invades from the exterior	Originates suddenly, without warning	Easy
Fear	Terror, psychological unease	A fear known by the patient, generated internally	Accumulates gradually	Difficult

Confucians' Duties to Parents: Volume 7, Internal Injuries, Fright (*Rú Mén Shì Qīn: Juàn Qī, Nèi Shāng Xíng, Jīng*, 儒门事亲·卷七·内伤形·惊): *"Fright belongs to yang emotions, being caused by extrinsic factors, the frightened person is unaware of it; fear (terror) belongs to yin emotions, being caused by intrinsic factors, the fearful person is self-aware of it."*

Improper Diet

Diet refers to the daily intake of food and drink. The human body transforms them into the essence of water and grain, and qi and blood as well, serving as the basis of life and maintenance of health. People's diet should be suitable for them individually in terms of quantity, diversity, and sanitation. Proper diet improves people's health while improper diet can function as a pathogen in causing various diseases.

Improper diets damage the body primarily by affecting the Spleen and Stomach that result in a series of pathological changes. Improper diet is one of the major endogenous pathogens that include the three aspects of eating and drinking without moderation, unsanitary diet, and incomplete diet.

① Eating and Drinking Without Moderation (Table 6-14)

A normal diet should remain in proper quantity. Uncontrolled diet without limitation or irregular

Table 6-14   Illness-causing characteristics of lack of dietary moderation

Dietary Pathogen		Illness-Causing Characteristics	Major Symptoms and Signs (examples)
Lack of dietary moderation	Excessive hunger	Injures the Stomach yin	gastric ulcers and pain, acid reflux
		Qi and blood deficiency	Qi and blood deficiency and failure of the viscera and tissues to be nourished with ensuing functional decline; children's physical growth and development may be affected
		Weak right qi	Susceptibility to exogenous pathogens
	Over indulgence	Injures the Spleen and Stomach	Abdominal distension and pain, belching, acid reflux, vomiting, diarrhea, and loss of appetite
		Internal generation of damp and phlegm	Formation of phlegmatic fluid, obesity, vascular obstruction, cough, and shortness of breath; "malnutritional stagnation" in children

dietary cycles of hunger and satiation may both lead to disease.

A. Excessive hunger

Long-term hunger with insufficient food intake may lead to damage in the following three ways:

First, the Stomach is injured. The Stomach dominates reception and digestion. Insufficient food intake may injure the Stomach yin, leading to symptoms like gastric ulcers and pain, Heartburn, etc.

Second, the generation of qi and blood is affected. Food and drink are the resources for the generation of qi and blood. Long-term dietary insufficiency will lead to the pathological changes of qi and blood deficiency. The viscera and tissues fail to be nourished and their physiological functions decline. In childhood, it may affect the growth and development of the body.

Third, the right qi is weakened. Suffering from long-term dietary insufficiency, leads to malnutrition, leading to emaciation and weak right qi, so the body becomes susceptible to externally contracted pathogens and develops disease rather easily.

B. Over indulgence

Eating and drinking more than necessary over a long period, or to eat and drink too much at one meal, may cause illness in the following two ways:

First, the food stagnates in the over-filled Stomach injuring it together with the Spleen.

The excess food affects the transformation and digestion of the Spleen and Stomach and often goes undigested. This leads to abdominal distension and pain, belching, acid reflux, vomiting, diarrhea, and loss of appetite.

Second, over-eating leads to the internal production of damp phlegm. The Spleen fails to transport and transform due to the long-term food stagnation, resulting in pathological generation of damp, which in turn, accumulates into phlegm. Phlegm may then transform into heat, and give rise to phlegmatic fluid, obesity, vascular obstruction, cough and shortness of breath. In children, long-term food stagnation may also cause "malnutritional stagnation" as a result.

Miraculous Pivot: Chapter The Five Flavors (Líng Shū: Wǔ Wèi, 灵枢·五味): "Without food intake, qi (of the body) gets declined in half a day, and prostrate in one day."

Plain Questions: Chapter Discussion on Bi-Syndrome (Sù Wèn: Bì Lùn, 素问·痹论): "Eating twice as much as usual leads to injury of the Stomach and Intestines."

Classic of Questioning: The Forty-nineth Question (Nàn Jīng: Sì Shí Jiǔ Nàn, 难经·四十九难): "(Improper) diet and over-strain hurts the Spleen."

Jǐng-yuè's Complete Works · Miscellaneous Syndromes: Internal Injury (Jǐng Yuè Quán Shū: Zá Zhèng Mó, Láo Juàn Nèi Shāng, 景岳全书·杂证谟·劳倦内伤): "Over hungry or fullness, or over strain or ease, can hurt people. Because people depend greatly on drink and food, which are dominated by the Spleen and Stomach, and abnormal alternations of hunger and fullness impair the Stomach qi; and the Spleen controls the extremeties, over-strain damages the Spleen qi."

② Unsanitary Diet (Table 6-15)

Taking in contaminated, cold and uncooked, rotten, or even poisonous food, may result in disease in the following three ways:

First, the Stomach and intestines are damaged. Unhygienic food invades the Stomach and intestines, resulting in gastrointestinal distress that manifests in symptoms like gastro-abdominal pain, belching, acid reflux, vomiting, diarrhea,

puss and blood stained stool, etc.

Second, it may cause food poisoning. The intake of poisonous or contaminated food results in food poisoning with signs such as gastro-abdominal pain, vomiting, diarrhea in mild cases, and unconsciousness and even death in severe cases.

Third, it may result in intestinal parasites that cause abdominal pain with an emaciated appearance and aphagia.

Synopsis of Golden Chamber: Volume 24, Dietary Taboos and Treatment of Disease (Jīn Guì Yào Lüè: Juàn Èr Shí Sì, Qín Shòu Yú Chóng Jìn Jì Bìng Zhì, 金匮要略·卷二十四·禽兽鱼虫禁忌并治): "Corrupted foods like foul rice, rotten fish, and putrid meat hurt people easily......livestock died from

Table 6-15   Illness-causing characteristics of unsanitary diet

Dietary Pathogen		Attacking Features	Major Symptoms and Signs (examples)
Unsanitary diet	Contaminated, cold and uncooked, rotten or poisonous food	Impairs the Stomach and intestines	Gastro-abdominal pain, belching, acid reflux, vomiting, diarrhea, puss and blood stained stool
		Food poisoning	Gastro-abdominal pain, vomiting, diarrhea in mild cases; coma and even death in severe cases
		Intestinal parasites	Abdominal pain with an emaciated appearance and aphagia

pestilence are poisonous and inedible."

③ Incomplete Diet and Addictions (Table 6-16)

An incomplete diet refers to favoring or abstaining from certain kinds of foods, including addictions to food of cold or hot nature, any of the five flavors, to certain categories, or alcohol addiction, etc.

A. Addiction to foods of cold or hot nature
Proper dietary habits require suitable food temperature. If one excessively favors cold or hot foods, it may cause an imbalance of the yin and yang of the body and lead to disease.

Cold food addiction: Excessive intake of cold or uncooked foods for a long period of time may impair the yang qi of the Spleen and Stomach, resulting in the internal generation of damp cold that manifests as abdominal pain, diarrhea, vomiting clear fluids, and cold extremities.

Hot food addiction: Excessive intake of hot,

spicy, or pungent foods may cause the accumulation of heat in the Stomach and intestines and injure the Stomach yin. Symptoms include thirst, bad breath, constipation, gastric ulcers and constant hunger, with red tongue and striped tongue coating.

Plain Questions: Chapter Major Discussion on the Theory of Yin and Yang and the Corresponding Relationships Among All the Things in Nature (Sù Wèn: Yīn Yáng Yìng Xiàng Dà Lùn, 素问·阴阳应象大论): "The cold or hot nature of the water and grain will affect the six fu-viscera."

B. Addiction to foods of any one of the five flavors
The five flavors of sour, bitter, sweet, pungent and salty have a certain affinity to the five zang organs respectively. Long-term addiction to food of any one of the five flavors may lead to unbalanced excess of the visceral qi and dysfunction of the viscera that leads to disease.

Plain Questions: Chapter Discussion on the Most Important and Abstruse Theory (Sù Wèn: Zhì

Table 6-16 Illness-causing characteristics of incomplete diet and addictions

Dietary Pathogen		Illness-Causing Characteristics	Major Symptoms and Signs
Incomplete diet and addictions	Addiction to food of cold or hot nature	Impairs the yang qi of the Spleen and Stomach	Abdominal pain, diarrhea, vomiting clear fluids and cold limbs
		Causes heat accumulation in the Stomach and intestines	Thirst, bad breath, constipation, gastric ulcers and constant hunger, with red tongue and striped tongue coating
	Addiction to food of any of the five flavors	Unbalanced excess of the visceral qi and dysfunction of the viscera	Causes various diseases
	Addiction to food of certain type	Promotes the generation of phlegm and transformation into pathogenic heat; causes nutrient deficiency	Obesity, dizziness, fainting, thoracic obstruction, apoplexy, diabetes, and intestinal furuncle (acute appendicitis or periappendicular abscesses), night blindness, goiter, rickets, beriberi
	Alcohol addiction	Alcohol toxins injure the Spleen and Stomach	Gastro-abdominal distension, lack of appetite, bitter taste and greasy feeling in the mouth, thick and greasy tongue coating, formation of abdominal masses or coma due to the alcohol poisoning

Zhèn Yào Dà Lùn, 素问·至真要大论): *"Each of the five flavors enters the Stomach and goes towards corresponding viscus, i.e. the sour flavor enters the Liver first, bitter enters the Heart, sweat enters the Spleen, pungent enters the Lung and salty enters the Kidney."*

Plain Questions: Chapter Discussion on Various Relationships Concerning the Five Zang-Organs (Sù Wèn: Wǔ Zàng Shēng Chéng Piān, 素问·五脏生成篇): "Over eating of salty foods causes obstructed vessel and abnormal complexion, over eating bitter foods leads to withered skin and baldness, over eating pungent foods makes for the tendon contraction and dry nails, over eating sour foods results in rough muscles and peeled lips, and over eating sweat foods brings on bone ache and loss of hairs."

C. Addiction to foods of certain categories

This means being partial or averse to food of certain categories, or to lack certain foods in one's diet. As time passes, disease may occur due to excess or deficiency of certain nutrients. For instance, addiction to sweet, greasy and rich foods can promote the generation of phlegm and transformation of pathogenic heat, leading to obesity, dizziness, fainting, thoracic obstruction,

apoplexy, diabetes, and intestinal furuncle (acute appendicitis or periappendicular abscesses). If a food addiction causes insufficiency of certain vital nutrients, it may bring about night blindness, goiter, rickets, beriberi, and so on.

Plain Questions: Chapter Discussion on the Interrelationship between Life and Nature (Sù Wèn: Shēng Qì Tōng Tiān Lùn, 素问·生气通天论): "Pathologic change caused by rich and fatty diet is manifested as furuncles."

Plain Questions: Discussion on Special Diseases (Sù Wèn: Qí Bìng Lùn, 素问·奇病论): "Overeating greasy food brings about internal heat, overeating food with sweet flavor brings about abdominal distension, thus the qi rises abnormally and transforms into diabetes."

D. Alcohol addiction

Extended addiction to alcohol may injure the Spleen and Stomach due to the alcoholic toxins, causing accumulation of damp and production of phlegm, which may then transform into pathogenic heat, resulting in gastro-abdominal distension, lack of appetite, bitter taste and greasy feeling in the mouth, with a thick and greasy tongue coating, in extreme cases, the formation of abdominal masses or coma due to the alcohol poisoning.

Treatise on Spleen and Stomach: On Injury Caused by Alcohol Addiction (Pí Wèi Lùn: Lùn Yǐn Jiǔ Guò Shāng, 脾胃论·论饮酒过伤): "Alcohol is of great heat and poisonous in nature, with both smell and taste belonging yang flavors......that damages original qi."

Inappropriate Work and Rest

A reasonable balance of work and rest is one of the necessary conditions for the maintenance of life and good health. Improper work and rest refers to long-term excessive strain and excessive rest, which may injure the body and bring on disease. (Table 6-17)

① Over-exertion

A. Excessive physical work
This means to engage in physical labor or exercise for long periods of time where the exertion impairs the constitution and leads to diseases. The illness-causing characteristics are as follows:

Table 6-17　Illness-causing characteristics of improper work and rest

Endogenous Pathogen		Illness-Causing Characteristics	Major Symptoms and Signs (examples)
Over-exertion	Excessive physical work	Consumes the right	Shortness of breath and unwillingness to speak, gasping, sweating, withered spirit, weakened limbs and emaciation
		Impairs the constitution	Hurts the bones and tendons, damages the tissues
	Excessive mental work	Depletes the Heart-blood and consumes the Heart-spirit	Palpitation, forgetfulness, insomnia and excessive dreaming
		Consumes the Spleen qi and leads to a loss of the Spleen's healthy transportation	Lack of appetite, abdominal distension and watery stool
	Excessive sexual activity	Consumes the essence and qi of the Kidneys	Pain and weakness in the lower back and knees, depressed spirit, dizziness, ringing in the ears, reduced sexual function, nocturnal emissions, premature ejaculation, impotence, or irregular menstruation, and vaginal discharge
Excessive rest		Stagnates the qi and blood circulation and leads to dysfunction of the *zang-fu* viscera	Lack of appetite, thoracic discomfort, abdominal distension, debilitation, weak muscles, deficient obesity, clumsiness; or palpitations worsened by movement, gasping, sweating; or being in low spirits, forgetfulness, and dull reactions; or dizziness, apoplexy, and pathological changes of qi stagnation and blood stasis, internal generation of water-dampness and phlegmatic fluid

Long-term physical exertion damages the essence and consumes the right qi of the internal viscera and leads to reduced physiological efficiency. Symptoms include shortness of breath and reduced speech, gasping, sweating, withered spirit, exhausted limbs and emaciation.

Over-exertion also impairs the constitution. Extended physical strain hurts the bones and tendons, damages tissue, and causes illness.

B. Excessive mental strain
Constantly over-working the brain through constant analytical thinking may gradually

lead to disease. Illness-causing characteristics are mainly reflected in injury to the Heart and Spleen. The Heart stores the spirit and dominates blood. Long term excessive mental work depletes the Heart blood and consumes the Heart-spirit, and manifests as palpitations, forgetfulness, insomnia and excessive dreaming. The Spleen governs transformation and transportation, and is associated with the emotion of contemplation. Excessive thoughtfulness consumes the Spleen qi and leads to the Spleen's loss of healthy transportation and manifests as a loss in appetite, abdominal distension and watery stool.

C. Excessive sexual activity

This refers to unrestrained sexual behavior or masturbation, early pregnancy and bearing multiple children in women. Excessive sexual activity consumes the essence and qi of the Kidneys. Symptoms of pain and weakness in the lower back and knees, depressed spirit, dizziness, ringing ears, reduced sexual function, nocturnal emissions, premature ejaculation, impotence or irregular menstruation, vaginal discharge, infertility and sterility, etc. may arise.

Plain Questions: Chapter Discussion on the Elucidation of Five-Qi (Sù Wèn: Xuān Míng Wǔ Qì Piān, 素问·宣明五气篇): "Impairments caused by five kinds of strain: Over watching hurts blood, excessive rest on bed impairs qi, prolonged sitting injures the muscles, unremitting standing injuring bones, constant walking injuring tendons, which are impairments with five kinds of strain."

Plain Questions: Pain (Sù Wèn: Jǔ Tong Lùn, 素问·举痛论): "Over-strain consumes qi……over-strain leads to dyspnea and sweating, internal and external qi are both discharged, thus qi is consumed."

Jǐng-yuè's Complete Works: Consumptive Disease (Jǐng Yuè Quán Shū: Xū Sǔn, 景岳全书·虚损): *"Excessive sexual lust leads to consumptive diseases."*

② Excessive Rest

Excessive rest or idleness is a long term state of leisure lacking in physical labor and exercise, with little mental work. They stagnate the qi and blood circulation and lead to dysfunction of the *zang-fu* organs, and thus bring about disease.

Clinical manifestations include anorexia, thoracic discomfort, abdominal distention, physical and muscular weakness, or deficient obesity and clumsiness; or palpitations worsened by movements, gasping, sweating; or being in low spirits, forgetfulness, dull reactions; or dizziness, apoplexy, and pathological changes of qi stagnation and blood stasis that leads to internal generation of water-damp and phlegmatic fluid, etc.

Section 3 Secondary Pathogens

Pathogens like phlegmatic fluid, blood stasis, and calculus are pathological byproducts of the disease process that are retained within the body and affect the body, causing new pathological changes and thus playing the role of a pathogen. Due to the nature of these pathological products, they are termed "secondary pathogens".

Phlegmatic Fluid Pathogen

① Basic Concept of the Phlegmatic Fluid Pathogen (Fig. 6-6)

The phlegmatic fluid pathogen is the pathological byproduct of metabolic dysfunction in the circulation of the body's water and fluids. It resides in the body and brings on new pathological changes and causes disease as a secondary pathogen.

The thick and turbid nature of the phlegmatic fluid is composed of phlegm, while the thin and clear portion is caused by fluid retention.

There are tangible and intangible forms of phlegm. The former refers to phlegm with material form, visible and tangible, or audible, like sputum, wheezing phlegm in the throat, and subcutaneous swelling. The latter, on the contrary, refers to phlegm disease which has no concrete form but only the phlegmatic signs. That is, invisible, intangible, and inaudible phlegm-induced pathological changes and their related syndromes. For example, satisfactory results may be obtained when treating symptoms of

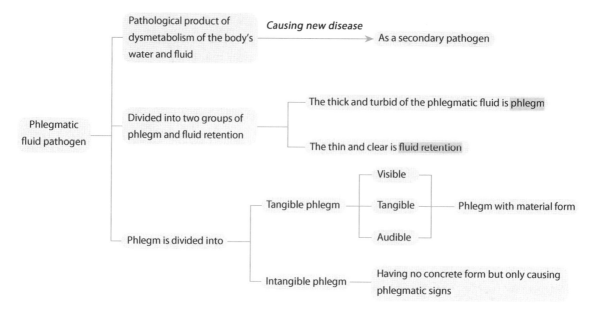

Fig. 6-6 Summary of the basic concepts of the phlegmatic fluid pathogen

dizziness, psychosis, mania, and dementia with the same method as that of treating material phlegmatic fluid.

This retained fluid has a relatively strong flowing nature and can accumulate in the interstitial spaces of the body. The clinical manifestations and nomenclature of the fluid retention varies with the different locations of retention. As raised in *Golden Chamber of Miscellaneous Diseases(Jīn Kuì Yào Luè,* 金匮要略）, there are four kinds of fluid retention，tan yin, or fluid retention in the gastro-intestinal tract; xuan yin, or fluid retention in the thorax; zhi yin, or fluid retention in the diaphragm; and yi yin, or fluid retention in the subcutaneous region.

There is another doctrine of "water, damp, phlegm, and fluid retention" which are all pathological products of metabolic dysfunction in the circulation of water and fluid, sharing the same origin and yet slightly different in nature. Generally speaking, damp accumulates and becomes water; water amasses and forms fluid retention; excessive fluid coagulates and generates phlegm. The thick and turbid is phlegm; the thin and clear is fluid retention. Water is thinner and clearer yet, and suffused water is dampness.

Feng's Brocaded Secret Records: Volume 12, Synthesized Reference on General Introduction of

Phlegmatic Fluid (Féng Shì Jǐn Náng Mì Lù: Juàn Shí Èr, Tán Yǐn Dà Xiǎo Zǒng Lùn Hé Cān, 冯氏锦囊秘录·卷十二·痰饮大小总论合参）: "*Disordered metabolism of body fluid results in the formation of phlegmatic fluid retention.*"

Jǐng-yue's Complete Works: Phlegmatic Fluid, Discussion On Syndrome (*Jǐng Yuè Quán Shū: Tán Yǐn , Lùn Zhèng,* 景岳全书·三十一卷·痰饮·论证): "*Phlegm and fluid retention are essentially different, though being in the same category. Fluid retention is of water-like nature......the difference between them lies in that fluid retention is thin and clear, whereas phlegm is thick turbid.*"

② Formation of the Phlegmatic Fluid (Fig. 6-7)

The formation of phlegmatic fluid is related to many factors, including the six exogenous climatic pathogens, the seven endogenous emotional pathogens, improper diet, as well as improper work and rest, which affect the metabolism of bodily fluids by disturbing the transformative function of qi on bodily fluids of the viscera of the Lungs, the Spleen, the Kidneys, and the *San Jiao.*

Jǐng-yue's Complete Works: Phlegmatic Fluid, Discussion On Syndrome (*Jǐng Yuè Quán Shū: Tán Yǐn , Lùn Zhèng,* 景岳全书·三十一卷·痰饮·论证): "*Dampness originates from the Spleen,*

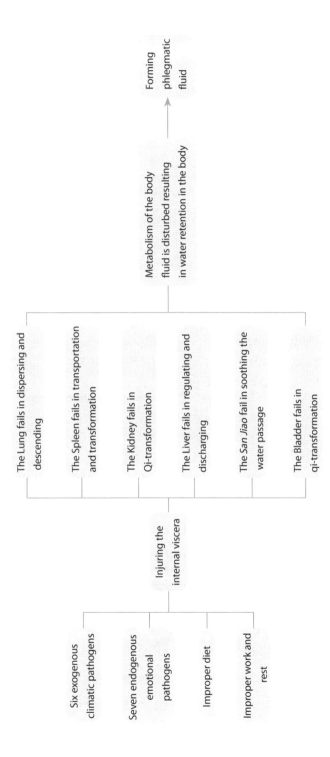

Fig. 6-7   Summary of the pathological formation of the phlegmatic fluid

the disturbed dampness is phlegm; the Kidney dominates water metabolism, and water also drift to transform into phlegm. So formation of phlegm is closely related to the Spleen and the root lies in the Kidney."

③ Illness-Causing Characteristics of the Phlegmatic Fluid Pathogen

Once phlegmatic fluid resides within the body, it causes visceral dysfunction and qi-flow disturbance. The qi and blood of channels and collaterals circulates unsmoothly, giving rise to new pathological processes. The general pathogenic features are:

A. Emerges and spreads throughout the entire body, resulting in extensive disease location

Once the phlegmatic fluid pathogen takes form, it spreads throughout the entire body, externally reaching the channels and collaterals, the muscles, bones and tendons, internally extending to the viscera.

B. Causes diverse and complicated syndromes

The phlegmatic fluid pathogen remains within the body, affecting the function of the viscera and the circulation of both qi and blood, as well as the metabolism of bodily fluids, leading to a diversity of pathological changes. The syndromes are divided into two categories of phlegm syndromes and fluid retention syndromes, with the former further divided into the tangible and the intangible. The progress of the phlegmatic fluid syndrome is extremely complicated. It may transform into yin cold and damage yang, or remain and transform into fire, or into dryness and injure yin, or attack together with wind or the heat, or even eclipse the Heart-spirit. Hence the theory of "various diseases originate from the aggravation of phlegm." Thus, its illness-causing nature is summarized as causing diverse and complicated syndromes.

Synopsis of Golden Chamber: On Pulse and Syndrome and Treatment of Phlegmatic Fluid and Cough (Jīn Kuì Yào Lüè · Tán Yǐn Ké Sòu Bìng Mài Zhèng Bìng Zhì, 金匮要略·痰饮咳嗽病脉证并治): "There are four kinds of fluid retention, what are they? The master said, there are Tan yin, Xuan yin, Zhi yin, and Yi yin. Tan yin, fluid retention in the gastro-intestinal *tract with emaciation and sthenic bowel sound; Xuan yin, fluid retention suspended in the chest and hypochondrium, causing pain when coughing or spitting; Yi yin, fluid retention in the subcutaneous region of the extremeties manifested as abscent sweat and heaviness of the limbs; and Zhi yin, diaphragm fluid retention leading to cough, dyspnea, edema and orthopnea."*

C. Lingering, persistent disease and extended course of treatment

Phlegmatic fluid comes from the accumulation of water and damp, being both a pathological byproduct and a pathogen that causes new pathological changes. Due to the lack of an easy cure and elimination of its pathogenic nature, full recovery from syndromes is difficult to achieve, so the disease course is usually prolonged and lingering.

④ Common Syndromes and Symptoms Caused by the Phlegmatic Fluid Pathogen

Clinical manifestations vary depending upon the location of invasion. (Table 6-18, Table 6-19)

Static Blood

① Basic Concept of Static Blood (Fig. 6-8)

Static blood refers to diminished blood circulation and includes the pathological product of extravascular blood retained in the body and the pathological changes of blood retained in the viscera and channels caused by unsmooth blood flow. It causes new pathological changes and is therefore classified as a secondary pathogen.

In the ancient classics, static blood is also referred to as "blood clotting", "fixed blood", "extravascular blood", "lochioschesis", "blood-retention", "corrupted blood", and "dead blood".

As a pathological byproduct and secondary pathogen, there are two related but different concepts of "stasis caused by disease" and "disease caused by stasis". The former focuses on the pathological course of blood stasis due to unsmooth blood circulation brought on by various diseases, or "stagnation of blood" while the latter refers to the secondary pathogen of the stagnated blood which

Table 6-18 Different disease locations and respective symptoms of the phlegm pathogen

Disease Location	Major Symptoms
Phlegm obstructs the Lungs	Cough, gasping, thoracic discomfort, profuse phlegm
Phlegm obstructs the Heart (unsmooth blood circulation)	Thoracic discomfort, palpitations
Phlegm eclipses the Heart orifice	Coma, dimensia
Phlegm-fire disturbs the Heart-spirit	Psychosis, mania
Phlegm rises to and aggravates the head and the eyes	Dizziness, unconciousness
Phlegm and qi congeal in the throat	Feeling of obstruction in the throat one is unable to cough up or swallow
Phlegm obstructs the channels	Numbness of the limbs, partial paralysis, Bell's palsy
Phlegm stagnates subcutaneously	Subcutaneous swelling and lumps
Phlegm retention in the bones and muscles	Deep tissue growths, fistulation and pyorrhea with blood (dorsal furuncle or multiple abscess)
Phlegm retention in the joints	Pain, swelling, rigidity, and deformity of the joints

Table 6-19 Different disease locations and respective symptoms of fluid retention

Diseased Location	Major Symptoms
Fluid retention in the Lungs	Thoracic discomfort, coughing and gasping with difficulty lying down, generalized swelling, vomiting clear sputum (retention of fluid in the diaphragm)
Fluid retention in the thorax	Fullness and swelling in chest, coughing that leads to pain in the ribs and thorax (fluid retention in the thorax)
Fluid retention in the gastro-intestinal tract	Gastro-abdominal distension and pain, intestinal gurgling, vomiting clear water and sputum (fluid retention in the gastro-intestinal tract)
Fluid retention in the skin and muscles	General edema, heaviness of the body, lack of sweat, reduced urine (fluid retention in the subcutaneous region)
Fluid retention in the abdomen	Drum-like swelling of the abdomen, reduced urine, varicose veins in the abdominal wall (ascites)

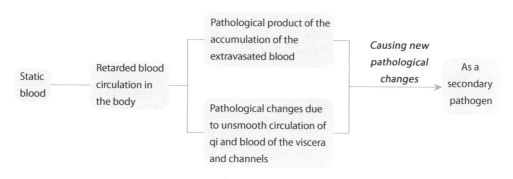

Fig. 6-8 Summary of Basic Concepts of Static Blood

causes new diseases, or "blood stasis".

Discussion on Blood Syndromes: Static Blood (*Xuě Zhèng Lùn: Yū Xuě*, 血证论·瘀血): "*The blood is still clear and fresh when it has just escaped from the vessels. Even though clear and fresh, it is extravasated blood, doomed to turn dark and become blood stasis.*"

② Formation of Static Blood (Fig. 6-9)

Various factors may lead to static blood, like invasion of exogenous pathogens, disharmony of emotions, injury due to improper diet, unbalanced work and rest, which cause dysfunction of the viscera and retard blood circulation, giving rise to static blood. The primary pathogeneses is as following:

A. Static blood due to bleeding

Trauma can break blood vessels and cause bleeding. The various causes of bleeding lead directly to extravascular blood, which cannot be properly digested or eliminated from the body and thus accumulates, forming static blood.

B. Static blood due to qi stagnation

Qi and blood circulate concomitantly, making harmonious qi flow one of the necessary factors for normal blood circulation, i.e. blood follows qi. If the qi flow becomes stagnant, then blood flows sluggishly. The static blood in the body forms blood stasis, that is, qi stagnation results in static blood.

C. Static blood due to qi deficiency

When deficient, qi is unable to drive the blood flow successfully, leading to sluggish circulation and forming blood stasis. Weakened qi may also fail in consolidating the blood and results in blood oozing extravascularly, then retained in the body and becoming static blood.

D. Static blood due to blood cold

Blood flows when warmed and coagulates when cold. The cold pathogen is coagulating in nature, so either invasion by exogenous cold evil or endogenous cold due to deficiency of yang may lead to abnormal blood circulation and the formation of static blood.

E. Static blood due to blood heat

When an invasion of heat evil reaches the blood phase, it intermingles with the blood, and burns the fluid component to cause thickness and stagnation of th e blood. The heat pathogen may also scorch the blood vessels causing the blood to flow extravascularly, leading to bleeding and the formation of static blood.

Among the above-mentioned pathogeneses of static blood, two general trends emerge. For reasons such as trauma, bleeding, qi-deficiency, and blood heat that cause static blood by driving the blood to flow extravascularly and be retained in the body; and those like qi-stagnation, qi-deficiency, blood cold and blood heat cause static blood by retarding the normal circulation of blood and lead to blood stasis in the viscera and channels.

Miraculous Pivot: Chapter On Carbuncle and Deep-rooted Carbuncle (*Líng Shū: Yōng Jū*, 灵枢·痈疽) : "*The cold evil stays in the channels and collaterals, leads to sluggish circulation of blood, finally resulting in blockage of the channels.*"

③ Illness-Causing Characteristics of Static Blood (Fig. 6-10)

After formation, static blood accumulates in the body and retards the qi flow, obstructing the vessels and affecting the circulation of both qi and blood as well as the functional activities of the viscera, leading to new pathological changes. In spite of the diversity of the syndromes and symptoms, the diseases caused by static blood have certain characteristics in common such as symptoms of pain, bleeding, and particular inspection and pulse manifestations.

A. Pain

The pain is mainly caused by static obstruction in the vessels and retarded qi and blood circulation. As the saying goes, the stagnation of qi and blood result in pain. The pain caused by static blood is usually stabbing and fixed, with tenderness that grows worse at night.

B. Growths and masses

Growths may be caused by blood stasis in the skin and channels due to trauma or by long-term accumulation of the static blood which forms an immobile abdominal mass. The position of the mass is characteristically fixed, with pain and usually with dark purple swelling around the area of trauma on the body surface; or with hardening and tenderness within the body.

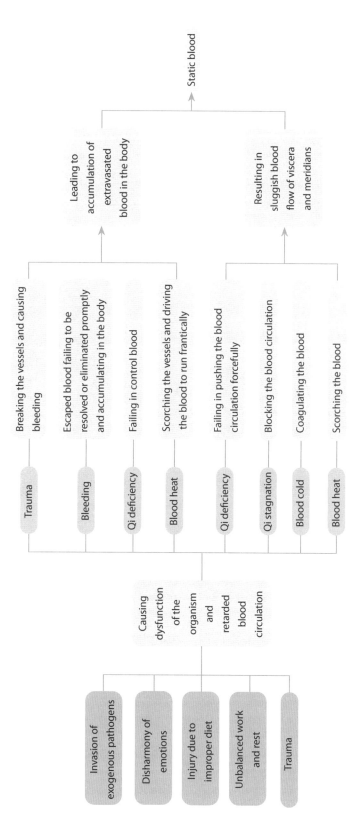

Fig. 6-9 Summary of the formation of static blood

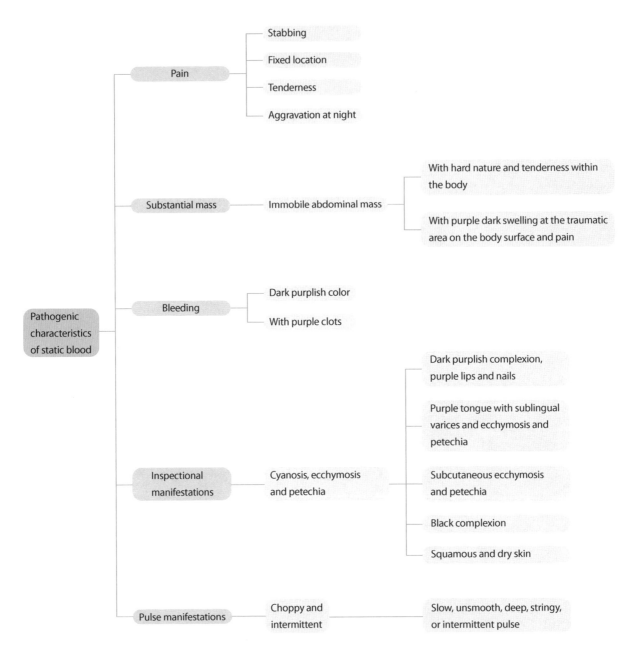

Fig. 6-10   General illness-causing characteristics of static blood

C. Bleeding

The obstruction of static blood in the vessels can cause extravascular bleeding characterized by dark purplish color, or with purple clots.

D. Inspection manifestations

The blood stagnates in the channels causing the hindrance of blood flow, manifested externally as a dark purplish complexion, purple lips and nails, purple tongue with sublingual varices or with subcutaneous ecchymosis and petechia. If the muscles, skin and channels go unnourished due to long term disease, there may be black complexion or dry and scaly skin.

E. Pulse manifestations

Vessel obstruction may result in a choppy and intermittent pulse due to the sluggish flow of blood. Patients with static blood syndromes tend to display slow, choppy, deep, wiry, regularly or irregularly intermittent pulses.

Discussion on Blood Syndromes: Blood Stasis (Xuě Zhèng Lùn: Yū Xuě, 血证论·瘀血): "In the middle Jiao, blood stasis leads to stabbing pain in the abdomen, hypochondrium, and lower back." "Blood stasis in the channels transforms into abdominal

mass."

Correction on Errors in Medical Classics: Agglomerate (Yī Lín Gǎi Còu: Jié Kuài, 医林改错·结块): "Qi is intangible and unable to agglomerate; that agglomerates must be tangible blood (stasis)."

④ Common Symptoms of Static Blood

Static blood causes various symptoms that manifest differently according to different positions. (Table 6-20)

Stones

① The Concept of Stones

Stones, or calculi, refer to hard, stone-like concretions that form in certain locations of the body. They are pathological byproducts that form under various

Table 6-20 Position and the correlating symptoms of static blood

Position of Stasis	Major Symptoms
Stasis in the Heart	Palpitations, thoracic discomfort, chest pain, purple lips
	Unconsciousness, mania
Stasis in the Lungs	Chest pain, hemoptysis of dark, purplish blood
Stasis in the Liver and Spleen	Bilateral growths in the thoracic and ribcage are with pain and tenderness
Stasis in the gastro-intestinal tract	Gastro-abdominal pain, haematemesis, melena
Stasis in the uterus	lower abdominal pain, irregular menstruation, dark purplish menstrous often with clots, dysmenorrhea, amenorrhea, metrorrhagia and postpartum metrostaxis
Stasis in the head	Intense or stabbing headache
Stasis in the chest and thoracic	Bilateral stabbing pain along the ribcage
Stasis in the extremeties	Cold limbs, with dark red or purple skin, and embolisms
Stasis in the interstitial space between the skin and muscles	Localized purple discoloration, subcutaneous swelling, and pain

conditions. They can lead to new pathological changes and are classified as a secondary pathogen (Fig. 6-11).

② Formation of Stones

The formation of stones is relatively complex and closely related to imbalance in dietary, emotional and lifestyle habits that lead to the accumulation of damp heat. Over a long period of time, this damp heat is further reduced to a solid formation. It is also closely related to factors like basic constitution, age and gender.

A. Improper diet

Addiction to pungent and spicy or sweat and greasy foods, or to certain other specific foods, may lead to accumulation of damp heat and form stones.

B. Internal injury from emotional factors

Unfulfilled intentions may cause Liver depression and failure of the Gallbladder to discharge bile. This long-term accumulation of bile may eventually lead to stones.

C. Improper drug administration

Over dose or long term administration of certain drugs may disturb the visceral functions and retard excretion, leading to the accumulation of pharmaceutical sediment in the body that may harden into stones.

D. Basic constitution

Certain types of people may be predisposed to metabolic abnormalities that lead to the formation of stones.

③ Illness-Causing Characteristics of Stones

A. Prone to formation in the Liver, Gallbladder, Stomach, Kidneys, and Bladder

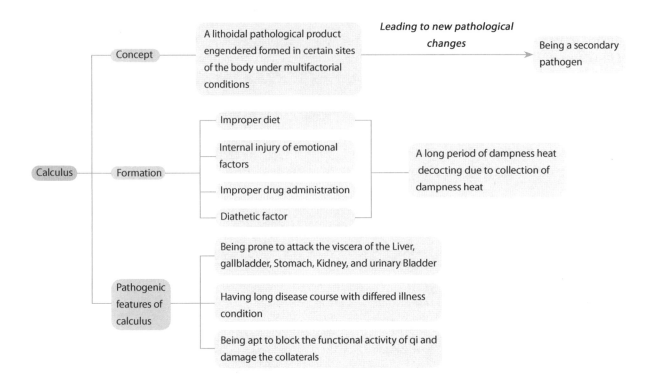

Fig. 6-11 Summary of the Formation and Illness-Causing Characteristics of Stones

The viscera of the Liver, Gallbladder, Kidney, and urinary Bladder are closely related to the generation and excretion of bile and urine while the Stomach governs food intake. This makes them the common location for the formation of stones, hence the diseases of Liver and Gallbladder stones, Kidney and Bladder stones, and gastric stones.

B. Long disease process with different levels of severity

The stones usually form through long term stewing of accumulated damp heat, with most calculus formations having a long course. Due to the difference sizes and positions, clinical manifestations vary greatly. Usually small stones have mild or no symptoms, while larger stones have more severe, more obvious symptoms and more frequent onsets.

C. Block the functional activity of qi and damage the collaterals

Being a substantial pathogenic factor retained within the body, the stones necessarily obstruct the flow of qi flow and affect the normal circulation of qi and blood and metabolism of the bodily fluids. Symptoms include localized aching pain and distention, usually paroxysmal, or vague, or distending, or acute, with fixed position. In addition, stones can also damage the vessels and cause bleeding.

④ Common Symptoms of Stones

Disease like the gallstones and urinary stones are commonly observed. Gallstones are solid formations in the biliary system including the gall Bladder itself and bile ducts. Urinary stones are solid formations in the urinary system, including renal stones, cystic stones and urethral stones. The clinical manifestations vary with the size, position, and existence of infection and blockage, etc. (detailed symptoms omitted)

Section 4 Miscellaneous Pathogens

In the etiology of Chinese medicine, there are other pathogens beside the exogenous, endogenous, and secondary pathogens, like trauma, parasites, congenital factors, toxic factors, etc. which also cause disease, referred to as the miscellaneous pathogens.

Trauma

Trauma refers to a variety of injuries caused by external forces such as physical violence of various types, e.g. external injury, scalds and burns, frostbite and animal bites (Table 6-21).

There is almost always a clear traumatic cause of injury and symptoms vary.

① External Injuries

External injuries refer to injuries caused by mechanical force, including injury from falls, fractures, and injuries from over-exertion, crushing injuries, impact injuries, gunshots, and stab wounds.

Table 6-21　Types of trauma and characteristics

Trauma		Major Symptoms
External injuries	Injury from falls, fractures, injuries from over-exertion, crushing injuries, impact injuries, gunshots, and stab wounds	Damage the skin and muscles in mild cases, leading to reduced localized blood circulation, swelling, haematoma, pain and bleeding; damage to the bones, tendons and internal organs, resulting in joint dislocation, fracture, ruptured skin and burst flesh, intense pain, excessive bleeding, unconsciousness, or even death
Scalds and burns	Burns from open flame, boiling water or oil, steam, or electric heat	Localized sensations of intense heat, redness and swelling, pain and blistering in mild cases; leather-like, waxy white, brown or even charred appearance of the affected area in severe cases; in extensive burn cases, the internal viscera may be invaded by the fire toxin, leading to coma
Frost bite	Prevailing cold of the environment together with a deficiency in body defenses	Localized frost bite; general frost bite, frozen rigor, or frozen stiffness
Animal bites	Bites from animals like ferocious beasts, poisonous snakes or mad dogs Stings by insects like scorpions, bees or wasps	In mild cases, the skin and muscles are injured, with localized swelling, pain and bleeding; in severe cases the internal viscera are damaged, the patient may die due to massive bleeding; those bitten by mad dogs may suffer from rabies, or hydrophobia; those bitten by poisonous snakes or stung by scorpions, bees, wasps, or centipedes, may suffer general symptoms of toxicity such as localized swelling and pain, dizziness, palpitations, sickness and vomiting, even coma and death

The external injuries can damage the skin and muscles in mild cases, leading to reduced local blood circulation manifested in swelling, haematoma, pain and bleeding; orthopedic damage and internal damage, may result in joint dislocation, fracture, ruptured skin and burst flesh, intense pain, excessive bleeding, unconsciousness, and may even be life threatening.

② Scalds and Burns

Scalds and burns indicate exposure to virulent fire, including open flames, boiling water or oil, steam, and electric heat, which burn the body.

In mild cases, the skin is burned resulting in localized sensations of topical heat, redness and swelling, pain and blistering. In severe burn cases, the muscles, bones and tendons may be burnt, the affected area appears leather-like, waxy white, brown or even charred. In cases of extensive burns, the internal viscera may be invaded by the fire toxin and then fall into loss of consciousness.

③ Frostbite

Frostbite is a general or localized injury caused by excessively low temperature.

Localized frost bite is caused by localized exposure of certain parts of the body, like the hands, feet, ears, nose and cheeks, to low temperature, and manifests in pale complexion and a cold numbness, followed by purplish swelling and itching pain, a scorching sensation, or blisters, ulcers and tissue necrosis.

General frost bite, frozen rigor, or frozen stiffness, is caused by prevailing yin-coldness of the environment and a deficiency in bodily defense, and manifests as chills, sudden drop in body temperature, pale complexion, cyanotic lips, tongue and finger nails, numbness, dull reactions, or unconsciousness, weak breathing and pulse, or even death.

④ Animal Bites

This refers to bites from animals like ferocious beasts, poisonous snakes or mad dogs, or stings by insects like scorpions, bees or wasps.

In mild cases, the skin and muscles are injured, with localized swelling, pain, and bleeding while the internal viscera may be damaged in severe cases, and the patient may die due to massive bleeding. Those bitten by mad dogs suffer from rabies, or hydrophobia. Those bitten by poisonous snakes or stung by scorpions, bees, wasps, or centipedes, may present general symptoms of toxicity such as localized swelling and pain, dizziness, palpitations, sickness and vomiting, even coma and death.

Parasites

This is a general name given to animal parasites that live within the human body and lead to disease by consuming the vital nutrients of qi, blood and bodily fluids, damage the viscera and tissues.

Parasitic infection refers to the intake of foods contaminated with parasite larva or external contact with water or earth contaminated with parasite larva that leads to parasitic disease.

The common parasites invading the human body include roundworm, hookworm, pinworm, tapeworm, blood fluke, etc. Clinical manifestations vary with the different pathways and location of infection. For instance, with roundworm there is abdominal pain around the naval region, and as it becomes more severe, may cause peripheral coldness, which is termed "roundworm limb-coldness"; pinworm is specifically characterized by unusual itching of the anus that grows worse at night; blood fluke is characterized by growths of the ribcage and swollen abdomen. (Syndrome differentiation and determination of treatment for parasite-induced illnesses is further discussed in courses on clinical medicine and so have been omitted here)

Congenital Factors

This refers to factors of hereditary origin often appearing during the fetal stages of development that lead to disease after birth. They include genetic factors inherited from parents and conditions that influence the health of the fetus during development in the womb and delivery and are usually divided into the two categories of fetal weakness and fetal toxicity.

Complete Work on Children's Diseases: Volume 2, Discussion on Fetal Disease (Yòu Yòu Jí Chéng: Juàn Èr, Tāi Bìng Lùn, 幼幼集成·卷二·胎病论): "Diseases of newborn infants are mostly of the kind like fetal deficit and inherited eruptions."

① Fetal Weakness

This refers to the insufficiency or abnormality of the essence and blood inherited from the parents, causing a naturally weak endowment to the baby.

The main causes of fetal weakness are twofold. The first is a deficiency or abnormality of the paternal essence and qi; the second, deficiency of the maternal qi and blood, both of which can influence the growth of the fetus and lead to fetal weakness.

Diseases of fetal weakness include both congenital diseases, like congenital anomaly or deformity, and inherent constitutional weakness, such as physical and mental growth defects of the infant baby.

Golden Mirror of Medicine: Knacks on Learning Miscellaneous Pediatric Disease, Volume 55,

Miscellaneous Syndromes (Yī Zōng Jīn Jiàn: Yòu Kē Zá Bìng Xīn Fǎ Yào Jué, Juàn Wǔ Shí Wǔ, Zá Zhèng Mén, 医宗金鉴·幼科杂病心法要诀·卷五十五·杂证门): *"Five lates (tardy growth,* 五迟*) in children (retardations of standing, walking, hair, denting, language) result from deficiency of the parents' qi and blood, which causes congenital deficit of Kidney qi and essence of the baby, leading to flaccid tendons and bones and retarded development of walking, denting, and sitting, etc.."*

② Fetal Toxicity

This refers to a heat toxin inherited from the mother, leading to sores, furuncles, and exanthematous diseases like small pox and chickenpox.

There are two main causes of fetal toxicity. The first is the contraction of contagious disease, such as congenital syphilis, by the parents. The second is improper diet or lifestyle habits or misuse of drugs and pharmaceuticals during pregnancy, e.g. an addiction to pungent and hot or greasy foods by a pregnant woman, may lead to concealed visceral fire in the mother's body that is passed on to the fetus and congeals into fetal toxicity.

Fetal toxicity leads to various diseases, including neonatal jaundice, infant thrush, ulcers and furuncles, chicken pox, measles, and congenital syphilis.

Complete Work on Children's Diseases: Volume 4, Syphilitic Lesions (Yòu Yòu Jí Chéng: Juàn Sì, Yang Méi Chuāng Zhèng, 幼幼集成·卷四·杨梅疮证): *"Syphilitic lesions are characterized by waxberry-like erythema and swelling, hence the name......infantile syphilis is due to the congenital toxins of the parents. Unlike the usual mentioned fetal toxin, it is mostly seen in prostitutes, being resulted from unsanitary sexual activities."*

In summary, congenital factors generally cause diseases of two categories, hereditary disease and inborn disease.

(1) Hereditary disease:

Inheritance is an important attribute of the biological system of reproduction, indicating the capacity for certain traits of the parental generation to be passed on to the filial generation. Likewise, pathological characteristics may also be handed down to offspring in much the same way, hence the occurrence of hereditary disease. i.e. certain abnormalities of the parents are passed on to the offspring through inheritance. For instance, hemophilia, schizophrenia, epilepsy, diabetes, hypertension, and color-blindness, and anaphylactic diseases, etc. are all genetic in nature.

(2) Inborn diseases:

Diseases that are born during the intrauterine period of development of the fetus, i.e. underdevelopment or deformity of certain parts of the fetus, are called inborn diseases. The occurrence of inborn diseases are related factors such as certain viral infections of the mother during pregnancy, administration of certain drugs that adversely affect the fetus, intense mental or emotional stimulus during pregnancy, contact with harmful physical or chemical materials, inbreeding, or inadvertent injury during delivery, may lead to diseases like congenital cardiovascular diseases, cleft palate, polydactyly, or aproctia, etc.

Various Poisons

This is a general term for the various diseases caused by ingested items. Besides the pestilential pathogens, food poisoning and fetal toxicity mentioned above, drug abuse, chemical poisoning and drug poisoning all fall into this category. Different poisonous pathogens have different natures and pathogenic features, resulting in various relevant clinical manifestations.

Chapter 7
The Onset of Disease

The theoretical system regarding the onset of disease is the study on the mechanisms, pathways, categories and influential factors in the onset of disease. It is a process of conflict between the damaging influence of pathogens and the restorative power of the right qi. The onset of disease is related to two aspects, one is the functional status of the body (the right qi), the other is the damage and influence of the pathogens on the body (the evil), which in turn affect the mechanisms, pathways, categories and influential factors in the onset of disease. This chapter will mainly discuss the basic mechanisms, influential factors, and the types of disease onset.

Section 1   Pathogenesis

Pathogenesis focuses on the relationship between the onset of disease and the vital (right qi) and pathogen (evil qi).

The Struggle between the Vital and the Evil and the Onset of Disease

The onset of disease is intimately related to both the right qi of the body and the invading pathogen. On the one hand, the invasion of the

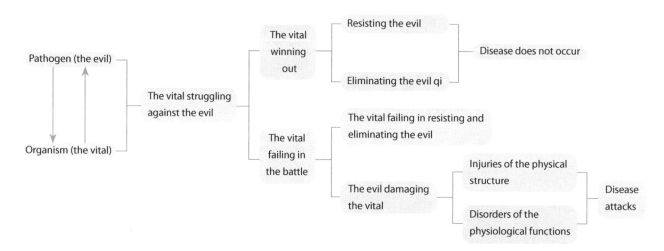

Fig. 7-1   The Struggle between the Right qi and the Pathogen and the Onset of Disease

evil qi causes damage to the body, while on the other; the right qi resists and drives the evil away. If the vital is superior in strength to the pathogen, disease will not occur, and vice versa. Thus the inferiority of the right qi and the invasion of the pathogen are taken to be the two basic factors in the onset of disease. (Fig. 7-1)

Miraculous Pivot: The Initiation of Various Diseases (*Líng Shū: Bǎi Bìng Shǐ Shēng*, 灵枢·百病始生): "*Evils such as wind, rain, cold, heat can only invade when the* right qi *of the body is deficient. Those who remain in condition when encountering sudden torrential rain must be strong enough to resist the evil. The occurrence of disease must be brought about by combination of deficient* right qi *and violent exogenous pathogen.*"

The Roles of the Right Qi and the Pathogen in the Onset of Disease

The right qi is the principle factor and the evil qi is the significant condition for the occurrence of disease.

① Deficiency of the Right Qi is the Internal Pathway to the Onset of Illness

(1) Definition of right qi

Right qi, relatively defined in opposition to evil qi, is a general term that refers to the vital functional activities of the body that govern life maintenance, including the ability of the body to heal itself, the adaptability to changing conditions, and the ability to fight off pathogens.

(2) Contribution of the right qi to onset (Fig. 7-2)

Right qi is responsible for the body's immune functions of resisting and dispelling pernicious influences. Chinese medical theory places great importance on the right qi in disease onset, maintaining that deficiency of the right qi is the prerequisite condition for illness as represented in the following aspects:

A. Strong right qi makes disease unlikely to occur

Powerful right qi can both resist the evil's invasion and remove adverse effects brought on by pathogens, thus making disease less likely

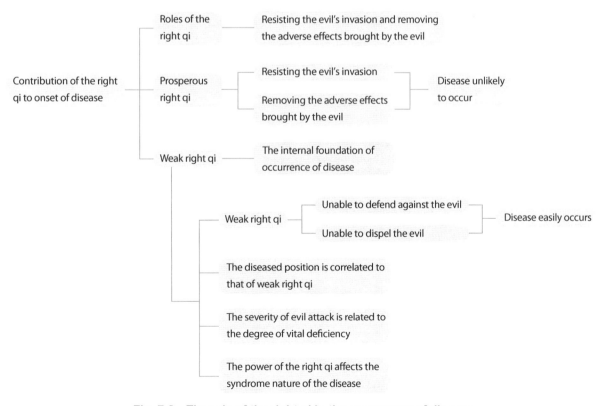

Fig. 7-2   The role of the right qi in the occurrence of disease

to occur, as the classical saying goes, "While the right qi is vigorous in the body, the evil is unable to invade."

B. Weak right qi facilitates the onset of disease

When the right qi of the body becomes relatively weak, it is unable to defend the body against evil qi or dispel pathogens, resulting in the structural and functional damage and the eventual onset of disease. This is keeping with the classical saying, "If the pathogen remains, the right qi must be deficient."

C. Disease position correlates to the specific weaknesses of the right qi

The evil tends to injure the body part or viscus with weak right qi, i.e. the evil invasion may indicate deficiency of the right qi of the affected location or viscus.

D. The severity of pathogenic attack is related to the degree of vital deficiency

Generally speaking, the severity of evil attack is related to the degree of vital deficiency. That is, mild weakness of right qi leads to slight evil invasion, and severe weakness of the right qi leads to severe evil invasion.

E. The power of the right qi affects the nature of the syndrome of the disease

When the pathogen attacks, if the right qi is vigorous and struggles intensely with the pathogen, the resulting syndrome is usually sthenic or excessive; on the contrary, a weak right qi being incapable of defending against the evil leads to a deficient, asthenic syndrome, or a deficient syndrome mingled with excess, even life threatening syndromes.

In conclusion, the power of the right qi determines whether an individual will fall ill or not, and is closely related to the location of attack, severity of invasion, and the nature of the syndrome of the disease. Hence the idea of the right qi being the primary factor and the pathogen the most important condition for the occurrence of disease.

Plain Question: Discussion on Acupuncture Methods (Sù Wèn: Cì Fǎ Lùn, 素问·刺法论): "With the right qi vigorous inside, the evil cannot invade."

Plain Question: Comments on Febrile Diseases (Sù Wèn: Píng Rè Bìng Lùn, 素问·评热病论): "Where evils converge, the right qi must be deficient."

2 The Pathogen as a Significant Condition for Onset

(1) Definition of pathogen

Compared to the right qi, the pathogen, or evil qi,

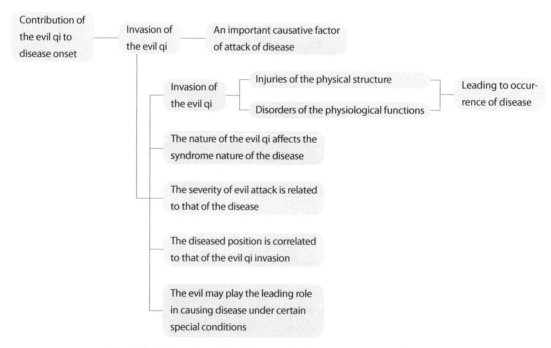

Fig. 7-3　The roles of pathogens in the occurrence of disease

is a general reference to various pathogenic factors, including exogenous and endogenous pathogens.

(2) Contribution of the pathogen to onset (Fig. 7-3)
Chinese medicine emphasizes the prerequisite role of the right qi in the occurrence of disease. However, the significance of the evil qi is also of great importance, represented as the following:

A. Evil qi is the causative factor of disease

Any disease has its special causative factors. The evil qi invades the body, damaging the body physically or functionally and causes disease. The organism will not suffer from diseases without pathogenic invasion or the resulting damage.

B. The nature of the pathogen affects the nature of the syndrome of the disease

Different evils attack the body and bring about different pathogenic features and syndrome characteristics accordingly. For example, yin cold pathogens cause cold syndromes, and yang heat pathogens cause heat syndromes; emotional pathogens cause emotional abnormalities; traumatic pathogens cause external injuries.

C. The severity of the pathogenic attack directly relates to the severity of the disease

The severity of disease is influenced by not only the strength of the right qi but also by the vigor of the pathogen. Slight attacks of evil qi lead to mild illnesses, and vice versa.

D. The disease location correlates to that of the invasion of the evil qi

The location of the invasion of evil qi influences the disease location. That is, pathogens remaining at the skin's surface cause external syndromes; evil directly invading the internal organs leads to internal syndromes. For instance, evil invading the lungs causes illness of the lungs, injury to the gastrointestinal tract results in gastrointestinal dysfunction.

E. Under certain special conditions, the pathogen may play the leading role in causing disease

When the evil is extremely overpowering, the right qi, though sufficient, fails to defend the body. Thus the evil plays the leading and crucial role in disease onset. Pathogens like pestilence, extreme temperature, high-voltage current, chemical toxins, and various traumas can injure the body in this way.

In summary, illness is caused by pathogens, and influenced by the pathogen's nature, vigor, and position of invasion, making it a significant factor in the onset of disease.

Confucians' Duties to Parents: Explanation on the Three Therapeutical Methods of Perspiration, Expectoration and Purgation (Rú Mén Shì Qīn: Hàn Tù Xià Sān Fǎ Gāi Jìn Zhì Bìng Quán, 儒门事亲·汗吐下三法该尽治病诠): "People are not born with disease. It is either caused exogenously or generated internally, due to pathogenic factors."

In addition, from the perspective of internal and external causes of disease, the right qi can be considered the internal factor and the pathogen the external. Therefore, it can also be said that a deficiency of the right qi is the internal basis of onset and the influence of the pathogen is the external condition.

The concept of internal and external factors in

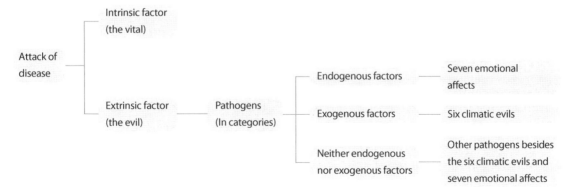

Fig. 7-4   Difference between the internal and external factors in pathogenesis and the endogenous and exogenous factors in etiology

the theory of pathogenesis is different with the endogenous and exogenous factors in the doctrine of triple pathogens in etiology. The former belongs to the realm of philosophical concepts, while the latter refers to the methodology for the categorization for pathogens, with the endogenous referring to the emotional pathogens, the exogenous indicating the climatic evils. (Fig. 7-4)

③ The Result of the Struggle between the Right Qi and the Pathogen Determines the Onset of Disease (Fig. 7-1)

As mentioned above, a deficiency of the right qi is the internal basis to onset, and the influence of the pathogen the external condition. In the course of onset, the right qi and the pathogen are in constant struggle, with the result of this struggle deciding whether the disease occurs or not.

A. The right qi emerges superior to the pathogen and illness does not occur

When the pathogen invades the body, the right qi rises to do battle with it. If the strength of the right qi succeeds in defending against and dispelling the pathogenic influence, the organism remains well protected with no injury or clinical symptoms and signs, and disease does not occur.

B. The evil overcomes the vital and results in disease

On the contrary, when the evil invades the body, the weak vital fails in defending against and dispelling the evil and the organism is injured or the physiological functions are disturbed, clinical symptoms and signs appear and disease occurs.

Section 2　Influencing Factors of Attack of Disease

The vital and evil qi are the two basic decisive factors in the onset of disease. However, other factors, both internal and external, also influence them, their struggle, and the onset of disease. These factors include the two main aspects of external environment and diathetic factors of the body.

The External Environment and the Onset of Disease

External environment is composed of the natural and social environments, both of which are inseparable from the existence of the human race. This includes climatic factors, geographic factors, and the conditions of everyday life and work. Humans depend on their natural and social environments in many ways, which in turn influence the physiological activities of the body and the onset of disease. Environmental factors mainly affect the onset in two ways of generation and transmission of evil qi.

① Seasonal and Climatic Factors

Abnormal changes in season or climate are good medium for the promotion and transmission of evil qi that can lead to various diseases. They are prone to cause commonly encountered seasonal illnesses or seasonal epidemics, like wind attack in spring, summer-heat stroke in summer, dryness impairment in autumn and cold damage in winter. The outbreak and spread of pestilence are also related to abnormalities in natural climate. In different seasons, there appear different evils and diseases accordingly.

② Geographic Factors

Climatic characteristics, the nature of the water and soil, and living customs vary with different regions and affect the physiological characteristics and disease onset of the local population. These differences combine simultaneously to form commonly encountered regional diseases. For instance, in the north, the cold evil and dryness evil are commonly observed, while in the south the heat evil and dampness evil arise more often.

③ Environmental Factors of Everyday Life and Work

An unfavorable living and working environment may also become a causative factor for disease. Living in a damp and dim place with foul air or mosquitoes and other pests may lead to the occurrence and prevalence of disease. Noxious gases, waste liquids, dust and unpleasant noise can all function as pathogens and cause disease, or acute or chronic toxicity.

④ Social Environmental Factors

Human beings live in a certain social environment, and the social, economic, cultural, marital and familial status, and interpersonal relationships are all related to the onset of disease to a certain degree. If one fails to adapt to the various stimuli of their social environment and the emotional activities are negatively affected, disease may result.

Diathetic Factors and the Onset of Disease

It also commonly referred to as the relationship of internal environment to the onset of disease. Generally speaking, people with sound diathesis are not prone to illness, while those with diathetic problems are. The body diathesis is related to a person's constitutional, mental, and nutritional status. It affects the vigor of the right qi of the body that is of crucial importance to the prevention or manifestation of disease.

① Constitutions and Onset

The body's basic constitution is dependent upon the right qi of the body. There are both strong and weak constitutions. People with sound diathesis have vigorous right qi and are not prone to illness, while those with a weak constitution have a somewhat weakened right qi that makes them more susceptible to illness.

There is an element of yin or yang predominance in a person's constitution. People of yang-predominance and yin-deficiency are susceptible to the invasion of heat evil causing heat syndromes (excessive and deficient heat). On the contrary, those who are yin-predominant and yang-deficient are susceptible to the invasion of cold evil causing cold syndromes (excessive and

deficient cold).

And there is the element of weight in constitution. Obese or overweight people tend to produce phlegm and damp, are prone to invasion from cold and damp evils, causing dizziness or apoplexy; skinny or underweight individuals are often deficient in yin fluid, susceptible to dryness and heat evils, resulting in pneumal tuberculosis and cough.

② Mental State and Onset

Mental status affects the onset of disease by influencing the right qi of the body. It is dependent upon emotional activities, so that a cheerful mental state leads to a pleasant mood, with a harmonious qi flow and the normal functioning of the viscera. As a natural result, the right qi is vigorous and able to resist and dispel evils. In contrast, a depressed mental state result in abnormal emotional activities with disordered qi flow and visceral dysfunction, leading to the decline of right qi and disease.

Different mental states affect the degree of severity and syndrome manifestation of a disease. Fervent emotional stimuli of great happiness, sorrow, rage and fright lead to acute onsets, such as sudden thoracic obstruction, cardialgia and apoplexy are often induced by violent emotional stimuli. Long term and persistent stimulation from grief, contemplation, and melancholy lead to the slow onset of disease. Examples are gastric pain and insomnia caused by long term mental overactivity.

③ Nutritional State and Onset

Nutritional status has significant influence on both the body's constitution and the right qi, consequently affecting the onset of disease. A favorable nutritional status and well-rounded diet helps the qi and blood be sufficient and the body constitution robust, thus the right qi is prosperous and illness rare. Malnutrition or an imbalanced diet may lead to deficiency of the qi and blood and a weak body constitution; the right qi is likely to fail in repelling evil qi, resulting in susceptibility to the attack of disease.

Section 3　Types of Disease Attack

The nature, type, pathogenic pathway, location of the pathogen, together with the difference in right qi and diathesis, and the outcome of the vital-evil struggle, result in various attacking forms of disease. Generally there are six types, or immediate attack, latent attack, slow attack, secondary attack, combined and complicated disease, and relapse (Fig. 7-5).

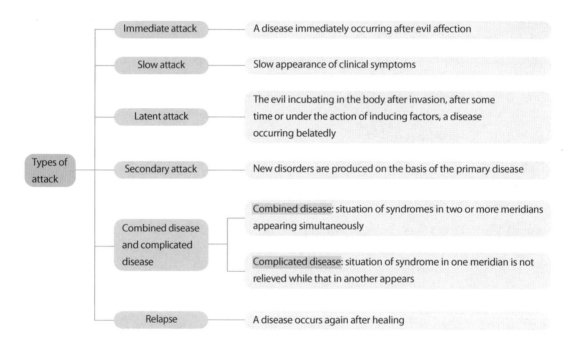

Fig. 7-5　Summary of type of disease attack

Immediate Attack

This refers to a disease that occurs immediately after contraction of evil qi. Also called "sudden attack", it is often seen in exogenous diseases and external injuries. It may be summarized as follows:

① Attack by Powerful Exogenous Evils

Invasion of the exogenous climatic evils of wind-cold, wind-heat, warm-heat, summer-heat, etc. lead to immediate onset.

② Attack by Pestilent Evils

Due to the strong infectious nature and virulence of the pestilent evils they cause immediate and acute onset.

③ Attack by Extreme Emotional Changes

Emotional changes like sudden rage or uncontrollable grief disorder the flow of qi within the body, leading to disharmony of qi and blood and visceral dysfunction, resulting in immediate onset.

④ Attack by poisonous substances

Unknowingly ingesting poisonous substances, being bitten by poisonous insects or snakes, or inhalation of toxic gases all lead to rapid onset of toxicity.

⑤ Attack by Various Traumas

A variety of trauma could cause immediate injuries.

Slow Attack

In opposition to immediate attack, slow attack is often seen in endogenous diseases. Pathological changes caused by excessive melancholy and sorrow, or dietary addictions, excessive strain or excessive rest, etc. accumulate gradually and lead to the slow appearance of clinical symptoms. In addition, exogenous diseases caused by damp invasion are also slow in onset.

Latent Attack

This means that the evil incubates in the body after invasion, and after some time or under the action of certain inducing factors, disease occurs. Examples are tetanus and rabies, both of which occur with delay following the initial invasion. In addition, the febrile disease of "insidious summer-heat" is also of this kind.

Plain Questions: Chapter Discussion on the Interrelationship between Life and Nature (Sù Wèn: Shēng Qì Tōng Tiān Lùn, 素问·生气通天论*): "Being attacked by pathogenic heat in summer leads to tertian malaria……being attacked by cold evil in winter results in febrile diseases in spring."*

Secondary Attack

This means that new disorders are produced on the basis of the primary disease, making the two closely related pathologically. For example, apoplexy resulting from hyperactivity of liver yang, pediatric stagnation that results as a secondary affleciton of malnutrition, the abdominal masses and drum-like swollen belly following liver disease, etc.

Combined and Complicated Disease

The terms of combined disease and complicated disease first appear in *Treatise on Exogenous Febrile Diseases (Shāng Hán Lùn,* 伤寒论*)*. The condition of syndromes appearing in two or more meridians simultaneously is called combined disease, usually seen under conditions of excessive evil and deficient right qi. Examples are combined febrile diseases of the greater yang and lesser yang meridians or of the greater yang and bright yang channels.

If the syndrome of one meridian is not relieved and another appears in a separate meridian, this is called complicated disease. This occurs mostly in the locational progression of a disease, and is essentially a relative transference of disease position in the disease course. Examples are complicated disease of greater yang and lesser yang meridians in the six meridians syndromes of febrile disease, and complicated disease of qi phase and nutritive phase in defensive-qi-nutritive-blood phase syndromes.

The difference between combined disease and complicated disease lies in the different sequence of onset, i.e. the former simultaneously and the latter successively.

Comments Collection of Treatise on Cold Pathogenic Diseases: Extended Understanding of the Theory of Treatise on Cold Pathogenic Diseases (Shāng Hán Lái Sū Jí: Shāng Hán Lùn Yì, 伤寒来苏集·伤寒论翼*): "Combined disease means syndromes in two or more meridians appearing simultaneously, and complicated disease refers to successive appearance of syndromes in one meridian then another."*

Relapse

When a disease occurs again after being successfully healed, it is known as a relapse, or "recurrence".

① Basic Characteristics of Relapse

A. The clinical manifestations of the relapsing disease are similar to that of the initial disease, however not a complete copy, and is usually more complicated.

B. The more frequent the relapse occurs, the more difficult complete recovery becomes during the stationary phase, and the worse prognosis becomes, as the disease becomes more likely to leave sequelae.

C. Most relapses have certain inducing factors.

(2) Major Types of Relapse

Due to the difference in the pathogen's nature and the vigor of the right qi of the body, there are different types of relapses. These include relapse after partial recovery, relapse with alternating intervals, and acute attack alternating with chronic remission (Fig. 7-6).

A. Relapse after partial recovery
This type is mostly seen in relatively serious exogenous febrile diseases. Improper diet and use of pharmaceuticals may further damage the weakened right qi and the residual evil qi then recrudesces to cause a relapse. For example, improper nursing and caring in the early recovery stage of a warm-damp syndrome may easily result in relapse.

B. Relapse with alternating intervals
Though the symptoms and signs of the initial attack are subdued with treatment, the root of the evil remains unexpelled from the body. Once the right qi becomes weak or some inducing factor appears, it causes a relapse. Like in asthma, the patient is no different from a healthy person during the intervals between attacks. However, the phlegm remains deeply rooted in the chest and diaphragm, and once the climate changes abruptly, or new evil affects the body, it causes a relapse. That is same for epilepsy and stone patients. Patients can live as normal, healthy people between attacks, while inducing factors may result in relapses.

C. Acute attack alternating with chronic remission
This is actually an alternation between remission with mild symptoms and acute attack of serious symptoms in chronic diseases. For example, in patients with symptoms such as drum-like swollen belly, cough and edema, their condition is relatively mild. However, when stimulated by

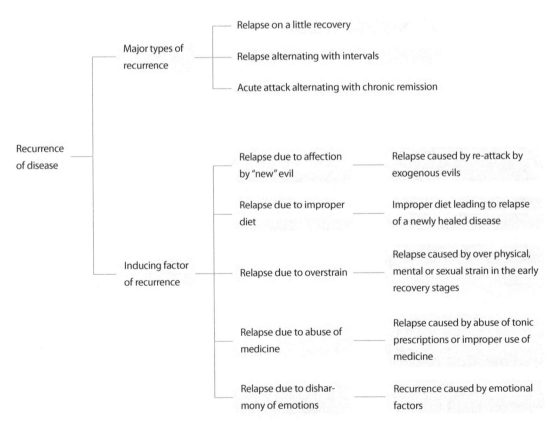

Fig. 7-6　Summary of the Types and Inducing Factors of the Relapse of Disease

inducing factors, it brings on an acute attack and the symptoms grow more severe.

③ Causes of Relapse

This refers to the inducing factors that assist the pathogen in damaging the right qi, leading to the break out of temporary pathological silence and a relapse of disease. The factors may be summarized as follows (Fig. 7-6):

A. Relapse due to affliction from "new" evil

This means that the relapse is caused by a new attack of exogenous evils. In the early recovery stage or the intervals between attacks, both the residual of evil and damaged right qi are weak. If at this time a new pathogen attacks, it is bound to aid the residual evil to further injure the right qi, leading to the activation of the pathological changes and resulting in relapse. It is commonly seen in both exogenous and endogenous diseases, especially in exogenous febrile diseases.

B. Relapse due to improper diet

When a disease is recently healed, improper diet may lead to relapse. For example, untempered diet may cause the relapse of spleen/stomach diseases; intake of seafood may lead to a relapse of hives or asthma; drinking alcohol and eating pungent and greasy foods may result in relapse of stranguria and hemorrhoids. Therefore, in the treatment of spleen/stomach and febrile diseases, dietetic restraint is of great importance to avoid relapse due to improper diet.

C. Relapse due to overstrain

This refers to relapse caused by over physical, mental or sexual strain in the early stages of recovery, seen in both exogenous and endogenous diseases. Examples such as chronic edema, asthma, hernia, apoplexy, thoracic obstruction and cardialgia, etc. all can relapse in this manner.

D. Relapse due to abuse of pharmaceuticals

This indicates a relapse caused by the abuse of tonifying prescriptions or improper use of medicine. In the early recovery stages, tonifying drugs can be used to assist and harmonize the healing process. However, the guideline of strengthening the right qi slightly without helping the evil, and eliminating the evil without harming the right qi must be followed. If one is overanxious to achieve a full recovery and uses intense tonifying methods, it will cause contrary deficiency that is unable to be replenished, or depress the right qi and assist the evil, with relapse as a result.

E. Relapse due to emotional disharmony

This refers to a recurrence caused by emotional factors. Diseases like hysteria, frightened epilepsy, goiter, globus hysteritis, psychosis and mania, etc. are prone to relapse in this way.

In addition, climatic and regional factors may also act as causes for relapse. For instance, asthma often reoccurs when the weather changes abruptly and with the chill of winter.

Chapter 8
Pathomechanism

Pathomechanism refers to the mechanism of the onset, development and transformation of a disease, also called pathology.

The study of pathomechanism is a theory investigating on the mechanism and law of the onset, development and transformation of a disease, which are of great significance for the diagnosis, prevention and treatment of the disease.

The main contents of pathomechanism in Chinese medicine include the mechanism of disease attack (pathogenesis, see chapter 7), the mechanism of pathological changes (focusing on the basic pathomechanism, the mechanism of the five pathogens produced by five *zang*-organs, and *zang-fu* organs' pathomechanism, which is omitted in this chapter) and the mechanism of the progress and transmission of disease.

Plain Questions: Discussion on the Most Important and Abstruse Theory (Sù Wèn: Zhì Zhēn Yào Dà Lùn, 素问·至真要大论): "Analyze pathogenesis with no violation of the natural law... cautiously grasp pathogenesis by recognizing what each symptom or sign is attributed to."[1]

Section 1   Basic Pathomechanism

The basic pathomechanism indicates the basic pathological reactions to invasion of the pathogens, being general rules of the pathological changes and the basis for the pathomechanism of various diseases and syndromes. It mainly includes the following aspects:

Superiority or Inferiority of the Vital or the Evil

It implies the rise and fall of the vital and the evil in the conflictive struggle of resistance and invasion. The result of the struggle influences both the attack and the development of the disease. In the course of a disease, the superiority or inferiority of the vital or the evil contributes to the changes of excess and deficiency of syndromes and the prognosis of the disease.

① The Relation between Superiority or Inferiority of either the Vital or the Evil and Change of either Deficiency or Excess (Fig. 8-1a, Fig. 8-1b)

(1) Pathomechanism of excess and deficiency
Excess and deficiency are a pair of opposite concepts in pathomechanism.

a. The pathomechanism of excess
Excess refers to the excess of evil qi, which is a pathological status with excess evil as the principal aspect of the contradiction. Right after the attack of the evil, the right qi is still not declined and can fight against the evil: the sharp conflict between them produces a series of

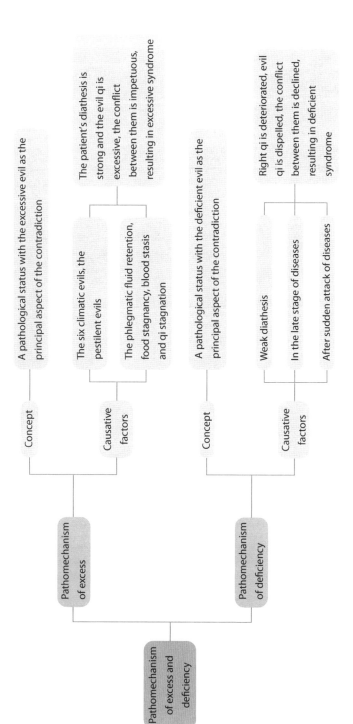

Fig. 8-1a   Relation between superiority or inferiority of either the vital or evil qi with changes of either deficiency or excess

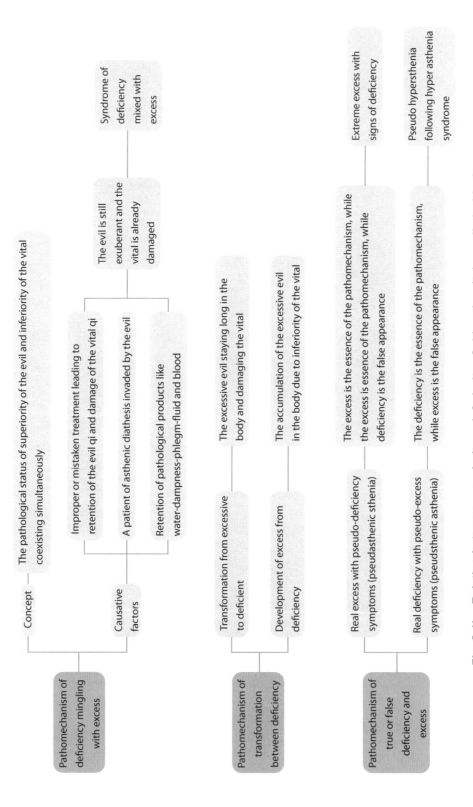

Fig. 8-1b Relation between superiority or inferiority of either the vital or evil qi with changes of either deficiency or excess

hyperactive pathological manifestations, called an excess syndrome.

An excess syndrome can be caused externally by the six climatic evils, the pestilent evils, or internally by phlegm-fluid retention, food stagnation, blood stasis and qi depression, etc., the patient's resistance is strong and the evil qi is excessive, the conflict between them is impetuous, resulting in an excess syndrome.

Excess syndromes often appear in the early and middle stages of disease, in exterior diseases, with symptoms of high fever, irritability and thirst, mania, delirium, loud voice and coarse breath, forceful pulse and thick and greasy tongue coating appearing; while in internal diseases caused by stagnation of phlegm, food, blood and qi, clinical manifestations of profuse phlegm and saliva, overflow of water-dampness, accumulation of food in the stomach and intestines due to indigestion, and qi and blood stagnation may appear.

b. The pathomechanism of deficiency

Deficiency refers to the deficiency of right qi, which is a pathological status with the deficient evil as the principal aspect of the contradiction. When the evil declines or is eliminated, the vital is also injured, and both sides are unable to struggle fiercely, so hypoactive pathological manifestations appear, called a deficient syndrome.

Deficient syndromes usually appear in people of weak resistance, or in the late stage of diseases, or after a sudden attack of vomiting and dysentery, over sweating, or exhaustion of blood, where the yin and yang are damaged and qi-blood-body fluid injured, organ function impaired and right qi deteriorated, hence the formation of a deficient syndrome.

A deficient syndrome is clinically manifested as spiritless, lassitude, emaciated face, shortness of breath, spontaneous sweating, night sweating, a feverish sensation of the five centers, or aversion to cold with cold limbs, weak pulse, etc.

Plain Questions: General Discussion on Deficiency and Excess (Sù Wèn: Tōng Píng Xū Shí Lùn, 素问·通评虚实论): "Pathogenic domination induces excess, consumption of essential qi causes

deficiency."

(2) Pathomechanism of deficiency mingling with excess

It refers to the pathological status of superiority of the evil and inferiority of the vital coexisting simultaneously.

The pathomechanism of deficiency mingling with excess can be caused by the following reasons: improper or mistaken treatment leading to retention of the evil qi and damage of the right qi; or evil qi invading a patient of deficient resistance whose right qi is too weak to dispel the evil; or the deficient right qi leading to the retention of pathological products like water-dampness-phlegm-fluid and blood.

It is clinically manifested as symptoms of both deficiency and excess syndromes, hence the name of syndrome as deficiency mixed with excess. There are two conditions of this pathomechanism: deficiency mixed with excess, and excess mixed with deficiency.

a. Deficiency mixed with excess

It refers to the pathological condition with deficiency as the principal aspect and excess of evil qi as a secondary condition. A syndrome of Spleen deficiency with dampness retention is of this kind, with the Spleen deficiency as the root (major factor) and the dampness retention the branch (minor factor).

b. Excess mixed with deficiency

It refers to the pathological condition with the excess as the principal aspect and the deficiency of the vital as the secondary condition. A syndrome of excessive heat injuring the body fluid is of this kind. The excessive heat is the root and the injury of body fluid is the branch.

(3) Pathomechanism of transformation between deficiency and excess

It refers to the transformation of the pathomechanism from excess to deficiency, or vice versa.

a. Transformation from excess to deficient

It is caused by excess of evil qi staying in the body, and damaging the right qi in the course of the disease. During the development of diseases with excess of evil qi as the principal aspect, when the evil is dispelled, the right qi is still damaged, and the deficient right qi takes the leading role, presented as a deficiency syndrome, hence the pathomechanism of transformation from excess to deficient. In the early and middle stages, the syndrome of excess evil is the major aspect, while with prolonged disease, in the late stage, a syndrome of qi-blood-yin-yang deficiency appears, indicating the transformation from excess to deficiency.

b. Development of excess from deficiency

In the disease course, the accumulation of excess evil in the body due to a deficiency of right qi may lead to the pathomechanism of development of excess from deficiency. In a deficient syndrome with deficiency of right qi as the principal aspect of the contradiction, the weak right qi and the hypofunctioning organs lead to water-dampness-phlegm-fluid retention and stagnation of qi and blood circulation. Alternately, if re-affected by the evil, forming pathological changes of the deficient right qi from the excess evil, this process is the pathomechanism of development of excess from deficiency. Examples are asthma from deficiency of the both Lung and the Kidney, where the right qi is deficient with the Lung-defensive qi unconsolidated, and when re-affected by wind cold evil, the asthma relapses and leads to an excess syndrome of cold evil restraining the body surface with profusion of phlegm in the body, indicating the development of excess from deficiency.

(4) Pathomechanism of true or false deficiency and excess

It is a pathological status of the lack of accord between the appearance of a disease and the essence of the syndrome of the disease under some special conditions, including two states of real deficiency with pseudo-excess symptoms, and real excess with pseudo-deficiency symptoms.

a. Real excess with pseudo-deficiency symptoms (pseudo-deficient excess)

It means the excess is the essence of the pathomechanism, while deficiency is the false appearance, mostly caused by failure of qi and blood to reach exteriorly due to the blockage of the channels as a result of the retention of excessive evil qi in the body. It is also termed as "extreme excess with signs of deficiency". For instance, in a case of rampant heat internally caused by heat retention in the gastrointestinal tract, there are excessive manifestations of constipation, abdominal fullness-firmness-tenderness, tidal fever, delirium; and deficient cold symptoms of yang qi depression like pallor, cold limbs, and listlessness also emerge as false appearance.

b. Real deficiency with pseudo-excess symptoms (pseudo-excess deficiency)

It means the deficiency is the essence of the pathomechanism, while excess is the false appearance, mainly caused by the failure of qi transformation due to the decline and dysfunction of organ qi and blood, resulting from weak right qi. It is also described as "pseudo-hyperexcess following hyperdeficiency syndrome". Take the syndrome of deficient Spleen unable to transport or transform vigorously as an example, where the pseudo excessive symptoms like abdominal distension and constipation may be seen.

Jīng-yuè's Complete Works: Deficiency and Excess (Jǐng Yuè Quán Shū: Xū Shí Piān, 景岳全书·虚实篇): "*Excess and deficiency means surplus and inadequacy. …… the deficient should be tonified, and the excess should be purged, that stands to reason. However, the situation of deficiency in excess or excess in deficiency is not as easy to understand, in details, in extreme deficient syndrome there may appear false excessive symptoms, and in extreme excessive syndromes there may be false deficient symptoms, which should be strictly distinguished.*"

② Relation between Superiority or Inferiority of both the Vital or Evil Qi and Prognosis of the Disease (Fig. 8-2)

In the process of the onset and development of a disease, the conflict between the right qi and the evil qi continuously affects the change in strength of decline or growth of the two sides, which is decisive in the developing tendency and conversion of the disease. Generally the superiority of the vital and inferiority of the evil leads to improvement and good prognosis of the disease; contrarily, the superiority of the evil and

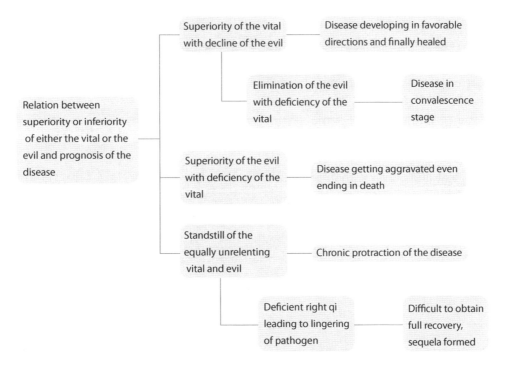

Fig. 8-2 Relation between superiority or inferiority of both the vital or evil
qi and prognosis of the disease

inferiority of the vital results in deterioration and a bad prognosis, even death; while the deadlock of the two sides leads to chronic protraction of the disease.

(1) Superiority of the right qi with decline of the evil qi
It means a pathological state of rising right qi of the body succeeding in fighting against the declining evil qi during the development of a disease, leading to a favorable turn towards recovery. It is caused by vigorous right qi, weak evil qi, or getting proper and timely treatment, which stops or diminishes the damage of the evil qi. As a result, the qi, blood and body fluid get restored and the organ's functions revived, and the disease develops in a favorable direction until it is finally healed. It is a commonly seen prognosis.

There is another condition of elimination of the evil qi with deficiency of the right qi, that although the evil qi is eliminated, the right qi is not easily recovered quickly. However its final direction is also favorable and leads to healing.

(2) Superiority of the evil qi with deficiency of the right qi
It refers to the pathological changes of excessive evil qi and deficient right qi when the organism fails to resist the evil qi, so that the disease gets aggravated and can even end in death. The appearance of this kind of prognosis always indicates the extreme deficiency of the right qi or over-excess of the evil qi, or failure in proper treatment, which results in a low level of evil-resistance function and the progressive damage to the body, with the proceeding deterioration of the disease; if the right qi is exhausted and the evil qi is still exuberant, the yin and yang will deplete and life will come to an end.

(3) Standoff of the equally unrelenting right qi and evil qi
It refers to the pathological process when the right qi and the evil qi are almost equal in strength with neither one able to defeat the other thoroughly, leading to a chronic protraction of the disease. The appearance of the standstill is caused by the slightly deficient right qi and appreciably excessive evil qi, where the former can't dispel the latter completely and the latter fails in invading deeply, hence the deadlock of the equally unrelenting two sides and a chronic protraction of the disease.

In the process of the stalemate between

the vital and the evil qi, if the vital gets further deficient and the remaining evil qi is still difficult to eliminate, it is called "deficient right qi leading to lingering of pathogen", being a special condition of the vital-evil struggle. It is caused by deficient right qi failing to dispel the evil qi completely, so a full recovery is difficult to obtain, and sequela occur.

The standstill status is only a pathomechanism of a relatively long period in the process of a disease, with the wane-and-wax change of the vital-evil struggle, since the disease usually develops ultimately towards recovery or deterioration.

Imbalance of Yin and Yang

Imbalance of yin and yang is an abbreviated

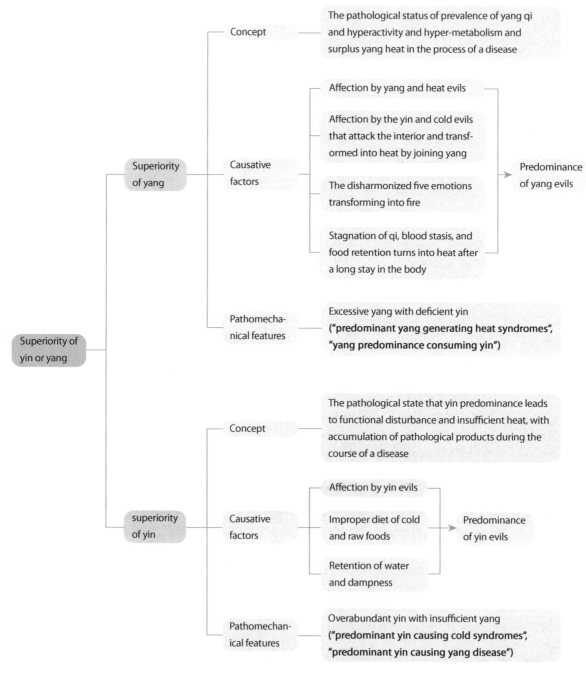

Fig. 8-3　Pathomechanism of superiority of yin or yang

version for discussing the loss of balance and harmony of yin and yang. Physically, the yin and yang of the body are in harmonious balance. While in the process of the onset and development of diseases, due to the influence of pathogens, the yin and yang fail to maintain balance to form pathological changes of superiority or inferiority of either yin or yang, mainly resulting in the following aspects:

① Superiority of Yin or Yang (Fig. 8-3)

It refers to the pathological changes of prosperity of either yin or yang, which belongs to the excessive pathomechanism where a "state of evil domination is considered as excess syndrome".

When the evil invades the body, the right qi rises to reject the evil, thus forming the pathological status of struggle between the evil and the vital. The evil has two aspects of yin and yang, the yin-evil invasion causing superiority of yin, while yang-evil invasion leads to superiority of yang.

The yin and yang of the body are in mutual restriction and are of a wane-and-wax relationship. In a disease course, an excess of yin leads to damage of the yang qi of the body, forming pathological changes of yin predominance with yang deficiency, and excess of yang results in damage of the yin fluid of the body, forming pathological changes of yang predominance with yin deficiency.

(1) Superiority of yang

It means the pathological state of prevalence of yang qi, hyperactivity and hypermetabolism, and surplus yang heat in the process of a disease.

The causative factors of a superiority of yang are either caused by yang and heat evils; or caused by yin and cold evils which attack the interior and transform into heat by joining yang; or lack of harmony with the five emotions transforming into fire; or stagnation of qi, blood stasis, or food retention turning into heat after a long stay in the body.

Superiority of yang is clinically manifested with excessive heat signs, like flushed cheeks, congested conjunctiva, restlessness, thirst, yellow urine, dry stools, yellow tongue coating, rapid pulse, etc..

The pathomechanical feature of yang superiority is termed as "predominant yang generating heat". Hyperactivity of yang heat for a long time consumes the yin fluid of the body, forming a pathomechanism of excessive yang with deficient yin. Thus an excessive heat syndrome of yang superiority is often accompanied by deficient yin fluid, termed as "yang predominance consuming yin".

(2) Superiority of yin

It refers to a pathological state where yin predominance leads to functional disturbance and insufficient heat, with accumulation of pathological products during the course of a disease.

It is often caused by yin evils like cold and dampness, an improper diet of cold and raw foods making cold evil stagnate in the middle *Jiao*, or retention of water and dampness.

Yin superiority is usually characterized by excessive cold, termed as "predominant yin causing cold syndromes". Long-term exuberance of yin cold evil damages the yang qi of the body, forming a pathomechanism of overabundant yin leading to insufficient yang, so that the excessive cold syndrome of yin superiority usually comes with symptoms of deficiency of yang, termed as "predominant yin causing yang disease".

Plain Questions: Major Discussion on the Theory of Yin and Yang and the Corresponding Relationships Among All the Things in Nature (Sù Wèn: Yīn Yáng Yīng Xiàng Dà Lùn, 素问·阴阳应象大论): "Predominant yin generates cold and causes yang disease, and yang predomination brings about heat and consumes yin."

② Inferiority of Yin or Yang (Fig. 8-4)

It refers to the pathological changes caused by deficiency of yin fluid or yang qi of the body in the process of a disease, belonging to the category of the deficient pathomechanism of "consumption of normal qi causing deficiency".

Insufficiency of either of yin or yang leads to an inability to restrict the other, causing relative excess of the other side, finally resulting in pathological changes of deficient yin causing

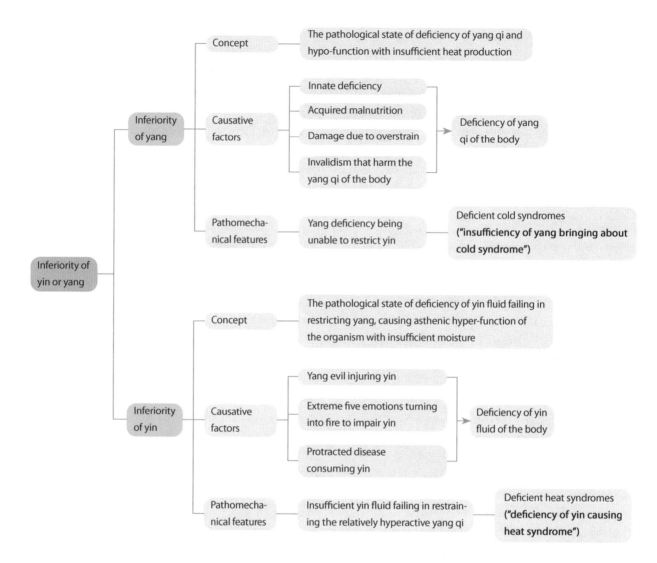

Fig. 8-4   Pathomechanism of inferiority of yin or yang

predominant yang, and yang deficiency causing yin excess.

(1) Inferiority of yang

Inferiority of yang, or yang deficiency, refers to a pathological state of deficiency of yang qi and resulting hypofunction with insufficient heat production.

The causative factors are innate deficiency, acquired malnutrition, damage due to overstrain, or invadilism harming the yang qi of the body.

Yang inferiority is clinically manifested as deficient cold with symptoms like a white complexion, an aversion to cold with cold limbs, gastro-abdominal cold pain, a pale tongue, slow pulse, a desire for lying quietly and crouched, profuse and clear urine, and watery diarrhea with indigested food in the stool.

The main pathomechanical characteristics of yang inferiority are mostly of deficient cold syndromes with yang deficiency that is unable to restrict yin, with relatively excessive yin, termed as "insufficiency of yang bringing about cold syndrome".

A cold syndrome brought about by superiority of yin is different from that brought on by inferiority of yang. Although both have cold manifestations, the former is an excessive cold syndrome, the latter deficient.

(2) Inferiority of yin

Inferiority of yin, or yin deficiency, refers to the pathological state of deficiency of yin fluid failing in restricting yang, causing deficient hyperfunction of the organism with insufficient moisture.

It is mostly caused by yang evil injuring yin, or extreme five emotions turning into fire to impair yin, or protracted disease consuming yin.

Inferiority of yin is clinically manifested with deficient heat signs like a hot sensation of the five centers, vexation, steaming bone feeling and tidal fever, flushed cheeks, emaciation, night sweats, a dry throat, a red tongue with little coating, and a thready and rapid pulse.

The pathomechanical characteristics of yin inferiority present as deficient heat signs of insufficient yin fluid with relatively hyperactive yang qi, termed as "deficiency of yin causing heat syndrome".

As for cold syndromes, a heat syndrome brought about by inferiority of yin is different from that brought about by superiority of yang. Although both have heat manifestations, the former is a deficient heat syndrome, the latter excessive.

Plain Questions: Discussion on the Regulation of Channels (Sù Wèn: Tiáo Jīng Lùn, 素问·调经论): "*Deficient yang causes external cold syndrome, and deficiency yin causes internal heat syndrome; excessive yang generates heat, and excessive yin generates interior cold.*"

③ Mutual Affection of Yin and Yang (Fig. 8-5)

Mutual affecting of yin and yang is a series of pathological changes of bilateral deficiency of yin and yang, resulting from the influence of specific consumption of either side on the other, including the two aspects of yin affecting yang and yang affecting yin.

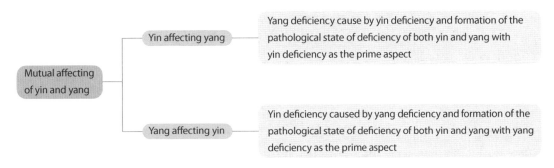

Fig. 8-5 Pathomechanism of mutual affecting of yin and yang

(1) Yin affecting yang

Due to yin fluid deficiency, yang qi is insufficiently generated, or is dissipated because yin fails to support yang, hence the result of yang deficiency cause by yin deficiency, and the formation of the pathological state of deficiency of both yin and yang with yin deficiency as the prime aspect.

(2) Yang affecting yin

On the other hand, due to the yang qi deficiency, yin fluid is insufficient in generation for lacking dependence, hence yin deficiency caused by yang deficiency, and the formation of the pathological state of deficiency of both yin and yang with yang deficiency as the prime aspect.

④ Blockage of Yin and Yang (Fig. 8-6)

It is a category of pathomechanism of true or false cold and heat due to the mutual rejection between yin and yang, including two aspects of yang being kept externally by superiority of yin internally and the opposite way.

(1) Yang kept externally by superiority of yin internally

It is also called "blockage of yang", referring to a pathological state that the extremely deficient yang qi fails to restrict yin, the superior yin jamming internally to keep the deficient yang float externally, leading to true internal cold with

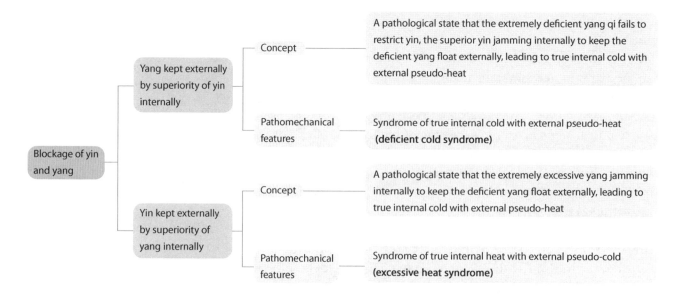

Fig. 8-6   Pathomechanism of blockage of yin and yang

external pseudo-heat.

The blockage of yang is presented as syndrome of true internal cold with external pseudo-heat, clinically manifested as deficient cold symptoms like pallor, cold limbs, watery diarrhea with indigested food in the stool, depression, desire for lying quietly and curled up, and feeble pulse, followed by pseudo-heat symptoms like flushed cheeks as if wearing makeup, general fever with a desire for clothing and quilts, thirst with desire for hot drinks, and a rootless large pulse. Hence the name of the syndrome is true internal cold with external pseudo-heat, the essence of which is deficient cold syndrome.

(2) Yin kept external by superiority of yang internally
It is also called "yin kept external". It refers to a pathological state where true heat hides inside, but false cold stays superficial. Extremely excessive heat stays so deep that it blocks the yang-qi's ability to disperse to the outside of the body and the four limbs. Therefore, yin is kept external.

The syndrome of yin kept external by excessive yang is true heat and false cold. It is clinically manifested as excessive heat symptoms like a high fever, flushed cheeks, coarse breath, restlessness, a red tongue and a rapid, large and forceful pulse, together with false cold symptoms like cold limbs, and a deep and hidden pulse, hence the name of true internal heat with external false-cold, the essence of which is excessive heat syndrome.

Jǐng-yue's Complete Works: *Record of Faith, True or False Cold and Heat Syndromes* (*Jǐng Yuè Quán Shū: Chuán Zhōng Lù, Hán Rè Zhēn Jiǎ Piān*, 景岳全书·传忠录·寒热真假篇): *"There are true or false heat and cold syndromes, that is, yin syndrome appearing as yang or yang syndrome as yin. Extreme yin can contrarily cause heat, i.e. real cold with pseudo-heat; and extreme yin results in cold, i.e. real heat with pseudo-cold."*

⑤ Transformation between Yin and Yang (Fig. 8-7)
It is a pathological process where the pathological nature of the imbalance of yin and yang changes into the opposite manifestation under certain conditions, transforming from yin to yang and from yang to yin.

(1) Transforming from yang to yin
It is a pathological process of an originally yang pathological nature transforming into yin under certain conditions, with the post-transformation pathology property belonging to yin. Like in some febrile diseases, yang heat symptoms of high fever, restlessness, thirst, cough, chest pain, red tongue with yellow coating, and rapid pulse appear in the early stage, due to the exuberance of the heat toxin consuming the right qi, and yin cold symptoms like pallor, cold limbs,

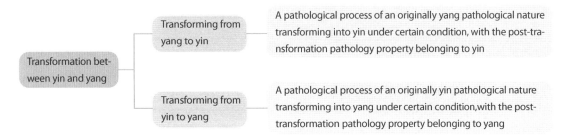

Fig. 8-7   Pathomechanism of transformation between yin and yang

profuse cold sweat, and feeble pulse may appear suddenly. Pathological changes like this are called "transforming from yang to yin".

(2) Transforming from yin to yang

It is a pathological process of an originally yin pathological nature transforming into yang under certain conditions, with the post-transformation pathology property belonging to yang. Like in the early stage of a common cold, there are exterior yin cold symptoms of aversion to cold relatively more severe than fever, a absence of sweat, general pain and headache, sniffling nose, a white and thin tongue coating, and a floating and tense pulse are presented. As the disease proceed, yang heat symptoms like fever, sweating, restlessness, thirst, a red tongue with yellow coating, and a rapid pulse appear. Pathological changes like this are called "transforming from yin to yang".

6 Depletion of Yin and Yang (Fig. 8-8)

Depletion of yin and yang is a pathological state of sudden and massive loss of both yin and yang of the body, leading to critical situations, including depletion of yin and depletion of yang.

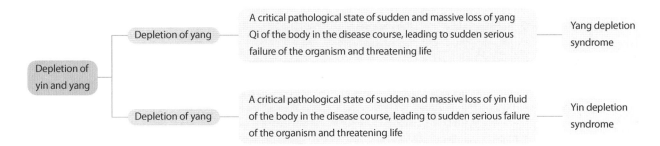

Fig. 8-8   Pathomechanism of depletion of yin and yang

(1) Depletion of yang

It is a critical pathological state of sudden and massive loss of yang qi of the body in a disease course, leading to exhaustion of the whole body's functions, and threatening life.

The causative factors may be summarized as the following: overwhelming evil defeating the vital, causing sudden collapse of yang qi; over-using diaphoretic, emetic, or purgative therapies, or over-sweating, vomiting and diarrhea, all of which leads to loss of yang qi following yin fluid loss; overstrain consuming the yang qi of one of yang-deficiency constitution; and chronic diseases consuming yang qi constantly, resulting in exhaustion of yang qi, thus causing yang depletion.

Yang depletion is clinically manifested as symptoms of yang qi collapsing with risk of death, like profuse sweat, pallor, cold limbs, aversion to cold, a desire for lying quietly with the body curled up, listlessness, and a feeble pulse, termed as yang depletion syndrome.

(2) Depletion of yin

It is a critical pathological state of sudden and

massive loss of yin fluid of the body in a disease course, leading to sudden serious failure of the all body functions and threatening life.

The causative factors may be summarized as prosperous heat evil, or prolonged detention of heat evil scorching yin fluid greatly, or other factors consuming yin fluid massively.

Yin depletion is clinically manifested as symptoms of yin fluid depletion with risk of death, like warm and sticky constant sweating, warm extremeties, dry and shriveled skin, deep-set eyes, restlessness or even coma, a forceless thready and rapid pulse or restless rootless pulse, termed as yin depletion syndrome.

Though there are pathomechanical and symptomatic differences between depletion of yin and depletion of yang, yin depletion can cause rootless yang to float externally, and yang depletion may result in sourceless yin becoming exhausted, thus they can transform into each other rapidly and cause divorce of yin and yang and even death, owing to their interdependence.

Treatise on the Headstream of Medicine:

Discussion on Depletion of Yin and Yang (Yī Xué Yuán Liú Lùn: Wáng Yīn Wáng Yang Lùn, 医学源流论·亡阴亡阳论): "How to distinguish the yin depletion from the yang depletion? Symptoms of sweating due to yin depletion are: warm limbs and skin, hot and salty sweat, thirst with desire for cold drink, coarse breath, and a great and forceful pulse; symptoms of sweating due to yang depletion are: aversion to cold, cold limbs and skin, cold and non-salty sweat, a desire for hot drinks without thirst, feeble breath, and a floating, rapid and hollow pulse."

Disorders of Qi and Blood

It means the dysfunctions of qi and blood caused by insufficiency of them, or the disturbance of their circulation.

① Disorders of Qi

(1) Qi deficiency (Fig. 8-9)

It refers to the shortage or hypofunction of qi.

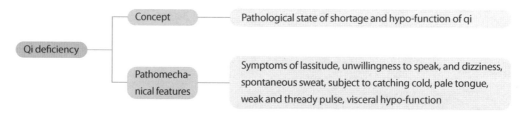

Fig. 8-9　Concept and syndromatic features of qi deficiency

Factors causing qi deficiency lie in the following aspects: congenital deficit; shortage of nourishment from acquired qi; dysfunction of the Spleen, Lung and Kidney causing deficiency of qi generation; internal injury due to overstrain and prolonged diseases; or aging or weak physique.

Clinically, it is manifested as symptoms of lassitude, unwillingness to speak, dizziness, spontaneous sweating, easily catching cold, a pale tongue, and a weak and thready pulse. Due to the qi deficiency of different organs, there may appear corresponding symptoms of hypofunction of that specific organ.

(2) Disturbance of qi flow (Fig. 8-10)

It refers to the disorders of qi circulation, including qi counterflow, qi sinking, qi blockage, qi desertion, and qi stagnation, caused by the abnormality of the movements of qi in ascent, descent, exit and entrance, etc..

a. Qi Stagnation

It refers to a pathological state of unsmooth or hindered qi flow, or stagnant qi.

It may be caused by depressed emotions, retentions of phlegm-dampness, food or blood stasis, or dysfunction of some organs and channels.

Clinically, qi stagnation is presented in many

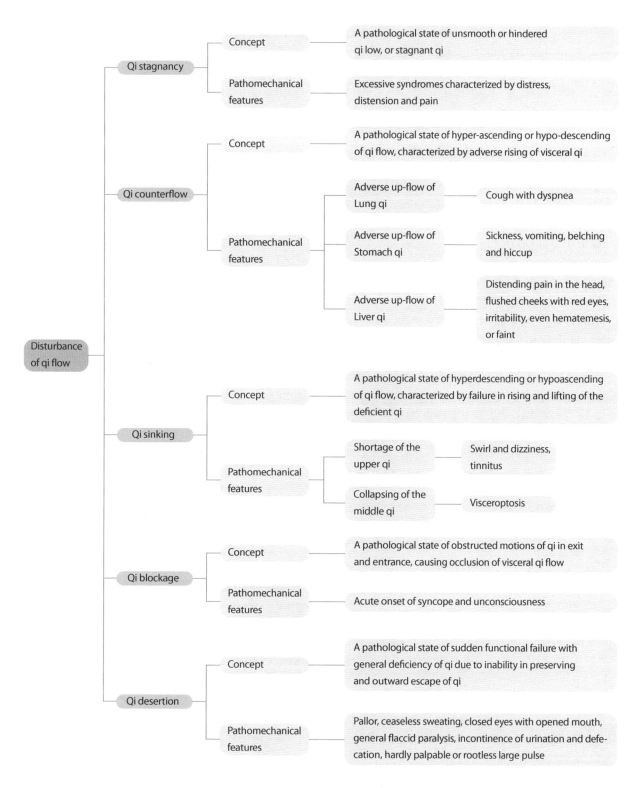

Fig. 8-10 Pathomechanism of disturbance of qi flow

ways. Local stagnation of qi in certain areas may cause distension and pain in the region. If the circulation of blood and body fluid is affected, blood stasis or water-dampness-phlegm-fluid retention may be formed. It usually affects the Lung, Liver, Spleen and/or stomach. Stagnated Lung qi leads to chest distress or cough and dyspnea; stagnated Liver qi causes emotional depression, and pain in hypochondrium or lower abdomen; stagnated Spleen and stomach qi results in paroxysmal distending pain in the gastro-abdominal region, relieved by belching or breaking wind.

Generally, qi stagnation usually causes excessive syndromes, while in some conditions, it may lead to deficiency syndromes. Pathomechanically, qi stagnation is commonly characterized by distress, distension and pain.

b. Qi counterflow

A pathological state of hyperascending or hypodescending of qi flow, was characterized by adverse rising of an organ's qi.

Causative factors of qi counterflow mainly lie in internal injuries from emotions, improper diet, or retention of phlegm-turbidity.

Clinically it is represented primarily as adverse up-flow of Lung qi, stomach qi, or Liver qi. In details, adverse Lung qi rising causes coughing with dyspnea; adversely rising stomach qi leads to nausea, vomiting, belching and hiccups; adversely rising Liver qi brings about distending pain in the head, flushed cheeks with red eyes, irritability, and even bleeding resulting from adverse flow of qi, in forms such as hemoptysis, hematemesis, or fainting due to hindrance of too much blood of the head.

Usually it occurs in excessive syndromes, but not absolutely.

Plain Questions: Chapter Discussion on the Interrelationship between Life and Nature (Sù Wèn: Shēng Qì Tōng Tiān Lùn, 素问·生气通天论): "Excessive anger leads to segregation of qi from the configuration, and blood stagnates in the upper part of the body, resulting in fainting due to extreme anger."

c. Qi sinking

This is a pathological state of hyper-descending or hypo-ascending qi flow, characterized by failure in rising and lifting of the deficient qi.

It is often caused by deficiency syndromes, weak constitution, or exhaustion by long-term diseases, which lead to weakness of Spleen qi, failure to ascend of clear yang and collapse of middle-*Jiao* energy, forming qi sinking.

The main clinical manifestations of qi sinking are described in two aspects. One is "shortage of the upper qi", i.e. deficient Spleen qi leading to the failure to ascend of clear qi, so that the head and eyes fail to be nourished, leading to symptoms of dizziness, tinnitus, or even a feeling like the room is spinning. The second is "collapsing of the middle qi", i.e. deficient Spleen qi causes inability of the body's qi to raise organs, brings about prolapse of viscera, like prolapse of stomach, prolapse of Kidney, prolaplse of uterus, prolapse of anus.

Since qi sinking is formed on the basis of qi deficiency and closely related to the deficient Spleen qi, it is usually accompanied by shortness of breath and lassitude, a low voice, and heaviness and distension in the lower back and belly, with constant desire for defecation.

Miraculous Pivot: Chapter The Treating Therapy from Oral Inquiry (Líng Shū: Kǒu Wèn, 灵枢·口问): "Insufficient of qi in the upper portion of the body being leads to chest distress, tinnitus, swirls and dizziness."

d. Qi blockage

A pathological state of obstructed movement of qi in exit and entrance, could cause blockage of organs' qi flow.

It is mainly caused by factors like emotional stimulation, or obstruction of qi circulation by exogenous pathogens or phlegm turbidity.

The clinical manifestations vary with the different organ that is blocked. For instance, qi blockage of the Heart leads to syncope and unconsciousness; qi blockage of the Lung causes dyspnea and asthma with a coarse voice; qi blockage of the urinary bladder leads to obstructed urination; and qi blockage of the large intestine brings about distending abdominal pain and constipation. The most commonly mentioned qi blockage refers to that of the Heart, characterized by acute onset of sudden syncope and unconsciousness, which usually alleviates spontaneously, but is occasionally unable to recover and can lead to death.

e. Qi desertion

A pathological state of sudden functional failure with general deficiency of qi, is induced by inability in preserving and outward escape of qi.

It can be caused by the inability of the right qi in fighting against evil qi, or consumption of right qi during the course of chronic diseases, or massive bleeding or sweating leading to qi exhaustion following a great blood loss or fluid outflow, causing qi to fail in internal concentration and escape.

Clinically it is manifested as pallor, ceaseless sweating, closed eyes with opened mouth, general flaccid paralysis, incontinence of urination and defecation, and a barely palpable or rootless large pulse.

Qi desertion shares much in common with depletion of yin and yang, clinically and pathomechanically, all belong to massive loss in pathomechanism and manifested as severe functional failure and a threat to the patient's life.

However, yang depletion has cold symptoms of dripping cold sweat and cold limbs, yin depletion has heat symptoms of warm and sticky sweating with warm extremities, while qi desertion itself usually is without these obvious heat or cold phenomenon. In other words, we can understand the relationship among them as qi desertion tending towards collapse of yang qi makes yang depletion, and that towards exhaustion of yin fluid forms yin depletion.

② Disorders of Blood (Fig. 8-11)

(1) Blood deficiency

It refers to an insufficient blood supply with a related decline in nourishing and moistening functions.

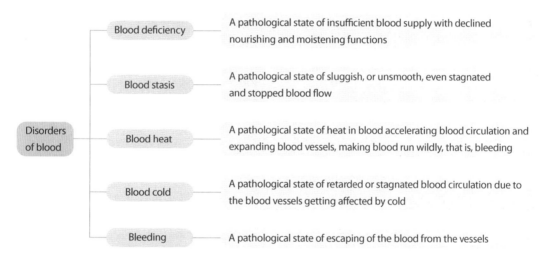

Fig. 8-11　Pathomechanism of blood disorders

Causes are: malnutrition due to improper diet and dysfunction of the Spleen and stomach in transforming water-food essence into blood can lead to insufficient blood production; or massive loss of blood fails to be replenished quickly enough; or an obstinate and chronic disease consuming the blood, can all be causative factors for blood deficiency.

Symptoms of declined organ and tissue functions like pale complexion, tongue, lips, and fingernails, lassitude, dizziness, a feeling like the room is swimming, and a thready pulse, are examples of clinical manifestations of blood deficiency, caused by the pathomechanism of failure of the blood in nourishing the organs and

tissues.

(2) Blood stasis

It is a pathological state of sluggish, unsmooth, or even stagnated and stopped blood flow.

Causative factors and syndrome characteristics are discussed in the section about "static blood" in chapter 6.

(3) Blood heat

It is a pathological state of heat in the blood, which can accelerate blood circulation and expand blood vessels, making blood run wildly, i.e. bleeding.

It is caused by exogenous warm-heat evils, or other evils turning into heat when invading deeply, or depressed emotions turning into fire, where internally generated fire and heat impairs the blood and leads to blood heat.

Besides the general excess heat syndromes, blood heat is also manifested as flushed cheeks with congested eyes, a red and crimson tongue, and a rapid pulse. If the vessels are 'burnt', there may be bleeding symptoms like hematemesis, macula, and hematuria. If the Heart spirit is disturbed, there may be restlessness, and even coma or unconsciousness, delirium, and mania. Finally, if the blood heat scorches the yin fluid of the body, it may lead to blood becoming sticky and thick and blocking blood circulation, eventually forming blood stasis.

(4) Blood cold

Blood cold is a pathological state of impeded or stagnated blood circulation due to the blood vessels being affected by cold.

Mostly it is caused by attack of exogenous cold evil, or internal generation of cold due to yang deficiency.

Common yin cold signs plus symptoms of stagnation of the blood vessels, such as coldness, like pain, or greenish-purple skin, hands and feet, fingernails, lips and tongue, clinically represent blood cold. If the cold coagulates in the Heart vessels and causes blockage, angina pectoris may appear; if it stagnates in the Liver channel, cold pain in the hypochondrium, lower abdomen and perineal region may occur, as well as menorrhagia or amenorrhea for women; if it accumulates in the blood vessels, it may cause frostbite.

(5) Bleeding

It is a pathological state of blood escaping from the vessels.

The overflow of blood from the vessels is brought on by factors such as: fire flaming up due to a disorder of qi and blood following an upwardly adverse flow of qi; fire heat forcing blood to flow frenetically; deficient qi failing in controlling the blood; extravasated blood obstructing in the vessels causing new bleeding; or injury of the vessels by trauma.

The escaped blood is also called "extravasated blood". If it fails to be eliminated in time and accumulates in the body, blood stasis is formed, which may induce various pathological changes. If bleeding is abrupt and copious, the qi will follow the blood in collapse, resulting in general functional failure.

③ Simultaneous Disorders of Qi and Blood

There is a physiological relationship of mutual generation, interdependence and mutual benefit between qi and blood. In other words, qi could generate, drive and control blood, and blood could generate and carry qi. Pathologically, qi disorders may affect blood disorders. Examples are: qi deficiency leading to blood deficiency, which is caused by qi failing to generate blood; deficiency or stagnation of qi causing blood stagnation due to qi fail to drive blood; bleeding due to the inability of deficient qi to control blood, or adversely-rising qi causing upwards flow of blood. On the other hand, blood disorders may affect qi disorders, as in: deficiency of blood causing qi deficiency due to qi's failure in generating blood; blood collapse resulting in qi desertion; and blood stasis causing stagnation of qi by retarding qi circulation. (Fig. 8-12)

Here we outline the concepts of simultaneous disorders of qi and blood in the following aspects.

(1) Qi stagnation with blood stasis

A pathological state in which qi stagnation leads to retarded blood flow and finally blood stasis.

(2) Qi deficiency with blood stasis

A pathological state is induced by the deficient qi fails in driving the blood circulation, leading to sluggishness of blood flow.

(3) Failure of qi in controlling blood

A pathological state in which the deficient qi is incapable of controlling the blood, thus allowing blood to escape outwardly, causing bleeding.

(4) Qi exhaustion following blood desertion

A pathological state in which qi follows blood in collapse when bleeding massively, forming a critical condition of prostration of both qi and blood.

(5) Deficiency of both qi and blood

It is a pathological state of coexistence of simultaneous qi and blood deficiency.

Plain Questions : Discussion on the Regulation of Channels (Sù Wèn · Tiáo Jīng Lùn, 素问·调经

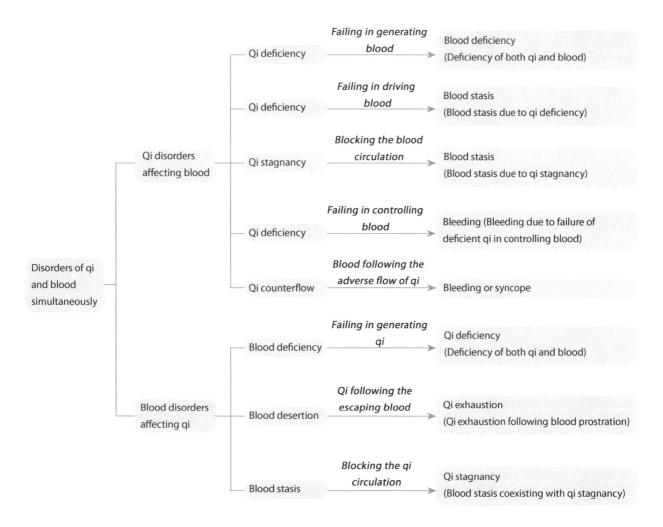

Fig. 8-12 Pathomechanism of simultaneous disorders of qi and blood

论): *"Disharmony of blood and qi may cause various diseases."*

Disorders of Body Fluid

It refers to a pathological state of insufficient production of body fluid, or disturbance in the transportation and distribution of body fluid.

1 Shortage of Body Fluid

A shortage of body fluid makes the organs and tissues fail to be nourished and moistened, producing a series of dry symptoms as a result.

The causative factors for shortage of body fluid can be summed up in the following aspects: attack of exogenous dry and heat evils or internally generated fire-heat damaging the body fluid; massive loss of body fluid due to profuse sweat, vomiting, urination and/or diarrhea; chronic disease consuming the body fluid; and decline of qi transformation of the organs causing insufficient generation of body fluid.

Owing to the lack of moisture and nourishment of organs and tissue, dry symptoms like dryness of the mouth, lips and nasopharynx, a red tongue with little moisture, deep-set orbits, dry and cracked skin, scanty urine, and constipation may appear.

From the point of degrees of injuries, there are two related concepts of *Jin* (thin fluid) consumption and *Ye* (thick fluid) consumption. The former is relatively mild and the latter serious. Generally, *Jin* (thin fluid) consumption focuses on the loss of water content, which is easily replenished, while *Ye* (thick fluid) consumption refers to loss of both water content and nutrient substance, which is relatively difficult to restore.

② Disturbance in the Distribution and Excretion of Body Fluid

It indicates a pathological state where abnormalities in the process of distribution and excretion of body fluid lead to retention of water-dampness in the body.

It is mainly caused by dysfunction of the Spleen, Lung, Kidney and *San Jiao*, which govern the distribution and excretion of body fluid, due to the exogenous or endogenous pathogens.

The disordered distribution and excretion of body fluid leads to retention of water-dampness in the body, causing various syndromes of turbid dampness blockage, phlegm-fluid accumulation, and water retention.

③ Disorders of Body Fluid and Qi and Blood Simultaneously

Disorders of body fluid and qi and blood simultaneously may lead to pathological changes of water-retention and qi stagnation, exhaustion of qi due to depletion of body fluid, depletion of body fluid causing lack of blood, blood stasis due to loss of body fluid, and the like (please examine the sections of the relationships of qi and blood to body fluid for reference).

Section 2   Five Endogenous Pathogens

The "five endogenous pathogens" is actually a concept of a series of pathological changes during the disease process. In it, the dysfunction of organs and channels, and disorders of qi, blood and body fluid, convert into wind, cold, dampness, dryness and fire, which are generated internally and share similar clinical manifestations of the exogenous pathogens of the wind, cold, dampness, dryness and fire, hence the term of the "five endogenous pathogens".

Though clinically similar to the six exogenous evils, the "five endogenous pathogens" conceptually belong to a pathomechanism, which is a different point than the six exogenous evils. The "five endogenous pathogens" usually cause interior syndromes, deficiency syndromes or syndromes of coexistence of both excess and deficiency. They seldom cause exterior syndrome, whereas the exogenous six climatic pathogens often cause exterior syndromes and excessive syndromes. (Table 8-1)

Table 8-1   The difference between the five endogenous pathogens and the six exogenous pathogens

	Six exogenous pathogens	Five endogenous pathogens
Conceptual category	Exogenous pathogens	A pathomechanical concept of a series of pathological changes during the disease process
Pathways attacked	Received externally	Generated internally
Clinical manifestations	Exterior syndromes, excess syndromes	Interior syndromes, deficient syndromes, or syndromes with a coexistence of excess and deficiency: seldom the cause of exterior syndromes

Internal Generation of Wind

① Definition of Internal Wind

It is also termed "wind stirring inside". During the disease process, both the excessive yang and hyperactive yang due to deficient yin failing in restricting can rise frenetically, leading to symptoms like dizziness, convulsions and tremors, which have pathological characteristics similar to the stirred wind. Since the internal wind is closely related to the Liver, it is called hepatic wind, or disturbing of Liver wind.

② Formation and Pathological Manifestations of Internal Wind

The pathological changes mainly lie in the following aspects: Liver-yang changing into Liver-wind; extreme heat causing wind syndrome; stirring-up of wind due to deficiency of yin, and blood deficiency generating wind.

(1) Liver-yang changing into Liver-wind

It is mostly caused by internal injuries of emotional factors. For instance, depressed Liver qi or too much rage causes overabundance and adverse rising of Liver qi and Liver yang; overstrain consumes the Liver and Kidney yin, leading to deficient yin failing to restrict yang; exuberant yang rises without control and transforms into wind, resulting in disturbing of Liver wind.

Clinically, besides the syndrome of hyperactivity of Liver-yang, symptoms like tremors, numbness of the limbs, dizziness, facial distortion, hemiplegia, and even sudden fainting due to adverse rising of blood following the adverse rising of qi.

(2) Extreme heat causing wind

It means overwhelming heat stirs up the wind, in a condition mainly seen in the worst stage of febrile diseases. The flaming heat evil scorches the yin fluid, damages nutrient blood, and burns the Liver channels and tendons which lose moisture, causing symptoms of high fever, tremors, convulsions, and neck rigidity, or even opisthotonus, eyes rolling back in the head, or coma to appear.

(3) Stirring of wind due to deficiency of yin

It is mostly seen in the late stage of febrile diseases or in chronic diseases when the body fluid is injured or consumed.

Clinically it is manifested as wind symptoms like tremors and convulsions, or restlessness of the limbs, together with low-grade fever, dry tongue with no coating or moisture, and a Chinese medicine, which indicates injury of body fluid.

(4) Blood deficiency generating wind

Due to insufficient blood generation, or massive blood loss, or chronic disease consuming nutrient blood, the Liver blood is deficient and fails to nourish the tendons, vessels, and collaterals, and deficiency wind is stirred up internally.

Symptoms like numbness in the limbs, tremors, and even convulsions of the limbs, as well as manifestations of deficiency of nutrient blood may appear.

Plain Questions: Discussion on the Most Important and Abstruse Theory (Sù Wèn: Zhì Zhēn Yào Dà Lùn, 素问·至真要大论): "Syndromes characterized by sudden onset of rigidity are related to wind."

Cold Originating from the Interior

① Definition of Internal Cold

Cold originating from the interior is also called "internal cold", referring to the weak yang qi of the body failing in warming and transforming, and leading to the internal generation of deficient cold, or suffusion of yin cold.

② Formation of Internal Cold

An innate condition of weak yang qi, yang injury in chronic disease, attack of exogenous cold evil, or over-eating cold and raw foods, can all impair yang qi of the body and lead to damage of yang qi, which then fails in restraining yin, resulting in exuberance of yin cold.

It is mainly related to yang deficiency of the Spleen and Kidney, especially the Kidney. The Spleen is the source of generating qi and blood, and Kidney yang serves as the root of yang qi of the whole body and warms up the organs and body. Thus deficient yang qi of the Spleen and Kidney leads to failure in warming, and easily results in deficient cold syndromes.

③ Pathological Manifestations of Internal Cold

First, failure in warming leads to internal generation of deficient cold, clinically manifested as a pale complexion, an aversion to cold with desire for warmth, cold limbs, a pale and swelling tongue with white and moist coating, deep, a slow and weak pulse, spasm of tendons and muscle, and arthralgia in the joints.

Second, the weak yang qi fails in transforming, leading to incorrect metabolism of the body fluid. Clinically, symptoms are frequent and clear urination, thin and clear sputum, saliva and nasal discharge, diarrhea, edema, and formation of phlegm fluid. Different organs have their own special clinical manifestation accordingly.

Plain Questions: Discussion on the Most Important and Abstruse Theory (Sù Wèn: Zhì Zhēn Yào Dà Lùn, 素问·至真要大论): "Cold syndromes characterized by contraction are related to the Kidney." "Syndromes characterized by discharge of thin, clear and cold fluid are related to cold."

Internal Generation of Dampness Turbidity

① Definition of Internal Dampness

It is also called "internal dampness", which is a pathological process where the governing and regulatory function of the Spleen, Lung and Kidney on water metabolism is disturbed, leading to obstructed distribution and excretion of body fluid, with resulting retention of water-dampness-phlegm-fluid formed.

② Formation of Internal Dampness

The formation of internal dampness mostly results from the factors which influence the governing and regulatory functions of the Spleen, Lung and Kidney on water metabolism, such as dietary factors like over-indulgence in uncooked, cold, greasy or sweet foods; over-indulgence in smoking and drinking alcohol; attack of the six climatic evils; or improper work and rest. The Spleen controls transportation and transformation of water-dampness, so the formation of internal dampness is mainly ascribed to a Spleen disorder.

③ Pathological Manifestations of Internal Dampness

The internal dampness causes different clinical manifestations when obstructing different places. If obstructed within the channels, it may cause a heaviness of the head that feels like it is wrapped, heavy limbs, and rigidity or impaired movement of the neck. In the upper *Jiao*, it causes chest distention and cough. In the middle *Jiao* it causes gastro-abdominal distention, loss of appetite, a greasy feeling or sweet taste in the mouth, and a thick and greasy tongue coating. In the lower *Jiao* it causes abdominal distention, loose stools, and difficulty in urination. In the skin and muscles, it causes edema.

Plain Questions: Discussion on the Most Important and Abstruse Theory (Sù Wèn: Zhì Zhēn Yào Dà Lùn, 素问·至真要大论): "Dampness syndromes characterized by edema and fullness are related to the Spleen." "Syndromes characterized by convulsion and stiff neck are related to dampness."

Internal Generation of Dryness due to Injury of Body Fluid

① Definition of Internal Dryness

It is termed as "internal dryness", which indicates a pathological state where the deficient or damaged body fluid cannot nourish and moisten the tissues and organs of the body, leading to pathological changes of a dry nature.

② Formation of Internal Dryness

It may be caused by body fluid consumption from chronic disease, over sweating, vomiting or diarrhea; massive loss of blood and essence leading to deficiency of body fluid; or exhaustion of body fluid due to overwhelming heat evil injuring yin. The yin fluid is insufficient, so dryness is generated internally.

③ Pathological Manifestations of Internal Dryness

It is usually accompanied by syndromes of yin deficiency with deficient heat due to the exhaustion of body fluid, and it occurs in various organs and tissue, but mainly seen in the stomach, Lungs and large intestine. Dryness-heat symptoms include: dry, peeling, or cracked skin; a dry mouth, pharynx and tongue, or even fissuring with little fluid; a dry nose and eyes with scanty tears; and brittle nails, constipation, and scanty and yellow urine may appear. If the fluid is mainly deficient in the Lungs, a dry cough with little sputum, or even hemoptysis may occur; if in the stomach, lack of appetite and a red tongue with no coating are symptoms; in the intestines, constipation.

Mysterious Truth of Etiology of Plain Questions:

Dryness (Sù Wèn Xuán Jī Yuán Bìng Shì: Zào Lèi, 素问玄机原病式·燥类): "All the symptoms of withered, arid, searing, and chapped, desquamative kinds, are results of dryness evil attack."

Fire–heat Generated Internally

① Definition of Internal Fire-heat

It is also named "internal fire" or "internal heat", meaning a pathological change where exuberance or hyperactive yang, or stagnation of qi and blood, can cause internal disturbance of fire-heat resulting in functional hyperactivity of the organism.

② Formation of Internal Fire-heat

It is mainly formed in the four ways as follows:

(1) Exuberance of yang qi turning into fire
Yang qi of the body physically warms the organs and tissues, which is called "minor fire" or "physical fire". While under pathological conditions, overwhelming yang qi leads to functional hyperactivity and consumes yin fluid, which is called "excess fire" or fire evil, also termed as "excessive qi produces fire".

(2) Accumulation of evils turning into fire
It includes two aspects. One is the accumulation of the six climatic evils transforming into fire, like heat transformed from stagnated cold, or production of fire due to stagnation of dampness. The other is the result of pathological products in the body stagnating the functions of qi and turning into fire, e.g. phlegm turbidity, blood stasis, food retention, and parasites, all of which can accumulate and transform into fire.

(3) Excessive five emotions turning into fire
It is also called "five emotions producing fire". Emotional stimulation affects the mutual balance among the organs, qi and blood, and yin and yang, leading to qi stagnation that finally turns into fire. If it is caused by depression of the Liver qi, it is called "Liver fire".

(4) Hyperactivity of fire due to yin deficiency
The deficient fire is caused by extreme yin injury and uncontrolled yang, leading to the production of deficient fire.

③ Pathological Manifestations of Internal Fire-heat

One is excess fire, e.g. fire caused by excess of yang qi, or extreme five emotions, manifested as high fever, flushed cheeks, thirst with desire for cold drinks, yellow urine, constipation, mania, a red tongue with yellow fur, and a large pulse. The other is deficient fire, presenting as a burning sensation of the five centers, steaming bones and tidal fever, flushed cheeks in the afternoon, emaciation, night sweating, a dry pharynx and mouth, a red tongue with little fur, and a thready and rapid pulse. Different invaded organs present their own respective symptoms.

Plain Questions: Discussion on the Most Important and Abstruse Theory (Sù Wèn: Zhì Zhēn Yào Dà Lùn, 素问·至真要大论): "Syndromes characterized by fever, fainting and convulsion are related to fire."

Section 3　Transmission and Change of Disease

Transmission and change of disease refers to the motion and variation of disease within the organs, channels and tissues. The pathomechanism of transmission and change is explained by the rules and patterns of disease evolvement and development.

Patterns of Transmission and Change

① Transmission in Location

Location refers to the diseased part of the body. The human body is an organic whole, and a disease in a certain part of it can affect and extend to other parts, leading to the involvement of the newly affected part. This is called "transmission".

The development tendency of a disease can be grasped once the locational transmission law is mastered, and the disease can be treated in a timely manner to prevent further development.

It includes the going outward and coming inward of the evil qi, and the transmission and change of both exogenous diseases and of endogenous disease.

(1) Going outward and coming inward of evil qi (Fig. 8-13)

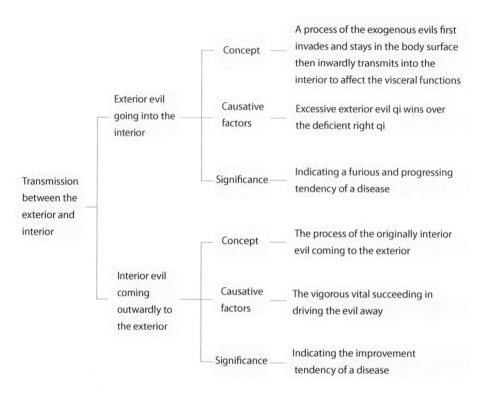

Fig. 8-13   Transmission and change between the exterior and interior

It is also called "transmission between the exterior and interior", or "transmission between the in and out", which is a pathological tendency of disease location.

The exterior and interior form pairs of opposite concepts. For instance, from the point of view of the whole body, diseases in the skin, muscle, channels and collaterals belong to the exterior, while those in the organs and deep in the marrow belong to the interior. As far as the skin, hair, and body hair and channels are concerned as a whole, the skin, hair, and body hair belong to the exterior and the channels belong to the interior. If *zang* organs and *Fu* organs are considered as a pair, the *zang* organs are the exterior and the *Fu* organs the interior; the three yang channels are the exterior, and the three yin channels the interior, and so on. The most frequently mentioned exterior and interior pair is that of the body surface and the organs.

Exterior syndromes are usually shallow and mild, interior syndromes are deep and serious. Thus, the exterior and interior can be taken as a concept of disease location and disease condition.

It includes two aspects of the exterior evil going into the interior, and interior evil coming into the exterior.

a. Exterior evil going into the interior

It refers to a process of the exogenous evils first invading and staying in the body surface, or defensive phase, and then inwardly transmitting into the interior to affect the organs' functions.

It occurs as a result of the vital-evil struggle, that is, when excessive exterior evil wins over the vital, and transmits to the interior, often indicating a furious and progressive tendency of a disease.

Plain Questions: Discussion on Contralateral Needling Therapy (Sù Wèn: Miù Cì Lùn, 素问·缪刺论): *"The evil invades the body, first impairs the skin and hair, then the minute collaterals, then the collaterals, then the channels, which connect the five zang viscera and distribute in the stomach and intestines, thus both yin and yang are affected and the five zang organs are injured. This is the transmission course of a disease starting at the skin and ending in the organs."*

b. Interior evil coming outward to the exterior

It indicates the process of the originally interior evil coming to the exterior as a result of the fight between the evil and the vital.

The resisting and evil-dispelling power of the

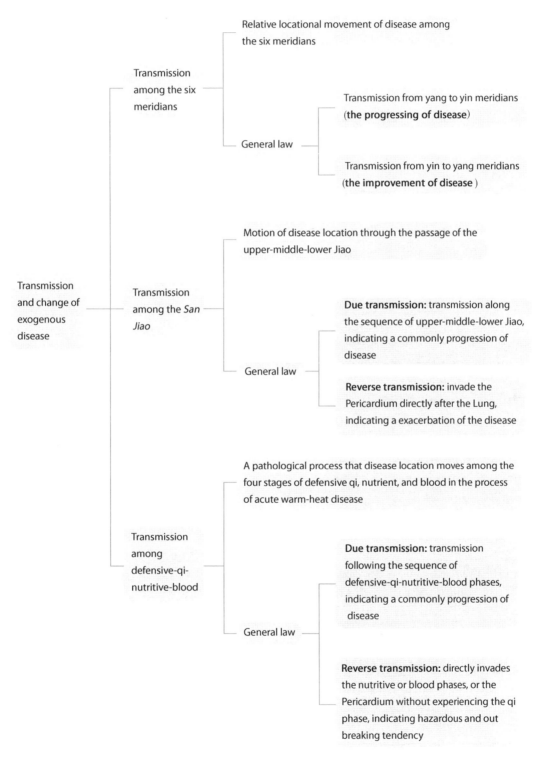

Fig. 8-14　Transmission of exogenous disease

right qi is decisive in this process, since once the vigorous right qi succeeds in driving the evil away, the disease transmits to the exterior, indicating the tendency towards improvement for a disease.

(2) Transmission and change of exogenous diseases (Fig. 8-14)

a. Transmission among the six channels

This is the relative locational movement of disease among the six channels, using the doctrine first established by Zhang Zhong-jing (Zhang Ji) in the *Han* dynasty in his *Treatise on Cold Pathogenic and Miscellaneous Diseases (Shāng Hán Zá Bìng Lùn, 伤寒杂病论)*, which is a recapitulation on the laws and nature of transmission among the six channels.

The general law of the six-channel transmission is from yang channels to yin channels, i.e. the sequence of *taiyang-yangming-shaoyang-taiyin-shaoyin-jueyin*, which implies the change of yang qi from vigorous to weak and the progression of the disease, and transmission along the opposite direction implying an improved disease condition with yang qi reinvigorated.

Additionally, transmissions between the yin and yang, exterior and interior, and hand and foot channels are other forms of six-channel transmission.

b. Transmission among the *San Jiao*

It means the motion of disease location through the passage of the upper-middle-lower *Jiao*, using the doctrine of *San Jiao* transmission established by Wu Ju-tong(Wu Tang) in the *Qing* dynasty in *A Piece on Warm-heat Diseases (Wēn bìng Tiáo Biàn, 温病条辨)*, which is a work on the laws and nature of the progression and development of febrile diseases.

The general law of *San-Jiao* transmission is: warm-heat evils come in through the nose and mouth, first invade the upper *Jiao* of the Lung and defensiveness, then further attack the middle *Jiao* of the Spleen and the stomach, and finally deeply disturb the lower *Jiao* of the Liver and the Kidney, which is also the pathway of the routine progression of the disease, called "due transmission". If the evils invade the pericardium directly after the Lung, it is a exacerbation of the disease progression beyond the general law, so it

is called "reverse transmission".

c. Transmission among *wei*-qi-*ying*-blood

It means a pathological process where the disease location moves among the four stages of *wei* (defensive qi level, 卫分), qi (qi level, 气分), *ying* (nutritive qi level, 营分), and the blood level (血分) in the process of an acute warm-heat disease. The theory of the *wei*-qi-*ying*-blood transmission and syndrome differentiation of warm-heat disease was first raised in *Writings on Warm-heat Disease (Wēn Rè Bìng Piān, 温热病篇)*, which explains the pathological regularity and nature of warm-heat diseases in different stages.

The law of *wei*-qi-*ying*-blood transmission reflects the progression process of going from exterior to interior, from outside to inside, from shallow to deep, and from mild to serious. Generally speaking, disease in the defensive phase is the early stage, characterized by fever and chills; the qi phase is the middle stage, with the evil having reached the Spleen, stomach, intestines, and gallbladder, characterized by aversion to heat but not to cold; the nutritive phase is the severe stage, with the evil having approached to the pericardium and Heart, characterized by a red and crimson tongue and restlessness with insomnia; and the blood phase is the late stage with the Heart, Liver, and Kidney affected, characterized by a red and crimson tongue, as well as blood consumption, blood disturbance, yin injury and wind stirring up.

The general law of the *wei*-qi-*ying*-blood transmission is following the sequence of *wei*-qi-*ying*-blood, reflecting the evil invading deeper and the disease condition worsening, which is "due transmission". If the evil directly invades the nutritive or blood phases without experiencing the qi phase, it is called "reverse transmission", indicating a hazardous and worsening tendency. Using common sense, transmission along the due sequence implies the progression of the worsening of the disease, and that along the converse sequence indicates alleviation or improvement.

In addition, the *wei*-qi-*ying*-blood transmission of a warm-heat disease may have different orders, such as simultaneous affection of both the *wei* and qi phases, or overabundant heat at both the *wei* and *ying* phases, or intense heat in both qi and blood systems, or even simultaneous attack of the four phases of *wei*, qi, *ying* and blood.

Systematic Differentiation of Warm-heat Diseases: Volume 2 (Wēn Bìng Tiáo Biàn: Juàn Èr, 温病条辨·卷二): "The reverse transmission of Lung disease affects the pericardium. The unhealed upper Jiao disease transmits to the Spleen and stomach in the middle Jiao, then to the lower Jiao of Liver and Kidney. This is the transmission course of disease starting at the upper Jiao, ending at the lower Jiao."

(3) Transmission of exogenous diseases

The basic transmission form of endogenous diseases is transmission among the organs, or between the organs and channels, or the body constituents.

a. Transmission among *zang* organs

It refers to the movement and variation of the disease among the five *zang* organs, owing to their close physiological relationship to one another (for details see the section regarding the relationship among the five *zang* organs).

b. Transmission between *zang* organs and *fu* organs

It means the transmission from *zang* organs to *fu* organs or the opposite. There are channels and collaterals between the *zang* and *fu* organs of the Heart and small intestine, Lung and large intestine, Spleen and stomach, Liver and gallbladder, and Kidney and urinary bladder, whose physiological functions are correlated closely. As a result, disease can transmit between them (for details see the section regarding the relationship between the *zang* organs and *fu* organs).

c. Transmission among *Fu* organs

It means the transmission in location among the six *Fu* organs. The six *Fu* organs, although they have different physiological functions, share the common physiological characteristics of "transferring and converting substance", that is, they individually take part in food digestion, essence and water absorption, and waste excretion. If one of them becomes affected, the related organ is doomed to be involved, and its physiological function is affected (for details see

the section on the relationship among the *Fu* organs).

d. Transmission between the organs and body constituents

The five *zang* organs are related to the five constituents, five organs and nine orifices physiologically and structurally. Thus, when the five *zang* organs are affected, the body constituents are influenced, and vice versa (for details see the section on the relationship between the *zang* organs and body constituents).

e. Transmission between the organs and the channels

The organs and channels are inter-related and a disease on either side can transmit to the other.

Plain Questions: Discussion on Bi-Syndrome (Arthralgia) (Sù Wèn: Bì Lùn, 素问·痹论): "Each of the five zang organs has its own body constituent. Lingering disease course of the body constituent is a sign of a problem with the correlated organ. Once re-affected by the evils, unhealed bone blockage affects the Kidney, unhealed tendon blockage affects the Liver, unhealed vessel blockage affects the Heart, unhealed muscle blockage affects the Spleen, and unhealed skin blockage affects the Lung. The classification of blockage is based on the season and location of evil attack."

Plain Questions :Discussion on Cough (Sù Wèn: Ké Lùn, 素问·咳论): "The Lung has the skin and hair as its body constituents. When the evil attacks the skin and hair, it affects the correlated organ of the Lung. When cold food and drink enter the stomach and impair the Lung through the Lung channel, it leads to Lung coldness, and both internal and external cold evils combine and cause Lung cough syndrome."

② Transformation of a Pathomechanical Nature (Fig. 8-15)

(1) Transformation between cold and heat

It is the pathological change of the pathomechanism from cold to heat or from heat to cold during the disease process.

a. Transforming from cold to heat

It means an originally cold syndrome transforming into heat, both being excessive syndromes, caused by cold evil invasion deep in the interior stagnating to become heat. For instance, in the early stage of an exterior syndrome, symptoms of

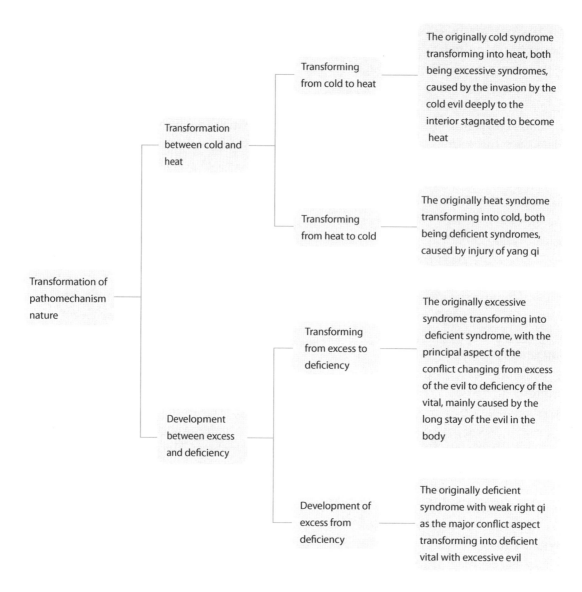

Fig. 8-15   Transformation of pathomechanical nature

serious chills with mild fever, absence of sweat, and a tense and floating pulse appear. Along with further invasion to the interior, the cold evil turns into heat and causes interior heat symptoms with high fever, aversion to heat but not cold, restlessness with thirst, and a large and rapid pulse.

b. Transforming from heat to cold

It means the originally hot syndrome transforming into cold, both being deficient syndromes, caused by injury of yang qi. For example, a patient with exuberance of yang-heat sweats profusely: the yang qi escapes with the sweat and leads to a pale complexion, cold limbs, cold sweat, and a feeble pulse, this is a process of transforming from excessive heat to deficient cold (yang exhaustion).

The transformation between cold and heat is related to differences in resistance, affected location and treatment. General laws are: diseases with the patient's condition being that of excessive yang and deficient yin, and affected in the yang organs and channels, are prone to transform heat and dryness; on the contrary, those with the patient's condition being that of excessive yin and deficient yang, and affected in the yin organs and channels, are prone to transform cold and dampness. Incorrect treatment that injures yang leads to the disease transforming to cold, while injuring yin causes transformation to heat.

The transformation between cold and heat

can be sudden or gradual. Usually exogenous diseases transform suddenly and rapidly, while endogenous diseases proceed slowly and gradually.

(2) Development between excess and deficiency

It is decided by the wane and wax between the vital and evil qi in the vital-evil struggle, including transforming from excess to deficiency and development of deficiency from excess.

a. Transforming from excess to deficiency

It means the originally excess syndrome transforming into a deficient syndrome, with the principal aspect of the conflict changing from an excess of evil qi to deficiency of the vital, mainly caused by the long stay of the evil in the body. The right qi is damaged even though the evil has been dispelled, so an excess syndrome transforms into a deficient syndrome. In the early and middle stages of exogenous diseases, the excessive syndrome is the major aspect, while if prolonged and in the late stage, the excessive syndrome transforms into deficiency syndrome due to deficiency of qi, blood, yin and yang.

b. Development of excess from deficiency

It refers to the pathological process where an originally deficient syndrome with weak right qi as the major aspect transforms into deficient right qi with excessive evil qi.

It is caused by evil accumulation due to the weak right qi in the disease course. That is, the weak right qi causes the organs' functions to decline, which leads to water-dampness-phlegm-fluid retention, qi stagnation, and blood stasis stay in the body; or a deficient syndrome of weak right qi becomes re-affected by an exogenous evil, both of which may lead to development of excess from deficiency. As in asthma from deficiency in both the Lung and the Kidney due to the weak right qi, the Lung-defensiveness is unconsolidated, and when re-affected by wind-cold evil, the asthma reoccurs, with an excessive syndrome of phlegm retention blocking in the Lung.

Influential Factors of the Transmission and Change of Disease

Many factors may influence the transmission and change of disease, such as the power of the right qi of the body, the nature of the evil qi, therapeutic measures taken, and the like. From the point of view of the wane and wax of the vital and evil qi caused by the vital-evil struggle: in the disease course, if the vital is strong and the evil weak, it transmits slowly or doesn't transmit at all, leading to improvement and recovery; on the contrary, if the vital is weak and the evil strong, the transmission is rapid, tending to be aggressive. If both the vital and the evil qi are vigorous, the clinical manifestations are severe; if both declined, the transmission is slow and the disease is in chronic recovery or in a lingering state. The patient's body state, psychological state, living environment, and regional and climatic conditions can all affect the strength of the right qi, while evil qi is influenced by climatic, regional, and living conditions (Table 8-2).

① Constitutional Factors

Whether a patient's susceptibility is strong or not affects the right qi directly, and therefore is influential in the transmission and change of disease, mainly in two aspects.

First, the strength or weakness of the body affects the disease transmission. People with strong constitution have a more acute disease onset, but fewer transmissions, and a shorter disease course; those with weak constitution have slower onset, and more and easier transmissions, especially invading the deeper parts, as well as a lingering course of disease.

Secondly, constitutional differences influence the transformation of the pathogens. This means that the characteristic of the pathogen changes to match the patient's constitution. Using common sense, pathogens invading a patient with yang-excess constitution tend to transform into fire, and the disease tends to develop into heat syndrome; while in a patient of yin-excess constitution, they tend to transform into cold and the disease tends to develop into cold syndrome. For example, dampness invading a yang-excessive body transforms into yang heat, forming dampness-heat; and it transforms into yin cold in a yin-excessive body, forming dampness-cold.

Table 8-2　Influential factors of transmission and change of disease

Influential factors		Influence on transmission and change of disease
Constitutional factors	Strong constitution	Acute disease onset, less risk of transmission, shorter disease course
	Weak constitution	Slower onset, more and easier transmissions
	Yang-excessive constitution	Tending to transform into fire and develop into heat syndrome
	Yin-excessive constitution	Tending to transform into cold and develop into cold syndrome
Pathogen-originated factors	Excess evils	Quick transmission
	Deficient evils	Slow transmission
	External yang evils	Quick transmission
	external yin evils	Slow transmission
Regional(geographical) factors	Living in topographically high places (tableland) with dry climate	Apt to transform into heat and dryness with yin injury
	Living in topographically low places (lowland) with humid climate	Apt to transform into dampness with yang injury
Climatic factors	Dry season with little rainwater	Apt to transform into heat and dryness with yin injury
	Humid season	Apt to transform into dampness with yang injury
Life factors	Pleasant mood, proper diet and work-rest rhythm	Diseases tend to improve
	Poor mood, improper diet and work-rest rhythm	Diseases tend to aggravate
Treatment factors	Proper treatment	Hindering and stopping the process of a disease, leading to a favorable result
	Improper treatment or mistreatment	Injuring the body's right qi or assisting the evil qi, resulting in deterioration of the condition or a negative prognosis

② Pathogen-related Factors

The evil forms of qi are important factors influencing the transmission and changes of disease. The power and nature of the pathogens affect the level of acuteness of onset. For the six climatic evils, relatively speaking, the stronger the evils are, the quicker the transmission would be; the weaker the evils are, the slower the transmission would be. As well, affection by yang evils transmits more quickly, by yin evils more slowly.

The transmission pathways vary with different pathogens. Exogenous diseases usually transmit between the exterior and the interior. Febrile diseases often transmit among the six channels, and warm-heat diseases mostly transmit among the *wei*-qi-*ying*-blood phases, or among the *San Jiao*. Endogenous diseases transmit among the organs.

The nature of the pathogen also influences the changes of the disease's nature. Since dryness evil is a yang evil, it transforms into heat easily, and since dampness evil is a yin evil, it transforms into cold frequently.

③ Regional and Climatic Factors

Changes of geographic environment, season and climate affect both the human body and the pathogens, and then influence transmission of disease.

Special constitutional characteristics and disease natures are formed under long-term action of geographical factors, which contribute to the transmission and transformation of disease. People living in topographically high places (tableland) with a dry climate are prone to heat and dry transformation, with body fluid injured; those living in topographically low places (lowland) are susceptible to dampness transformation with yang qi damaged.

Seasonal factors may also affect the transmission and transformation of disease. People in a dry season with little rainwater easily to get heat, or dryness transformation, with yin injured; those in a humid season may suffer from dampness transformation with yang affected.

④ Life Factors

This mainly includes the emotions, dietary factors, rhythm of work and rest, etc., which affect the transmission and changes of disease by acting on the right qi of the body. In general, a pleasant mood and proper diet and work-rest rhythm are beneficial to the recovery of the vital, contributing to recovery; while a poor mood and improper diet and work-rest rhythm are harmful to the right qi, leading to aggression.

Additionally, whether the treatment is proper or not affects the transmission of disease directly. Proper treatment can hinder and stop the process of disease, leading to a favorable result; but improper treatment, or mistreatment, may injure the body's right qi or assist the evil qi, resulting in a deterioration of the condition, or a negative prognosis.

Chapter 9
Principles for Prevention and Treatment

The theoretical system of prevention and treatment includes basic principles for preventing and treating diseases, which are two different theories and methods to combat diseases, both aiming at the elimination of diseases, thus promoting the health and longevity of people.

Section 1   Prevention

Prevention is to apply certain measures to prevent the occurrence and development of diseases.

Early in *The Yellow Emperor's Internal Classic* (*Huáng Dì Nèi Jīng*, 黄帝内经) the idea of "treating before the onset of disease" is raised, which is the earliest record of prevention in CM theoretical system, emphasizing on the prevention of disease (following the prognosis of a disease). For healthy people, the aim of prevention is to stop the occurrence of disease by enhancing the body constitution; for sick people, the aim is avoid allowing the disease to develop, change, and transmit. (Fig. 9-1)

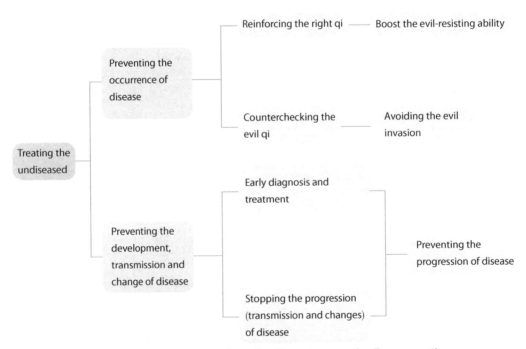

Fig. 9-1   "Treating before the disease occurring"—prevention

Prevention includes preventing diseases from attacking as well as preventing diseases from changing after disease onset.

Plain Questions: Major Discussion of Regulation of Spirit According to the Changes of the Four Seasons (Sù Wèn: Sì Qì Tiáo Shén Dà Lùn, 素问·四气调神大论): *"Wise men insist on prevention rather than treatment after disease occurs, and governing rather than counterattacking. Once the disease has taken shape, or the chaos has burst out, either the treatment or the counterattack is too late, like digging a well after thirst is felt, or casting weapons after a battle breaks out."*

Preventing Disease from Occurring

It means to apply various measures before the onset of a disease to prevent it from occurring.

In ancient classics, it is called "health preservation", "health cultivation", and "health regulation", meaning to adjust the healthy status of body for conserving life, which is of great importance to building body constitution, preventing against disease onset, and lengthening life.

The occurrence of disease is mainly related to two kinds of factors, the right qi and the evil qi. For disease, insufficiency of right qi is the internal reason and invasion by evil qi is the external reason. Therefore, the basic principles of prevention (health preservation) are to increase the right qi, and to prevent the evil qi from invading.

① Reinforcing the Right Qi (Fig. 9-2)

Enhancing the constitution and raising the right qi to boost the ability to resist evil qi, occurrence of disease may be avoided. The basic methods of raising the right qi are as follows:

(1) Conforming to the natural law

That is, to use the laws of nature to preserve health. Human life is closely related to the changes in the natural world, so people must understand and grasp the laws of nature and adapt themselves to the changes in order to obtain coordination between the human life

rhythm and natural rhythm. The daily life of a person must be in synch with the natural changes of the seasons and days and nights, clothing must be appropriate, diet be proper, work and rest be regular, in this way health is preserved, the right qi is raised, and invasion of evil qi is avoided. Ideas like "obeying the wane-wax law of yin and yang", "preserve yang in spring and summer, and foster yin in autumn and summer" in *The Yellow Emperor's Internal Classic (Huáng Dì Nèi Jīng,* 黄帝内经) are examples of keeping harmony between the internal and external environment of the body.

Plain Questions: Major Discussion of Regulation of Spirit According to the Changes of the Four Seasons (Sù Wèn: Sì Qì Tiáo Shén Dà Lùn, 素问·四气调神大论) says: *"The yin and yang of the four seasons are the basis for all things. Therefore wise men cultivate yang in spring and summer, and take good care of yin in autumn and winter, to comply with the natural law of qi generation and storage which guides health preservation. So we hold that the yin and yang of the four seasons are the basis for all things. If the law is disobeyed, the root of life and death is subjugated, giving birth to disasters; if the law is abided, diseases have nowhere to run riot, this is called wisdom achievement."*

(2) Emphasizing mental health care

Emotional activities are presentation of the visceral functions. Uncontrolled seven emotions may injure the viscera directly and lead to disorders of qi flow, destroy the balance of yin-yang-qi-blood, damage the right qi and cause disease. So, mental health care is an important aspect of health preservation and prevention of diseases.

A cheerful and pleasant mood, and a quiet mind without greedy desires are required for mental health care, that is, the "tranquilized mind" as raised in *The Yellow Emperor's Internal Classic (Huáng Dì Nèi Jīng,* 黄帝内经). Thus the qi flow is easy and smooth, qi-blood-yin-yang is in harmony, the right qi is vigorous to prevent disease from occurring, and people enjoy health and longevity.

Plain Questions: Ancient Ideas on Flow to Preserve Natural Healthy Energy (Sù Wèn: Shàng

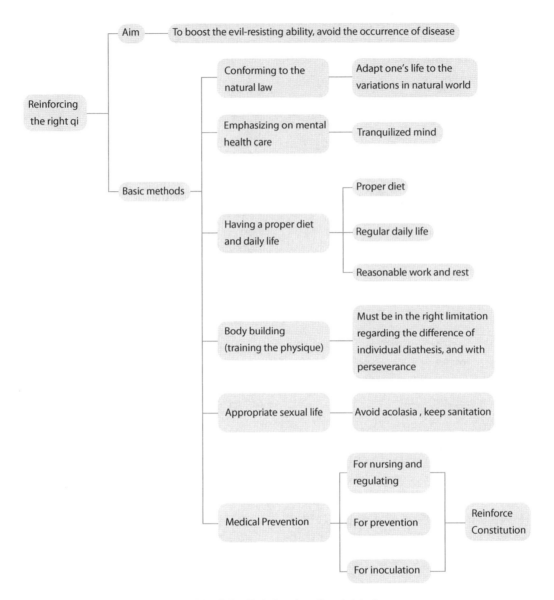

Fig. 9-2 Reinforcing the right qi

Gǔ Tiān Zhēn Lùn, 素问·上古天真论): "*Having a tranquilized mind, the right qi in the body flows normally; keeping a sound mind in the interior, diseases have nowhere to occur.*"

(3) Having a proper diet and daily life

It includes keeping eating properly, have a regular schedule in daily life, and having reasonable amounts of work and rest.

a. Proper diet

Food and drink provide the body's nutritive substance. A proper diet can build up the physique, raise resistance to evil qi, and prevent disease from attacking. On the other hand, an improper diet can easily impair the spleen and Stomach, consume the right qi, and cause various diseases. A proper diet includes: first, eating and drinking at the right time and in the proper amount; second, avoiding consuming contaminated, poisonous or rotten foods; and last, to have a balanced diet of the five flavors, and avoid overindulgence in or addiction to any special kind of food.

b. Regular daily life

People's daily life should have a certain amount of regularity, and be in accordance with the seasonal changes. A regular daily life contributes to the vigorous spirit and health of the body.

c. Reasonable work and rest

This means that physical exertion should have certain limitations, and work should be alternated with rest, thus allowing the qi and blood to circulate smoothly, which in turn promotes body health. Otherwise, overstrain consumes circulation of the qi and blood, and too much rest stagnates it, bringing about diseases.

Plain Questions: Ancient Ideas on Flow to Preserve Natural Healthy Energy (Sù Wèn: Shàng Gǔ Tiān Zhēn Lùn, 素问·上古天真论*): "Those ancient people who are aware of the rules of health preservation, emulate yin and yang, and comply with the health-cultivation method, having proper diet and daily life with regular work and rest, can achieve rest and spiritual harmony and gain longevity. Present-day people do not act like that: they drink alcohol instead of normal drinks, lead an abnormal life instead of a normal one, and even have sex while drunk, resulting in essence exhaustion due to self-indulgence and right qi consumption due to addiction. They only seek temporary happiness, without knowing how to keep vitality or use spirit properly, and this kind of irregularity of life finally brings on premature senility before fifty years of age."*

(4) Body building (training the physique)

"Life is motion." Physical training can promote qi and blood circulation, strengthen the muscles, bones and tendons, raise the body constitution, and increase disease resistance, thus resulting in health and longevity. Sports like gymnastic exercise, traditional Chinese shadow boxing (Tai Ji Quan, 太极拳), and martial arts are all good approaches to body building. The exercise must be in the right amount regarding the differences in individual constitution, and should be done with perseverance, while overstrain and trauma must be avoided.

Master Lu's Annals: Relieving Depression (Lǔ Shì Chūn Qiū: Dá Yù, 吕氏春秋·达郁*): "Moving water never stagnates, and a door-hinge is never worm-eaten: both are results of motion."*

(5) Appropriate sexual life

An appropriate sexual life for a couple is conducive to their individual and mental health. Being a physiological need, it does no harm to people. However, sexual life consumes the kidney essence, which is the material basis for growth, development and reproduction, so too much sexual activity must be avoided to preserve the kidney essence, in case over-consumption of the essence causes premature senility or susceptible to diseases.

In addition, cleanliness of the sexual life must be paid attention to: when either of the couple is sick or unwell, sex should be avoided. Too much sexual activity must be abstained from, otherwise, various diseases will come forth and could even threaten a person's life.

(6) Using herbs as prevention

This includes herbs used for nursing a person back to health, regulating a condition, prevention, or inoculation. That is, to achieve the aim of improving constitution, right qi invigoration and disease prevention through the actions of herbs.

What herb application for nursing and regulating means to apply some certain herbs which is beneficial to the body, to assist the right qi and achieve the goal of prevention.

Herb application for prevention is also an effective method, e.g., applying isatis root and dyers woad leaf to prevent influenza and mumps, and pussley to prevent bacillary dysentery, are convenient and effective preventative approaches.

Herb application for inoculation is of predominance significance in prevention for some diseases. Early in the 16th century, Chinese people invented variolization, a process of inoculation a susceptible person with material taken from a vesicle of a person who has smallpox. This is regarded as a pioneering effort for artificial immunization, which opens up a road for the late vaccinoprophylaxis science, which is prevention by vannication.

Plain Questions: Discussion on Acupuncture Methods (Sù Wèn: Cì Fǎ Lùn, 素问·刺法论*): "Yellow emperor said, 'I heard that when the five kinds of pestilential evils come, people are all susceptible to infection regardless of age, and the symptoms are similar. If no prevention or treatment is applied, why do some people not contract it?' Qi Bo said, ' those people who do not contract it have vigorous right qi to resist the evil, so the invasion of the pestilential evils is avoided......another method is taking in ten pills of Xiao Jin Dan (Small Golden Pills) as herb prevention, so no evil will invade.'"*

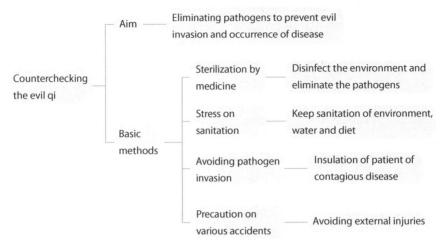

Fig. 9-3   Counterchecking the evil qi

② Counterchecking the Evil Qi (Fig. 9-3)

Invasion of evil qi leads to diseases. Besides reinforcing the right qi, it is also important to countercheck the evil, including:

(1) Sterilization by medicine

Eliminating the pathogen by using some specific medicine also contributes to the prevention of some diseases. In ancient times, people use a fumigant of atractylodes rhizome and realgar to disinfect the air; nowadays, people use herbs in an aerosol form to remove toxins from the body and kill toxins in the body, as an effective sterilization method for prevention and treatment of disease.

(2) Stress on sanitation

This includes maintaining a sanitary environment as well as ensuring that water and food are sanitary, in order to prevent pathogens from invading through the mouth, nose and body surface, which is of great importance in preventing diseases of the respiratory and digestive systems.

(3) Avoiding pathogen invasion

Isolating a patient with a contagious disease is one of the key measures to prevent the spread of the disease.

(4) Preventing accidents

Various injuries from falls and animal bites must be avoided in daily life as much as possible.

Plain Questions: Ancient Ideas on Flow to Preserve Natural Healthy Energy (Sù Wèn: Shàng Gǔ Tiān Zhēn Lùn, 素问·上古天真论): "Climatic

pathogens should be avoided in conformation with the different seasons."

Prevent the Development, Transmission and Change of Diseases

This refers to the application of effective methods to prevent a disease that is already present from developing, transmitting and changing, in order to achieve early recovery. The basic principles are early diagnosis and treatment, and stopping the progression of disease. (Fig. 9-4)

① Early Diagnosis and Treatment

Generally speaking, in the early stages of disease, the location is superficial, the condition is mild, and the right qi is not seriously damaged. Thus, diagnosis and treatment in the early stage contributes to the elimination of the evil qi and protection of the right qi: the disease seldom transmits and usually is easy to recover from.

Plain Questions: Major Discussion on the Theory of Yin and Yang and the Corresponding Relationships Among All Things in Nature (Sù Wèn: Yīn Yáng Yīng Xiàng Dà Lùn, 素问·阴阳应象大论): "The coming of pathogenic factors is like the wind and rain. The best doctors treat disease when it is in the skin and hair, then the tendons and vessels, then the six Fu organs, then the five zang organs. Those treated in the five zang organs are confronted with an unfavorable prognosis, since

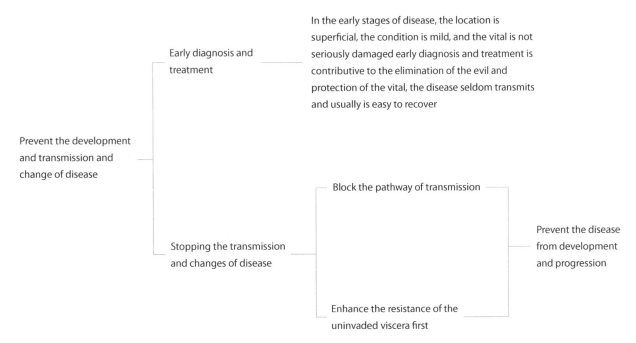

Fig. 9-4 Prevent the development, transmission and change of disease

the disease has already reached a critical point."

② Stopping the Progression (Transmission and Changes) of Disease

This is preventing a disease from developing by means of early diagnosis and treatment on the basis of understanding both the law of onset and development, and the transmission pathways.

(1) Block the pathway of transmission

Disease transmission has certain pathways and laws, such as six meridian transmission, defensive-qi-nutritive-blood phase's transmission, and triple Jiao transmission for exogenous diseases, and viscera transmission and meridian transmission for endogenous diseases. Once the laws and pathways are understood, early measures can be taken to prevent the disease. For instance, the Taiyang (太阳) stage of cold attack is the key stage for early diagnosis and treatment to impede its progression; and in the early stage of measles, the blocked measles toxin can easily transmit into the organs and lead to a more severe case, so treatment by sweating and letting the rash erupt must be applied in a timely manner to avoid transmission into the internal organs.

(2) "Enhance the resistance of the uninvolved organs

first"

Ye Tian-shi (叶天士) first raises this in the *Qing* dynasty, and it means to apply support and enrich the unaffected locations or organs before the disease transmits to them, according to the law of transmission. As the saying goes, "a liver problem is doomed to affect the spleen due to the subjugation of the liver wood on the spleen earth, so the spleen must be replenished in advance", that is, to nourish the spleen qi so that is strong enough to resist evil attacks by administrating spleen-replenishing medicine in the treatment of liver problems, thereby preventing the liver problem from transmitting. Similarly, in warm-heat disease, when the Stomach yin is injured, it will affect the kidney yin as it progresses. Therefore, Ye Tian-shi states in the above-mentioned theory that it is important to add kidney yin replenishing herbs to prescriptions for Stomach yin nourishment, in order to prevent the consumption of kidney yin. These are all examples of "enhancing the resistance of the uninvolved organs first".

Synopsis of Golden Chamber: On Syndrome and Pulse Manifestation of Various Viseral and Meridional Diseases in Different Transmission Sequences(Jīn Kuì Yào Lüè: Zàng Fŭ Jīng Luò Xiān Hòu Bìng Mài

Zhèng, 金匮要略·脏腑经络先后病脉证): *"Once a liver problem is recognized, it is doomed to transmit to the spleen, so the spleen should be tonified first."*

Section 2   Treatment Principles

A treatment principle is the general rule for treating disease. It is a theoretical system formulated under the concepts of holism and syndrome differentiation, which play an important guiding role in the clinical method for prescription herb determination.

Principle is different from method, however. The former is the general rule for guiding the latter, and the latter, directly related to the determination of prescriptions, herbs and acupoints, is the concrete treatment measures established under the guidance of the former.

There is also a difference between the concepts of general method and concrete method. The former aims at a series of syndromes of the same pathomechanism with wider applicability; while the latter is the treatment method within the general method established to treat a certain syndrome. For instance, "assisting the vital to eliminate the evil" is a principle, "perspiration"

is the general method, and "dispelling the evil in the superficial layer with herbs of pungent taste and warm nature" is a concrete treatment method. The concepts are related but different, and the difference is not absolute.

The treatment principle determination in CM theory takes the predominant idea of treating the root of the disease, which means the root must be explored to treat the essence of the disease.

The key points of treating the root of disease are "seeking the root" and "treating the root". "Seeking the root" is to analyze the information regarding the pathogen, location, course, nature, vital-evil condition of the disease and organism reaction, etc., to figure out the syndrome, which is the pathological nature of acertain stage of the disease process, and the pathomechanism, which is the summary of the syndrome nature. So the nature of the disease lies in the pathomechanism; "to treat the root" is to treat the disease according to the syndrome nature, thus "seeking for the root" and "treating the root" form an inseparable entirety, with the former as the prerequisite for the latter, and the latter as the purpose of the former, and the method to remove disease. Therefore treating the root of the disease is an incarnation of the concepts of holism and syndrome differentiation. (Fig. 9-5)

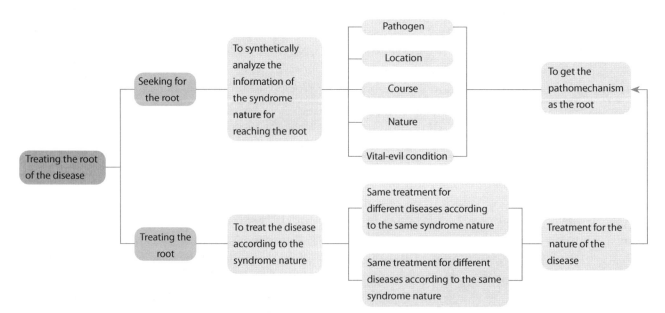

Fig. 9-5   Treating the root of the disease

Under the guidance of the idea of "treating the root of the disease", the treatment principle includes: routine treatment and paradoxical treatment, treating the branch and the root, strengthening the vital and dispelling the evil, regulating yin and yang, regulating the organs (omitted in this section), regulating qi-blood-body fluid, and suiting treatment to the time, place and individual.

Plain Questions: Major Discussion on the Theory of Yin and Yang and the Corresponding Relationships Among All the Things in Nature (Sù Wèn: Yīn Yáng Yīng Xiàng Dà Lùn, 素问·阴阳应象大论): *"Treat the root of the disease."*

Routine Treatment and Paradoxical Treatment

The nature and manifestation of a disease might be either in accordance or contradictory. Therefore there are routine treatments and paradoxical treatments, which are two principles respectively aiming at whether the disease has false signs or not, referring to the relationship (accordant or contradictory) between the nature (cold or heat, replenishing or discharging) of administrated herbs and the disease.

Plain Questions: Discussion on the Most Important and Abstruse Theory (Sù Wèn: Zhì Zhēn Yào Dà Lùn, 素问·至真要大论): *"Apply the routine treatment by going against the nature of the syndromes and symptoms, and paradoxical treatment by going along with the nature of external false signs of the disease."*

① Routine Treatment (Fig. 9-6)

(1) Definition

It is a commonly used treatment principle of going against the nature of the syndromes and symptoms, also called "reverse treatment", i.e. the nature of formulas and herbs are opposite to that of the syndrome.

(2) Indications

It is indicated for syndromes with their nature and manifestation in accordance. Examples are heat syndromes with heat symptoms, cold syndromes with cold symptoms, excess syndromes with excess symptoms, deficient syndromes with deficient symptoms.

(3) Common treatment methods of this principle

a. Heating the cold

A case of cold nature with cold signs should be treated with warm or hot herbs, and a cold syndrome should be treated with hot herbs. For instance: treating an exterior cold syndrome with

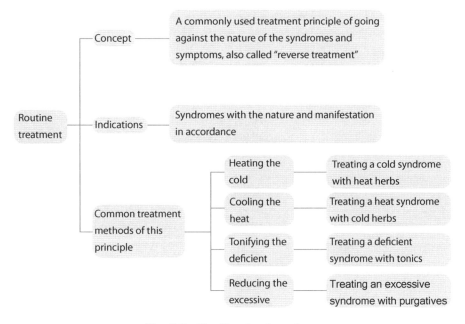

Fig. 9-6 Routine treatment

pungent-warm herbs, or treating and interior cold syndrome with pungent-hot herbs.

b. Cooling the heat

A case of heat nature with heat signs should be treated with herbs of cold or cool nature, just like treating a heat syndrome with cold herbs. E.g. treating an exterior heat syndrome with pungent-cold herbs, or treating an interior heat syndrome with bitter-cold herbs.

c. Tonifying the deficient

A case of deficient nature with deficient signs should be treated with herbs of tonification or invigoration, just like treating a deficient syndrome with tonics. E.g. treating a blood deficiency syndrome with blood-replenishing herbs for tonification, or treating a qi deficiency syndrome with qi tonifying herbs to supplement the qi, etc..

d. Reducing the excessive

A case of excess nature with excess signs should be treated with herbs to induce sweating, vomiting, or purgation, to reduce the excess, or treating an excess syndrome with purgatives. E.g. treating a food retention syndrome with digestion-promoting herbs, or treating a blood stasis syndrome with blood-activating herbs, etc.

Plain Questions: Discussion on the Most Important and Abstruse Theory (Sù Wèn: Zhì Zhēn Yào Dà Lùn, 素问·至真要大论): *"Heat the cold, cool the heat." "Purge the exuberant and replenish the insufficient."*

② Paradoxical Treatment (Fig. 9-7)

(1) Definition

It is a treatment principle of going along with the nature of external false signs of the disease, also called "conforming treatment", i.e. the nature of recipes and herbs are consistent with that of the false manifestations.

(2) Indications

It is indicated for syndromes with the nature and manifestation not in absolute accordance or in contradictory, such as heat syndrome with pseudo-cold symptoms, cold syndrome with

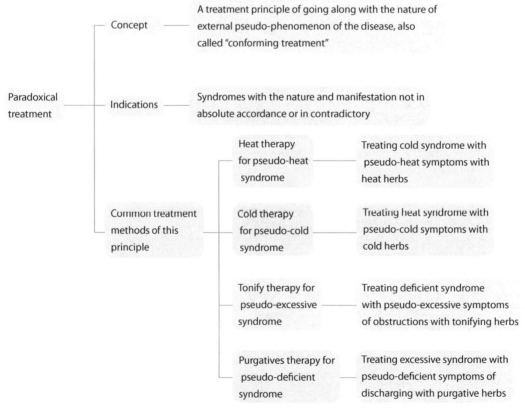

Fig. 9-7   Paradoxical treatment

pseudo-heat symptoms, excessive syndrome with pseudo-deficient symptoms, and deficient syndrome with pseudo-excessive symptoms.

(3) Common treatment methods of this principle

a. Heat therapy for pseudo-heat syndrome

It is also called "treating heat with heat", indicated for cold syndromes with pseudo-heat symptoms caused by excessive yin rejecting yang. The yin cold being excessive internally leads to real-cold symptoms like watery diarrhea with indigested food in the stool, cold limbs and feeble pulse, however, the yang being rejected externally causes pseudo-heat symptoms like fever and flushed cheeks. With the real cold nature and false heat manifestations, it should be treated with warm-heat herbs to treat the root of cold syndrome. The usage of heat herbs on pseudo-heat symptoms is regarded as "treating heat with heat".

b. Cold therapy for pseudo-cold syndrome

It is also called "treating cold with cold", indicated for heat syndromes with pseudo-cold symptoms caused by excessive yang rejecting yin. The yang heat being excessive internally leads to real-heat symptoms like high fever, restlessness with thirst, yellow and scanty urine, a red and crimson tongue and rapid pulse, however, the yin being rejected externally causes pseudo-cold symptoms like cold limbs and deep and hidden pulse. With the real heat nature and false cold manifestations, it should be treated with cold herbs to treat the root of heat syndrome. The usage of cold herbs on pseudo-cold symptoms is regarded as "treating cold with cold".

c. Tonic therapy for pseudo-excess syndrome

It is also called "treating obstructions with tonics", indicated for deficiency syndromes with pseudo-excess symptoms of obstructions caused by deficiency. Examples are the suppression of menstruation due to blood deficiency being treated by blood nourishing method; blockage of urine due to kidney yang deficiency failing to transform water being treated by warming and replenishing kidney yang, and once the kidney yang is strengthened the urination is normal; and constipation due to spleen qi deficiency failing to transform and transport being treated by tonifying the spleen qi.

d. Purgative therapy for pseudo-deficient syndrome

It is also called "treating openness with purgatives", indicated for excess syndromes with pseudo-deficient symptoms of discharge caused by internal blockage of the evil. Examples are metrorrhagia and metrostaxis caused by blood stasis, where the bleeding due to the blood stasis blocks the channels and blood can not move in the channels. It needs to be treated by promoting blood circulation to resolve blood stasis, so once the stasis is resolved, the bleeding stops. As well, it includes cases of stranguria due to dampness-heat, symptoms of frequent urination with urgency and pain caused by accumulation of dampness-heat in the urinary bladder, so that methods of inducing urination for treating stranguria, and clearing away dampness-heat of bladder should be applied. It is of the same reason in case of using digestion-promoting methods to treat diarrhea due to food accumulation.

Plain Questions : Discussion on the Most Important and Abstruse Theory(Sù Wèn: Zhì Zhēn Yào Dà Lùn, 素问·至真要大论): "*Apply tonics therapy for pseudo-excessive syndrome, and purgatives therapy for pseudo-deficient syndrome.*"

Appendix: Relationship between Routine Treatment and Paradoxical Treatment (Fig. 9-8)

a. Common points:

Both aim at treating the nature of the disease, and are classified in the category of "treating the root of disease".

b. Different points:

Routine treatment goes against the nature of the syndromes, and is indicated for syndromes with the nature and manifestation in accordance with each other.

Paradoxical treatment goes along with the nature of external false signs of the disease, and is indicated for syndromes with the nature and manifestation either not in absolute accordance or actually in contradiction to each other.

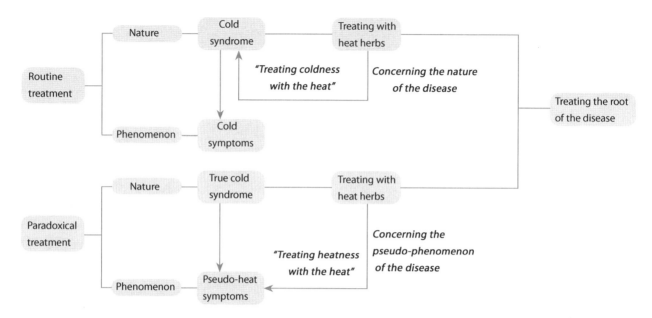

Fig. 9-8   Relationship between routine treatment and paradoxical treatment (examples)

Treating the Branch or Root of Diseases, and Acute or Chronic Diseases

① Definition

The root and the branch are a pair of opposite concepts with multiple meanings, which are often used to summarize the relation of essence and phenomenon, primary and secondary, cause and effect, etc. of a disease process. The acute or chronic problems of the root and branch refer to the difference between fundamental and incidental, and the treatment should be in certain process accordingly.

The division of the root and branch is relative according to the concrete condition in the disease process. For example, the vital is the root whereas the evil is the branch; the pathogen is the root whereas the symptom is the branch; the primary or original condition is the root whereas the secondary or complicated is the branch; the visceral portion is the root whereas the meridian or external portion is the branch, and so on and so forth. Thus clinically, distinguishing the root and the branch is conducive to seeking and treating the principal contradiction or the principal aspect

of the contradiction.

Jǐng-yuè's Complete Works: Record of Faith, Branch and Root(Jǐng Yuè Quán Shū: Chuán Zhōng Lù, Biāo Běn Lùn, 景岳全书·传忠录·标本论): "The branch and root of a disease means that the root is the origin of the disease, and the branch is the development."

② Principle for Application and Indication (Fig. 9-9)

(1) Treating the root for chronic diseases

This is a commonly used principle when the disease condition is moderate (the branch is not emergent), to treat the root of the disease. It is mainly suitable for the following two conditions:

Concerning the nature and phenomenon of disease, the nature is the root and the phenomenon is the branch. The branch (symptom) originates from the root (nature), when the branch is not urgent, the root should be treated, and once the root is relieved the branch is automatically alleviated. Examples are a case of cough due to yin deficiency, where the cough is the branch and the yin deficiency is the root. If treated by the method of nourishing the lung yin, once the yin is sufficient, the cough is diminished.

Concerning the primary and secondary conditions of a disease, the primary is the root and the secondary is the branch. When the

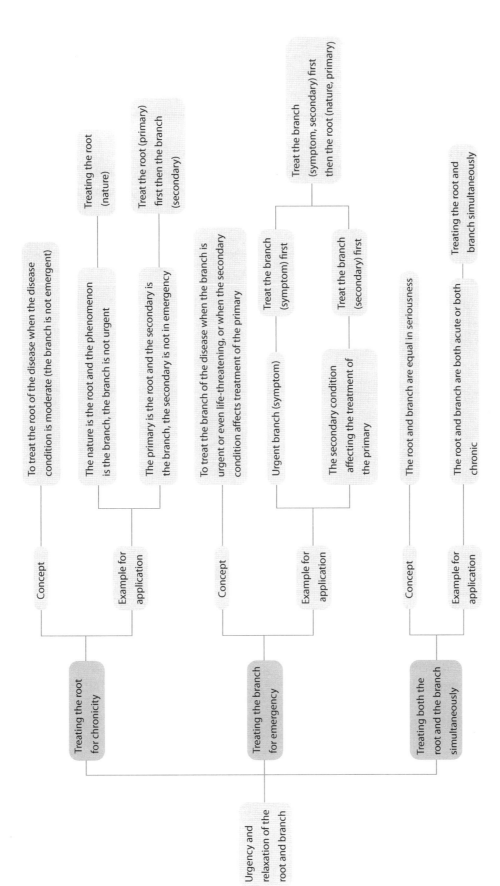

Fig. 9-9 Principles for application and indication of treating the acute or chronic state of the branch or the root

secondary is not an emergency, the primary should be treated first and then the secondary. For instance, in the case of a cough caused by an external pathogenic factor, symptoms like palpitations, insomnia and too many dreams may appear secondary to the cough. If they are not urgent, the cough should be treated first, while the palpitations, insomnia and many dreams should be treated second after the external evil is relieved and the cough stops.

(2) Treating the branch for acute diseases

When the branch is urgent or even life-threatening, or when the secondary condition effects the treatment of the primary, the branch should be treated first.

In case of an urgent branch (i.e. symptom) like high fever, convulsions, severe pain, drastic vomiting, dyspnea or wheezing, massive bleeding and lack of urine, it should be treated first.

In a case of the secondary condition effecting the treatment of the primary, such as a common cold secondary to a chronic Stomach ailment, the common cold should be treated first.

Treating the root must follow treating the branch for an emergency situation.

(3) Treating both the root and the branch simultaneously

When both of the root and branch are equal in seriousness, they should be treated simultaneously.

If the root and branch are both acute or both chronic, dealing with either of them alone wouldn't meet the demand for treatment, so the principle of treating them simultaneously should be applied. As in the case of cold for a patient with deficient qi, the qi deficiency leads to recurrent attacks of cold, with the vital is the root and the evil as the branch. However, if only the right qi is replenished, the evil easily lingers on; if only a sweating method is applied, the vital is prone to be damaged. Therefore, in this kind of condition, simultaneous treatment of the root and branch should be applied.

In conclusion, the application of treating the root and the branch should be under the guidance of "treating the root of disease", and according to analysis on the concrete condition, the principal contradiction should be grasped and treatment should be administered flexibly.

Plain Questions: Discussion on the Transmission of Biao (Branch) and Ben (Root) (Sù Wèn: Biāo Běn Bìng Chuan Lùn, 素问·标本病传论): "*Those who understand the law of the root and branch of disease always have appropriate treatment, while those who don't usually misbehave…*"

Classified Classic: Category of Biao(Branch) and Ben(Root) (Lèi Jīng: Biāo Běn Lèi, 类经·标本类): "*Emergency should be treated instantly though it might be the branch of a disease, that is, treating the branch in urgent condition.*"

Strengthening the Vital and Dispelling the Evil

① Basic Concepts of Strengthening the Vital and Dispelling the Evil(Fig. 9-10)

It is the principle indicated for treating deficient syndromes and excess syndromes, including two aspects of strengthening the vital and dispelling the evil.

(1) Strengthening the vital

It is a principle of strengthening the right qi of the body, building up the physique and raising the resistance against the evil, obtaining a recovery from disease.

Commonly used methods are: tonifying qi, nourishing blood, fostering yin and warming yang, according to different deficiencies of the qi-blood-yin-yang, in order to replenish the organs. Additionally, methods of food therapy, acupuncture and moxibustion, *tui na* and physical training can also strengthen the right qi.

The principle of strengthening the right qi is indicated for various deficiencies.

(2) Dispelling the evil

It is a principle of driving out the evil qi to eliminate or alleviate injury caused by pathogens, aiming at the recovery of health.

Commonly used methods are as follows: diaphoresis (sweating), emesis (vomiting), purgation, heat-clearing, cold-dispelling, dampness-resolving, phlegm-dissipating, qi-flow-invigorating, blood-flow-activating, and digestion-promoting, etc. according to the nature

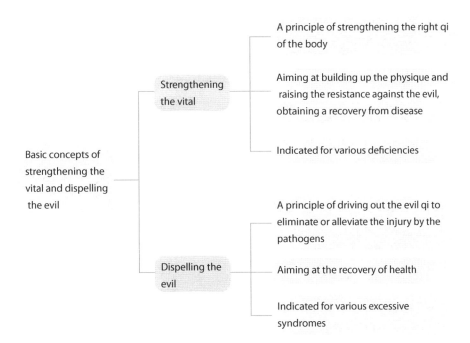

Fig. 9-10　Basic concepts of strengthening the vital and dispelling the evil

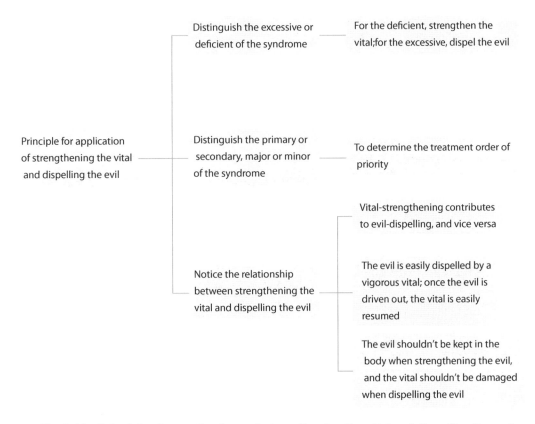

Fig. 9-11　Principles for applications of strengthening the vital and dispelling the evil

of the pathogen and the disease location.

It is indicated for various excess syndromes.

Plain Questions: Discussion on the Three Regions and Nine Divisions (Sù Wèn: Sān Bù Jiǔ Hòu Lùn, 素问·三部九候论): "For excess syndromes, purging methods should be used, and for deficient syndromes, replenishing methods should be applied."

Miraculous Pivot: Retention of the Evil (Líng Shū: Xié Kè, 灵枢·邪客): "Tonify the deficiency, reduce the excess."

② Principles for Application of Strengthening the Vital and Dispelling the Evil (Fig. 9-11)

(1) Distinguish the excess or deficiency of the syndrome: for the deficient, strengthen the vital; for the excess, dispel the evil.

The syndrome differentiation should be precisely based on the proper premises; otherwise the misuse of tonics or purgatives will lead to serious results of further damage of the vitality in cases of deficiency, or further tonification of the evil in cases of excess.

(2) Distinguish the primary or secondary syndrome, to determine the treatment order of priority.

It is indicated for syndromes of deficiency mingling with excess. The treatment order of priority should be determined in accordance with the primary or secondary syndrome.

(3) Notice the relationship between strengthening the vital and dispelling the evil: the evil shouldn't be kept in the body when strengthening the vital, and the vital shouldn't be damaged when dispelling the evil.

The two aspects of strengthening the vital and dispelling the evil are mutually dependent and complementary. Vital-strengthening contributes to evil-dispelling, and vice versa. At the same time, misuse of this principle may lead to assisting the evil or damaging the vital mistakenly.

③ Methods of Application of Strengthening the Vital and Dispelling the Evil (Fig. 9-12)

(1) Single application

Strengthening the vital only: suitable for various deficiency syndromes, or false excess with real deficiency syndromes.

Dispelling the evil only: suitable for various excess syndromes, or false excess with real deficiency syndromes.

(2) Combining applications

The simultaneous application of purging-tonifying therapy is suitable for syndromes of excess & deficiency that are mutually included. Neither the vital-deficiency nor the evil-excess is in a crucial state, so simply strengthening the vital may assist the evil, simply dispelling the evil may damage the vital. The combined usage of both of them is suggested here.

a. Vital-strengthening assisted by evil dispelling:

It is to mainly strengthen the vital and dispel the evil secondarily. The indication is a deficient syndrome complicated with excess.

b. Evil-dispelling assisted by vital-strengthening:

It is to mainly dispel the evil and secondarily strengthen the vital. The indication is an excess syndrome complicated with deficiency.

For instance, the case of a common cold from qi deficiency syndrome should be treated with combining application of strengthening the vital and dispelling the evil, since the single use of either is inappropriate. When the treatment proceeds, the syndrome nature of the two aspects should be distinguished.

(3) Successive application

The successive usage of strengthening the vital and dispelling the evil is an application of treating the two aspects according to the order of priority of deficiency and excess in a mingled syndrome. The vital should not be damaged nor should the evil be tonified mistakenly.

a. Strengthening the vital before dispelling the evil:

It is also called "tonification before elimination", indicated for a deficient syndrome complicated with excess, in which the right qi is too deficient to stand the attack upon the evil. Therefore the vital should be strengthened first until it is restored enough to bear the attack, and then the evil should be dispelled. For instance, "drum-belly" is caused by water retention due to qi deficiency, where the deficiency of the vital is the major aspect of the contradiction. The extremely

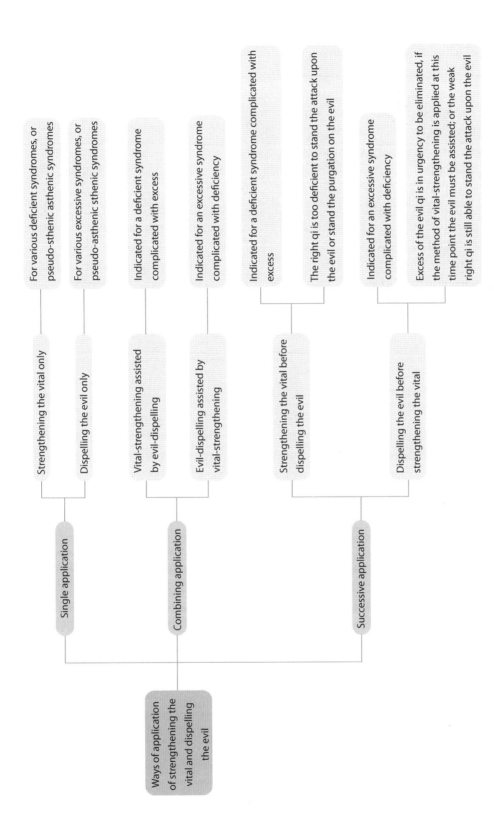

Fig. 9-12 Ways of application of strengthening the vital and dispelling the evil

deficient vital cannot stand the purgation on the evil, so we must strengthen the vital first then purge the evil of water retention to avoid mistakes.

b. Dispelling the evil before strengthening the vital:

It is also called "elimination before tonification", indicated for an excess syndrome complicated with deficiency, in which the excess of the evil qi is in the most important thing to be eliminated. If the method of vital-strengthening is used at this time, the evil qi will be assisted; even if the right qi is weak, it can still tolerate elimination. Thus, the evil must be dispelled first and then the vital should be strengthened. For instance, in the case of metrorrhagia and metrostaxis due to blood stasis, under the prerequisite of right qi which is not seriously damaged, the blood flow should first be activated to remove the stasis, and then the blood should be replenished.

Regulating Yin and Yang

It is to remedy defects and rectify errors to restore the relative balance between the yin and yang of the body.

Plain Questions: Discussion on the Most Important and Abstruse Theory (Sù Wèn: Zhì Zhēn Yào Dà Lùn, 素问·至真要大论): "Yin and yang should be distinguished and regulated prudently, aiming at mutual balance between them."

① Eliminating the Excess (treatment for excess of either yin or yang)

It is to treat a case with excess of yin or yang with reducing methods, or "reducing what is excessive".

For an excess cold syndrome due to exuberance of yin, the method of dispelling the yin-cold with warm-hot herbs is used, i.e. "warm what is cold". If the excessive yin damages yang, presenting yang deficiency at the same time, then the yang should be replenished simultaneously, that is, eliminating the evil with strengthening the vital.

For an excess heat syndrome due to exuberance of yang, the method of clearing up the yang-heat by cool-cold herbs is used, i.e. "cool down what is hot". If the excessive yang damages yin, presenting yin deficiency at the same time, the yin should be nourished simultaneously, that is, again, eliminating the evil with strengthening the vital.

② Supplementing the Deficiency (treatment for deficiency of either yin or yang)

It is also called "tonifying what is deficient", meaning treating a deficient syndrome by methods of tonification.

A deficient heat syndrome due to hyperactivity of yang resulting from yin deficiency should be treated with yin-nourishing methods to restrict yang, also called "treat yin for yang-illness", or "checking the hyperactivity of yang by nourishing the kidney yin, the origin of water".

A deficiency cold syndrome due to overwhelming yin caused by yang deficiency should be treated with yang-replenishing methods to restrict the predominance of yin, also called "treating yang for yin-illness", or "expelling the excess of yin by supporting the kidney yang, the source of fire".

Based on the theory of mutual dependence between yin and yang, in treatment of deficiency of yin, herbs of yang-strengthening actions may be added to a yin-nourishing prescription as a subsidiary, this is called "seeking yin from yang"; on the other hand, in treatment of deficiency of yang, herbs of yin-nourishing actions may be added to a yang-replenishing prescription as a subsidiary, this is called "seeking yang from yin". Methods of this kind can reach a mutual generation of yin and yang and restrict the bias and side effects of the pure tonification of either yin or yang.

Plain Questions: Major Discussion on the Theory of Yin and Yang and the Corresponding Relationships Among All the Things in Nature (Sù Wèn: Yīn Yáng Yīng Xiàng Dà Lùn, 素问·阴阳应象大论): "treating yin for yang disease, treating yang for yin disease".

Jǐng-yue's Complete Works: Eight New Strategies on Prescriptions(Jǐng Yuè Quán Shū: Chuan Zhōng

Lù, Xīn Fāng Bā Lüè, 景岳全书・新方八略): *"Those who are adept in replenishing yang must know to seek for yang from yin, with the aid of yin, yang prospers and flourishes endlessly; and those who are adept in nourishing yin must know to seek for yin from yang, with the backup of yang, yin thrives and blooms infinitely."*

③ Applying Paradoxical Treatment (for treating mutual rejection between yin and yang)

As discussed in the previous section on "paradoxical treatment", a cold syndrome with pseudo-heat symptoms caused by exuberant yin rejecting yang should be treated with the method of "treating heat with heat"; and a heat syndrome with pseudo-cold symptoms caused by overwhelming yang rejecting yin should be treated with the method of "treating cold with cold".

④ Combination of Replenishing Yin and Yang (for treating mutual effect and damage between yin and yang)

A deficient syndrome of both yin and yang due to mutual effect between yin and yang should be treated with the method of replenishing both yin and yang, but distinguishing between the primary and secondary syndromes.

For a deficient syndrome of both yin and yang with yin deficiency in the leading place which is caused by yin-deficiency affecting yang,

yang-replenishing method should be applied subsidiarily to yin-nourishing treatment.

For deficiency syndrome of both yin and yang with yang asthenia as the most apparent, which is caused by yang-deficiency affecting yin, a yin-nourishing method should be applied secondarily to the yang-replenishing treatment.

⑤ Emergency Treatment of Consolidation (for treating depletion of yin or yang)

Depletion of yin or yang is a crucial state where massive loss of the right qi of the body causes general functional failure and threatens life, which should be immediately treated with emergency treatment of consolidation. For yin-depletion syndrome, emphasize restoring yin and consolidating qi from collapsing; for yang-depletion syndrome, emphasize restoring yang and consolidating qi from collapsing.

Regulating Qi–Blood–Fluid

① Regulating Qi (Fig. 9-13)

Pathological changes of qi mainly include qi deficiency and disorders of qi flow. Thus, regulation of qi includes replenishing qi and regulating qi flow.

(1) Replenishing qi

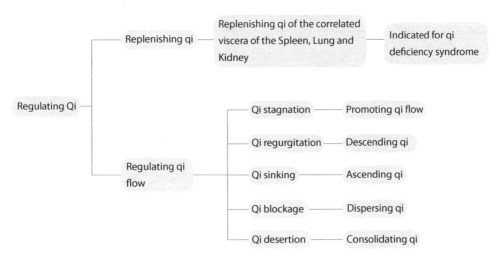

Fig. 9-13 **Regulating qi**

It is indicated for qi deficiency syndromes. qi deficiency caused by insufficient generation of qi is closely related to the spleen, lung and kidney. Thus replenishing qi means mostly to replenish the qi of the three organs. Qi deficiency caused by consumption of qi during a disease course can be related to any organ, clinically, so qi of the related organ should be tonified.

(2) Regulating qi flow

It is mainly indicated for disorders of qi circulation, including qi stagnation, qi counterflow, qi sinking, qi desertion, and qi blockage. The respective treatment methods are: promoting qi flow, lowering qi, raising qi, dispersing qi and consolidating qi. Clinically, qi flow should be regulated according to the different characteristics of qi flow in certain organs.

② Regulating Blood (Fig. 9-14)

The pathological changes of blood include blood deficiency, blood stasis, bleeding, blood heat, and blood cold, which should be regulated

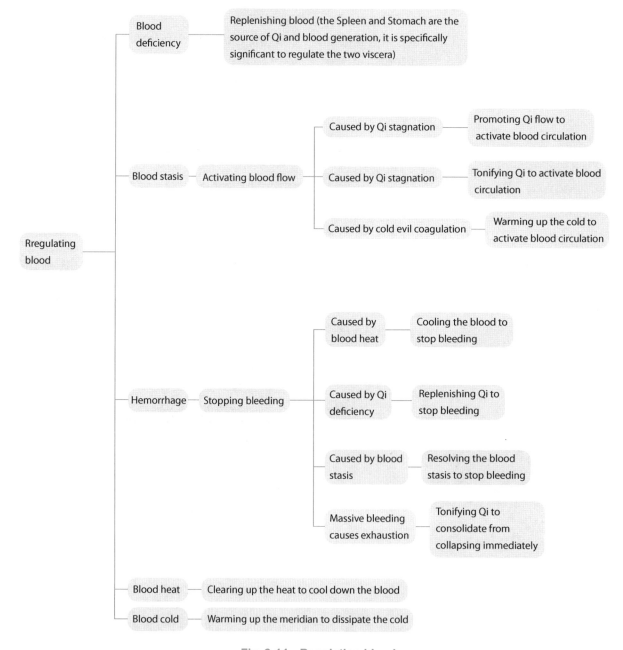

Fig. 9-14   Regulating blood

respectively according to the causes clinically.

(1) Replenishing blood for treating blood deficiency

Blood originates from the essences of water and food, so it is closely related to the functions of the spleen, Stomach, heart, liver and kidney. To regulate the functions of the related organs it is of certain importance to replenish blood, and, since the spleen and Stomach are the source of qi and blood generation, it is specifically significant to regulate these two organs.

(2) Activating blood flow for treating blood stasis

Blood stasis is caused by diverse factors: if from qi stagnation, it should be treated by promoting qi flow to activate blood circulation; if from qi deficiency, by tonifying qi to activate blood circulation; if from cold evil coagulation, by warming up the cold to activate blood circulation.

(3) Stopping bleeding for treating hemorrhage

If the bleeding is caused by blood heat, it should be treated by cooling the blood to stop bleeding; if from qi deficiency, by replenishing qi to stop bleeding; if from blood stasis, by resolving the blood stasis to stop bleeding; if massive bleeding causes exhaustion, the metho d of tonifying qi to consolidate it & save it from collapse must be taken immediately.

(4) Clearing up the heat to cool down the blood for treating blood heat

(5) Warming up the channels to dissipate cold for treating blood cold

③ Regulating Body Fluid

(1) For treating deficiency of body fluid, the method of nourishing yin to produce fluid should be undertaken.

(2) For treating retention of body fluid, the method of resolving dampness and discharging water should be applied.

Water-dampness retention has various pathological changes. Those with excessive dampness should be treated with methods of dampness resolving, dampness-discharging or dampness-drying; those with edema should be treated with inducing urination to alleviate edema; those affected by phlegm-fluid should be treated with dissipating phlegm and expelling fluid retention. As far as the organs are concerned, the Water-dampness retention is caused by many factors but mostly related to the functions of the spleen, lung, kidney and *San Jiao* in governing water metabolism, so the visceral functions should be simultaneously regulated.

④ Regulating Relationships among Qi, Blood and Fluid

(1) Regulating relationships between qi and blood (Fig. 9-15)

Disorders of qi and blood often affect each other, with the result of simultaneous illness of qi and blood, so the relation between them must be regulated.

a. Qi disorders affecting treatment of blood disease

Blood deficiency caused by deficient qi failing to generate blood should be treated by qi-replenishing aided by blood-nourishing, or by nourishing both qi and blood; blood stasis caused by deficient qi failing to push blood should be treated with qi-replenishing aided by blood-flow-activating; blood stasis caused by stagnated qi obstructing blood flow should be treated with qi-flow-promoting aided by blood-flow-activating; bleeding caused by deficient qi failing to control blood should be treated with qi-replenishing aided by blood-astringing (invigorating qi to control blood).

b. Blood disorders effecting treatment of qi disease

Qi deficiency caused by deficient blood failing to generate qi should be treated by blood-nourishing assisted by qi-tonifying, or replenishing both qi and blood; excessive bleeding followed by exhaustion of qi should be treated by reinforcing qi to consolidate the qi and blood from collapsing.

(2) Regulating the relationship between qi and body fluid (Fig. 9-16)

Replenishing qi to promote the production of body fluid should treat insufficiency of body fluid generation due to qi deficiency. If disorders of distribution and excretion of body fluid due to qi deficiency or qi stagnation cause water-dampness-phlegm-fluid retention, it should be treated by tonifying qi to promote fluid circulation or to discharge water. Loss of body fluid caused by unconsolidation of the deficient

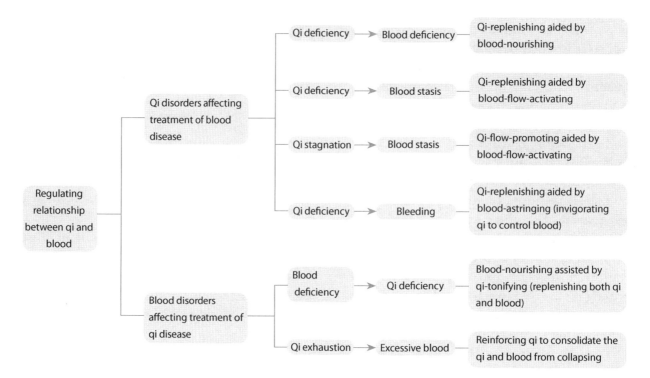

Fig. 9-15　Regulating the relationship between qi and blood

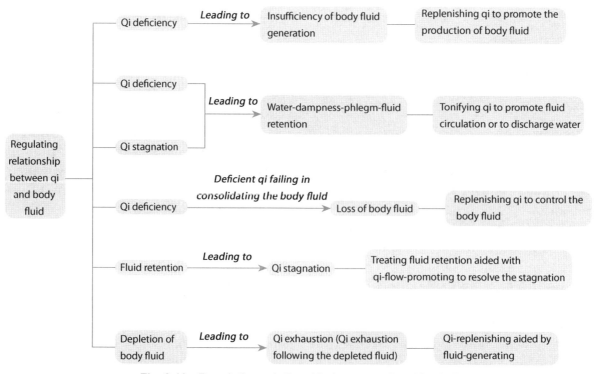

Fig. 9-16　Regulating relationship between qi and body fluid

qi should be treated by replenishing qi to control the body fluid;. Treatment of qi stagnation caused by fluid retention should be aided by qi-flow-promoting to resolve the stagnation. Finally, qi-replenishing aided by fluid generating should treat exhaustion of qi due to depletion of body fluid.

(3) Regulating the relationship between blood and body fluid (Fig. 9-16)

Blood and body fluid often affect each other pathologically: massive loss of blood consumes body fluid, and massive loss of fluid leads to empty blood vessels (depletion of body fluid causing lack of blood). Thus, the method of

nourishing blood to promote the production of body fluid should be applied alongside the etiological treatment.

Suiting Treatment to the Time, Place and Individual

1 To Suit Treatment to Time (Fig. 9-17)

(1) Definition

It is the principle of choosing the appropriate method and herbs according to the climatic

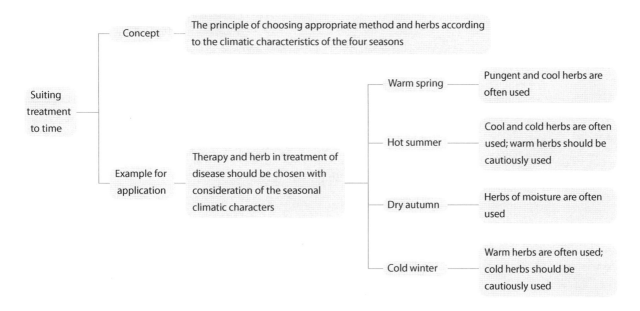

Fig. 9-17 Suiting treatment to time

characteristics of the four seasons.

(2) Application

The weather changes in the four seasons of the year, and the warmth, heat, coolness and cold affect the human body physiologically and pathologically. Therefore therapies and herbs for the treatment of diseases should be chosen with consideration of the seasonal climatic characters. In summer, the yang qi of the body goes upward and the striae loosens and opens, therefore people easily sweat and easily get attacked by wind-cold evil. For this condition, herbs of a pungent and warm nature should be carefully used to

avoid over-dispersion consuming qi and body fluid. In winter, the yang qi of the human body is kept internally and the striae is compacted, so if attacked by wind-cold evil, pungent and warm herbs can be used relatively freely for dispersion; while if attacked by heat evil in winter, cold herbs should be cautiously used to avoid damage of yang qi. So, in conclusion, pungent and cool herbs are often used in spring which is warm; cool and cold herbs are often used in hot summer days, but not warm or hot herbs; in the autumn, the weather is dry, so herbs of a moist nature are usually used; in freezing winter, pungent and warm herbs are more favorable than the cool and cold ones.

Plain Questions: Major Discussion on the Progress of the Six Climatic Changes (Sù Wèn: Liù Yuán Zhèng Jì Dà Lùn, 素问·六元正纪大论): "Keep away from the cold climate when using the cold herbs, keep away from the cool climate when using the cool herbs, keep away from the warm climate when using the warm herbs, keep away from the hot climate when using the hot herbs: this principle is also suitable for diet."

② To Suit Treatment to Place (Fig. 9-18)

(1) Definition

It refers to the principle of choosing the appropriate method and herbs according to the local characteristics of the different geographic

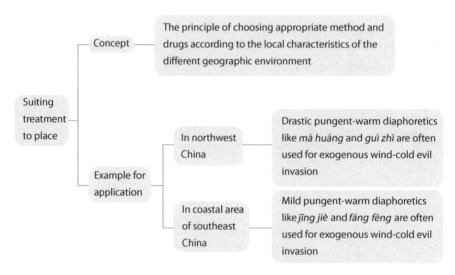

Fig. 9-18 Suiting treatment to place

environment.

(2) Application

Different places vary in topography, climate, quality of water and soil and living habit and style. As a result, people in different places have different physiological and pathological characteristics. When determining treatment, factors of geographic characteristics should be considered. In northwest China, the terrain is high, the climate is cold and dry with little rainfall, people have a diet of milk products, meat, and grain crops, with strong constitution and compacted striae. If attacked by exogenous wind-cold evil, drastic pungent-warm herbs to induce sweating like *má huáng* (Herba Ephedrae, 麻黄) and *guì zhī* (Ramulus Cinnamomi, 桂枝) are often used. In the coastal area of southeast China, the climate is warm and moist, people have a relatively delicate dietary structure of fish, shrimp and fine rice, with delicate constitution and loose striae. If attacked by exogenous wind-cold evil, mild pungent-warm herbs to induce sweating like *jīng jiè* (Herba Schizonepetae, 荆芥) and *fáng fēng* (Radix Saposhnikoviae, 防风) are often used.

Plain Questions: Discussion on Different Therapeutic Methods for Different Diseases (Sù Wèn: Yì F ǎ Fāng Yí Lùn, 素问·异法方宜论): "Treatment of the same disease in different patients may be different, all come to recovery, how comes this? Qi Bo answered, geographical difference contributes to it."

③ To Suit Treatment to Individual

(1) Definition

It is the principle to choose the appropriate method and herbs according to the characteristics of a patient's age, gender, constitution, and so on.

(2) Application

a. Age

People of different ages have different physiological and pathological characters, so the application of therapy and herbs should be flexible. As for children with a vigorous nature but delicate organs and insufficient qi and blood, illness status is changeable, easy to get heat or cold, deficiency or excess. Thus the treatment of a child patient should be mild and not drastic, and in small dose. For elderly patients, vitality fades, qi and blood are deficient, organ functions decline, and the illness presents mainly as a deficient syndrome, or deficiency mixed with excess, the treatment should be in strengthening the vital and cautiously purging. Young adults are full of right qi with strong resistancee and plenty of qi and blood, the visceral functions are vigorous, and they usually present excess syndromes. The treatment should be purging the excess, and the dose could be relatively large.

b. Gender

Women have different physiological and pathological characters from men. Women take the blood as the foundation; they suffer from disorders of menstruation, leucorrhea, pregnancy and birth giving, and illnesses of the breasts and the uterus. Drastic cathartics, blood-breaking herbs, lubricating and exciting methods, or orifice-opening or poisonous herbs should be used in prudence or prohibited in menstrual or in gestational periods. As well, in postnatal periods of a female patient, conditions like qi and blood deficiency and lochia should be paid attention to. Men have essence as their root, so pathologically there may be impotence, postcoital protrusion, premature ejaculation, emission, spontaneous emission and dyspermatism. The kidney stores esscence and dominates reproduction, so treatment determination should be on the basis of regulating the kidney function in addition to the concrete pathomechanism of the disease.

c. Constitution

Owing to the difference of innate endowment and acquired factors, each individual has different physical resistance to disease, and a different body constitution. Different resistance means special susceptibility to different pathogens, leading to pathological changes of cold-hot-warm-cool natures. The treatment should be accordingly different in some degree. For instance, a patient of strong resistance is prone to excessive syndromes, and the body is strong enough to stand treatment by reduction, so the herbs could be in larger dose if necessary. Adversely, a patient of weak resistance is susceptible to deficient syndromes, and the body is not strong enough to stand reduction treatments, so the herbs should be in smaller doses. A patient of yang-excess or yin-deficient constitution usually shows heat syndromes, which should be treated with cool and cold herbs; and a patient of yin-excess or yang-deficient constitution usually shows cold syndromes, which should be treated with warm and hot herbs.

The principle of suiting treatment to these three factors reflects the sense of regularity and flexibility in the practice of treatment determination based on syndrome determination, and it incarnates the concept of holism. Clinically, any problem should be treated with all aspects considered, thus a constantly effective therapeutic effect could be achieved.

Miraculous Pivot: On Pains (Líng Shū: Lùn Tòng, 灵枢·论痛): "Those with strong Stomach qi and robust and muscular physiques are resistive to evils and those of weak Stomach qi and scrawny figures are liable to pathogenic factors."

Bibliography

1. Sun Guang-ren. Basic Theory of Traditional Chinese Medicine (textbook series of new century programmed by national Chinese medicine academies). Beijing: China Press of Traditional Chinese medicine, 2002

2. Li De-xin. Basic Theory of Traditional Chinese Medicine (programmed textbook series of national medicine textbook construction seminar of China). Beijing: People's Medical Publishing House, 2001

3. Liu Yan-chi, Guo Zhenxia. Basic Theory of Traditional Chinese Medicine (21st century textbook series for medical academies). Beijing: Science Press, 2002

4. Zhang Deng-ben. Basis for Traditional Chinese Medicine (new century textbook series programmed for national Chinese medicine academies). Beijing: China Press of Traditional Chinese Medicine, 2003

5. Li De-xin. Basic Theory of Traditional Chinese Medicine (textbook series for national adult education of Chinese medicine academies). Changsha: Hunan Scientific and Technical Press, 2001

6. Wu Dun-xu. Basic Theory of Traditional Chinese Medicine (Chinese medicine textbook series programmed for general higher education). Shanghai: Shanghai Scientific and Technical Publishers, 1995

7. Wang Xin-hua. Basis for Traditional Chinese Medicine (Chinese medicine textbook series programmed for general higher education). Shanghai: Shanghai Scientific and Technical Publishers, 1995

8. Yin Hui-he. Basic Theory of Traditional Chinese Medicine (integrated compiled textbook series, 5th edition). Shanghai: Shanghai Scientific and Technical Publishers, 1984

Index

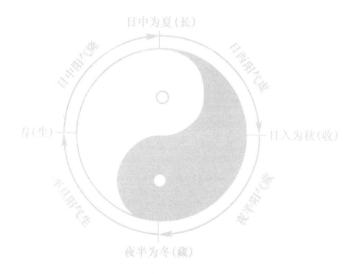

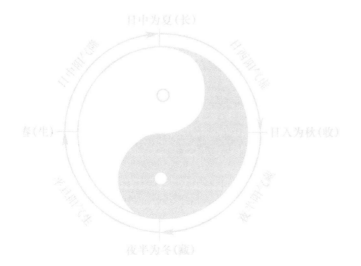

图书在版编目（CIP）数据

中医基础理论图表解（英文）/周学胜编著. —北京：
人民卫生出版社，2007.10
（中医基础学科图表解丛书）
ISBN 978-7-117-09240-1

Ⅰ. 中⋯　Ⅱ. 周⋯　Ⅲ. 中医医学基础–中医学院–
教学参考资料　Ⅳ. ①R22

中国版本图书馆CIP数据核字（2007）第 140972 号

人卫智网	www.ipmph.com	医学教育、学术、考试、健康，购书智慧智能综合服务平台
人卫官网	www.pmph.com	人卫官方资讯发布平台
人卫智慧服务商城	www.pmphmall.com	人卫官方自营电商平台

中医基础理论图表解（英文）

编　　著：周学胜
出版发行：人民卫生出版社
地　　址：北京市朝阳区潘家园南里 19 号
邮　　编：100021
网　　址：http://www.pmph.com
E - mail：pmph @ pmph.com　zzg@pmph.com
发　　行：zzg@pmph.com.cn
购书热线：010–59787340　010–59787413
经　　销：新华书店
开　　本：889×1194　1/16
版　　次：2007 年 10 月第 1 版　　2018 年 10 月第 1 版第 3 次印刷
标准书号：ISBN 978-7-117-09240-1/R・9241

打击盗版举报电话：**010-59787491**　E-mail: WQ @ pmph.com
（凡属印装质量问题请与本社市场营销中心联系退换）

28